THE Duality of the Mind

A New View of Insanity:

THE

Duality of the Mind

PROVED BY THE

Structure, Functions, and Diseases of the Brain

AND BY THE

Phenomena of Mental Derangement, and Shown to be Essential to Moral Responsibility

by A. L. Wigan, M.D., 1844

Foreword by Joseph Bogen, M.D., F.A.C.S.

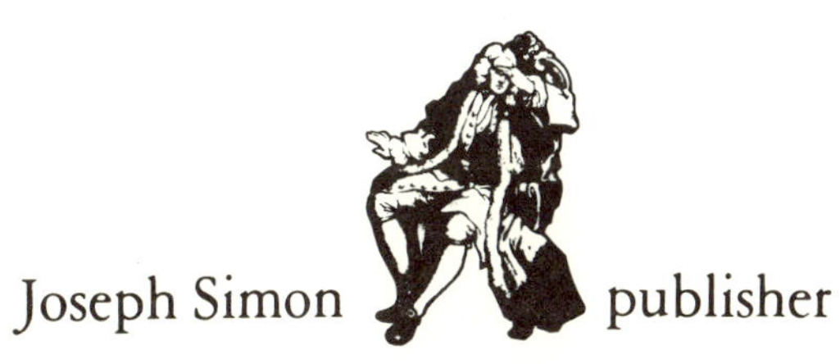

Joseph Simon publisher

Printed in the United States of America
Designed by Joseph Simon
Printed on Long-life Paper

Library of Congress Cataloging in Publication Data

Wigan, A. L. (Arthur Ladbroke)
A New View of Insanity.

Reprint. Originally published: London : Longman, Brown, Green, and Longmans, 1884.
Bibliography: p.
1. Mental illness. 2. Mind. 3. Brain. I. Title. II. Title: The Duality of the Mind.
[DNLM: WN W654n 1844a]
RC454.4.W54 1985 616.89 85-50042
ISBN 0-934710-11-2
ISBN 0-934710-12-0 (lim. ed.)

CONTENTS

PAGE

FOREWORD ix

PREFACE xix

CHAPTER I: *Introduction; Unsettled State of Mental Philosophy; A new Instrument for its Investigation; Mind and Soul* 3

CHAPTER II: *Origin of the Work; Rev. J. Barlow on Man's Power over himself to prevent and control Insanity; High Intellectual Cultivation of the Clergy; There can be no discrepancy between the Word and the Works of God* 8

CHAPTER III: *Description of the Brain adapted to Non-Medical Readers; Functions of the Brain* 12

CHAPTER IV: *The Duality of the Mind; Propositions to be proved; Results if proved* 19

CHAPTER V: *Disclaimer of Materialism; Mind in its popular sense connected with the Material World by means of our Physical Organization; Use of the Ganglionic System* 25

CHAPTER VI: *Progress of my own Convictions; Proofs that one Cerebrum may be destroyed yet the Mind remain entire; Examples from Conolly, Johnson, Cruveilhier, Abercrombie, Ferriar, O'Halloran, and others; Reflections; Case of Cardinal, from Dr. Bright's Work; Early Remarks of Dr. Gall* 30

CHAPTER VII: *Quotation from Quarterly Review; Comparison with a Theatre; Pinel; Double Volition from Cerebral disturbance, caused by great anxiety* 42

CHAPTER VIII: *False Perceptions; Errors of the Organs of Sense; Example of Delusion; My own Delusion; Case of Nicolai and Dr. Bostock; Case of Cerebral disturbance from diffused Gout; Double Mind; Self-Restraint; Case of Moral Insanity* 50

CHAPTER IX: *Sentiment of Pre-existence; Explanation; Princess Charlotte's Funeral; Impressions on the Senses; Phrenology; Clergyman with opposing Convictions; Remarks of Mr. Solly; Cerebellum; Antagonism of the two Brains* 64

CHAPTER X: *Examination of the Opinions of Dr. Holland; Comparison of the Theory with a new Railway; The Brain as a Double Organ; Examples of the Double Mind; Inferences; Mode in which alone they can be drawn from Examination after death of the Insane* 76

CHAPTER XI: *Power of resting one Brain; Castle Building; Case of Delusion from Pride; Another from Reverse of Fortune; Equivocal Hallucination; Case of a Painter; Gentleman who saw his own self; Lady who thought herself Mary Queen of Scots* 89

CHAPTER XII: *Dr. Abercrombie's Treatise on the Mental Powers; Cases of Hallucination; Cerebral disturbance without Disease; Morbid appearances on Dissection; Hallucination confined to a single point; Nature and Causes of Insanity; Circumstances in which argument may be addressed to the Insane* 101

CHAPTER XIII: *Two Processes carried on together; Counting Steps; Objections to the Explanation; The animal is created Dual at first; Gradually joined; Moral Responsibility; Considerations on Phrenology; Differences in Form and Texture at the base of the Brain* 112

CHAPTER XIV: *Phrenology continued; Case of Spectral Illusions, and commencement of Moral Insanity, cured by Bleeding; other Cases; Mental Pictures by an Artist; Inability to remember Faces; Inability to distinguish Dreams from Realities; Robert Hall and Cowper* 123

CHAPTER XV: *Diffused Disorder affects only one side; Death of Dr. Wollaston; Imbecility compatible with high Moral qualities; Story of the two Children; Character changed by a Spicula of Bone; Case of antagonist Convictions in a Clergyman* 132

CHAPTER XVI: *Case of Mr. Percival; Reflections; Diseased Volitions* 146

CHAPTER XVII: *Definition of Insanity; Comparison of the Watch; Dr. Conolly's Inquiry into the Indications of Insanity; Proofs of Double Mind in that Work; Examples of rapid Transition of Thought; Of two concurrent Trains of Thought; Forms of Mental disturbance; Mr. Barlow; Examples of two antagonist Volitions; Moral and Medical objects of Dr. Conolly's work* 157

CHAPTER XVIII: *Apology for quoting largely from established Writers; Long case of Moral Insanity from Dr. Pritchard; Remarks thereon; Danger of allowing large latitude to equivocal Responsibility; Progress of Depravity; Other Cases from Dr. Pritchard; Dr. Hawkins; Early Inference drawn by myself from similar cases* 181

CHAPTER XIX: *Progress of Insanity; Unimportance of the Mode in which it is manifested; Varieties in the condition of the Blood; Miracles; False Perceptions; Nature of Insanity; Catalepsy; Ganglionic System; Rarity of Insanity; Moral Reflections* 193

CHAPTER XX: *Difficulty of deciding the Point at which Insanity begins; Mathematicians and Artists; Increase of Mental Powers; Madness of Volition; Negligent Volition; Power of controlling Hereditary tendency to Insanity; Self-control of Lunatics; Medical Jury* 205

CHAPTER XXI: *Distinction between Folly and Imbecility; Possibility of cultivating an imperfect Brain into average Intellect; Education not to be hurried; Frauds of Tutors; Precocious Intellect; Examples of Cruelty in forcing premature Development; A peculiar form of Cerebral Irregularity; Dr. Haslam on Sound Mind and Insanity; Power of selecting or discarding a subject of Thought; Associations* 219

CHAPTER XXII: *Hysteria; Hypochondriasis; Hydrophobia* 239

CHAPTER XXIII: *Difficulty of obtaining information of the early Pathological State; Dr. Greding's Reports; Impropriety of classing Idiots with the Insane; Attempts to educate Idiots; Opinions of Georget on Disease of the Brain as the cause of Insanity* 246

Chapter XXIV: *Change in the Brain from exercise of its Fibres; Instinct and Reason; Jacobi's Remarks on the Intellect of Insects; Ratiocination of an Elephant and of Spiders* 254

Chapter XXV: *Dr. Macnish, on the Philosophy of Sleep; Argumentative Dreams; Conscience; Somnambulism; Absence of Mind; Moral Apoplexy; Speech given by Terror; Coma; Sudden Restoration of the Faculties* 267

Chapter XXVI: *Dr. Brigham on the Effect of Mental Cultivation; Mind and Soul; Gradual extinction of Faculties by Pressure on the Brain; Restoration on removing it; Summary of the Argument on the distinction between Mind and Soul* 282

Chapter XXVII: *Double or alternate Consciousness; Double Identity; Four States of the Brain from Injury; Explanation of the alternate Consciousness; Action of the Cerebral Fibres; their number; Powers of the Microscope* 289

Chapter XXVIII: *Rev. J. Barlow on the connexion between Physiology and Intellectual Philosophy; State of the Brain when its higher Faculties are not called into action; Reason why there should be Two Organs of Thought; Mr. Hewitt Watson's Essay on the use of the Double Brain* 295

Chapter XXIX: *Power of abstaining from Evil; Calvinistic Doctrines; Great Concert of Nature; Effect of the new Theory, if adopted; Quotation from J. B. Rousseau; Change by Conversion; Proposal of early restraint in Insanity; Amendment of the Criminal Law; Concluding Parable* 305

Appendix I: *On the Influence of Religion on Insanity* 317

Appendix II: *Conjectures on the Nature of the Mental Operations* 326

Appendix III: *On the Management of Lunatic Asylums* 336

Foreword by Joseph Bogen, M.D.

THE AWARD of the Nobel Prize in Physiology to Roger Sperry[15] in 1981 brought widespread recognition to the concept of the dual brain, for which the split-brain research under Sperry's aegis provided the most important evidence.[16,17] But the concept of the dual brain (that we each have two brains and that they can work to a significant extent independently) had engaged scientists, physicians, and philosophers for well over a century. Of the many who wrote on this subject, Arthur Ladbroke Wigan was not only the most ardent enthusiast, but among the most readable as well. And he may have been the most thoughtful, since he only published his delightful book, "The Duality of the Mind," after more than two decades of consideration and investigations. He wrote: "The mind is essentially dual, like the organs by which it is exercised;" and then: "The idea has presented itself to my mind, and I have dwelt on it for more than a quarter of a century, without being able to find a single valid or even plausible objection."

Wigan's selections and interpretations of evidence, sometimes amusingly archaic by modern standards, were on a par with the medical writings of his time, of which his is a particularly good example. He was almost always eloquent even when over-reaching the facts (of which he had collected more than any of his peers). Although he was excessively discursive at times, with a frequent appeal to anecdote and cameo asides, he made up in liveliness of style and literary interest whatever was lost in redundancy. Two examples from "The Duality of the Mind":

> "Each man knows his own bad volitions, which he has been able to suppress; but he knows not which of his neighbours, whom he thinks so pure, have had the same difficulties to encounter; still less does he know those who have indulged their evil propensities undetected of all but One."

> ". . . it is safer for society to punish than to give extensive impunity; just as it is safer and more extensively beneficial to mankind that the marriage tie should be indissoluble, although the enforcement of the bond is often accompanied by the most cruel tyranny and injustice."

It is perhaps more to the point to quote at length what may well be the pithiest statement of his creed, to which I have referred[3] as "Wiganism."

> If, for example, as I have so often stated, and now again repeat, one brain be a perfect instrument of thought—if it be capable of all the emotions, sentiments, and faculties, which we call in the aggregate, mind—then it necessarily follows that man must have two minds with two brains; and however intimate and perfect their unison in their natural state, they must occasionally be discrepant, when influenced by disease, either direct, sympathetic, or reflex. (Chap. XIX)

Not only the opinions of Wigan but even the fact of his existence barely survived into the 20th century. Forty years after Wigan's death Maudsley[12] referred in a footnote to him and to "his original and suggestive book on The Duality of the Mind (1844), a book which has never perhaps obtained the attention which it deserved . . . ." And Hunter and MacAlpine[10] gave him six pages. But his name does not appear in standard reference works on the history of medicine. In a brief note on Morton Prince, Harms[9] wrote:

> Holland, a fashionable court physician of his time . . . speculated that "there could be two states of consciousness side by side or following one another according to changes of conditions."

> A more impressive presentation of earlier observations of "dual consciousness" came from a contemporary and countryman of Holland, Arthur Ladbroke Wigan. History has treated this important man rather strangely. Although referred to in contemporary literature as ingenious and celebrated, nothing about his life has come down to us, except the date of his death, December 7, 1847.

The interest in Wigan that has recently emerged is due in part to my article in 1969 entitled "The Other Side of the Brain,"[2] particularly because this article was republished (in an abbreviated form) in a widely read collection assembled by Robert Ornstein.[13]

In my 1969 article I suggested that the demise of the two-brain view (and with it the neglect of Wigan) could be attributed to the emergence of the concept of left hemisphere dominance in the late 19th century, the result not only of work by Broca and subsequent aphasiologists but also the work of Liepmann on apraxia. According to Goldstein (1953) it was Liepmann who made ". . . the important discovery of the dominance of the left hemisphere." Isler and Regard[11] suggest that some credit should go to Wigan, since he considered the possibility of left hemisphere dominance (see Chap. XXI) on the basis that most people are right-handed. But it seems clear that to the extent he held such views, he influenced few if any others. The rise of the concept of cerebral dominance has been expertly reviewed by Benton.[1] And the reappearance of the two-brain view is reviewed in my recent chapter on "The Callosal Syndromes."[4]

Isler and Regard suggest that Wigan's near oblivion was also attributable to his own "hard headed, stubborn and extremely aggressive" character. They particularly single out his denunciation of Dr. Holland's insistence on the "Oneness of the Mind" in spite of his belief in the doubleness of the brain. Wigan wrote as follows:

> To me it seems that Dr. Holland's fixed notion on that subject is like the fixed notion of the opponents of Galileo,

> that the earth was stationary in the centre of the system; and that had his mind been free from prepossession on this subject, he could not have resisted the influence of such evidence as he has himself accumulated. (Chap. X)

Wigan's stubborness (or perhaps his independence) is reflected in his criticism of Holland, in spite of the fact that he dedicated his book to Holland (possibly in the hope of currying favor?). As pointed out by Isler and Regard:

> Sir Henry Holland (1788–1873), physician in ordinary to the Royal couple, was "one of the best-known men in London society, the friend and advisor of almost every man of note," says the Dictionary of National Biography from whose pages Wigan is conspicuously absent. Holland's answer to the insult was as final as it was elegant: In a new edition of his writings on the nervous system, "Chapters on Mental Physiology" of 1852, he acknowledged Wigan's dedication in a footnote, at the same time quashing his opinions with the remark that he found it "unwise and injurious to push speculation beyond the closest induction from . . . observations (of facts)."

And so it is that radical innovators, right or wrong, are in the main easily shrugged off by those whose social superiority is accompanied by a confident assertion of received doctrine, sufficiently embellished here and there to give them, among their peers, the appearance of originality.

Whatever the causes either for the eclipse of the two-brain view (and with it Wigan) or for the more recent revival, there is again an interest in it and him. So it has often happened that people have asked me, "How did *you* ever hear of Wigan?"

In 1966 while considering that the co-occurence in the human of cerebral duality (also true in cats and monkeys) and of hemispheric specialization must surely have a variety of remarkable implications, I was searching for any relevant evidence. I chanced upon an excellent article by Robert Efron.[6] Toward the end of this article he suggests that a slight delay in perception by one cerebral hemisphere with respect to the other might afford a physiologic explanation for the phenomenon of *déja vu*. Added later, in galley proof, was a footnote on page 423 beginning as follows:

> "Prof. O. L. Zangwill has kindly called to my attention a monograph ("The Duality of the Mind" by A. L. Wigan, 1844, published by Longman, Brown and Green, London) in which the author suggests an explanation of déja vu superficially resembling the one proposed in this paper."

Efron was at some pains to dissociate himself from Wigan's radical ideas on duality of cognition, volition, etc. On reading this I thought, well *he* (Efron) may think Wigan foolish, but it sounds like *just* the sort of thing I have come to believe myself! So I made my highest priority then to learn more of Wigan and especially to read his book. None of this was easy as he seemed to have all but vanished. To this day no one has been able to locate a photograph, painting, or even a sketch of the man. This included the Bettman Archive in New York City, the Royal College of Physicians in London, and the Wellcome Institute in London. It also includes Basil Clarke, whose investigation of Wigan's life[5] is probably the most thoroughgoing so far. I was eventually able to borrow a copy of the 1844 book from the National Library of Medicine in Washington and I had it long enough to use it in the 1969 article.[2]

What remains difficult to explain is how I came to omit any mention of Efron from this 1969 article. Since that time I have cited him often, collaborated with him[7] and enjoyed immensely the pleasure of his company, inspite of the fact that he still stubbornly clings to his Hollandish view.*

There is, I am told, a copy of Wigan's book at Cambridge University and apparently another used by Isler and Regard, but I have heard with certainty of no other original copy. Several persons in England, among them Oliver Zangwill,

*In any event, as J. Johnstone said, "Wigan seems to have spent a lot of time in other peoples footnotes."

have attempted to purchase a copy for me, but without success so far. It was a happy chance that Joseph Simon and I met, and that we became well acquainted. One day, on a sudden impulse, I called to suggest that he undertake the labors of republishing a nearly extinct item, adding it to his list of largely unavailable classics in literature and philosophy. Since he needed to read it before agreeing, our first step was to obtain it from the National Library of Medicine; they sent us a microfilm of the same volume which I had borrowed in 1967 (there were identical marks in the margins). His reading enjoyment made him an enthusiast; and it is to his skilled efforts that we owe the appearance of this beautifully rendered volume.

Only a few editorial changes have been made in the original text, the most obvious being the change in page numbers resulting from a complete resetting in new type. (In the original, page 196 is followed by page 101, and the original pagination resumes at page 241). Since our principal purpose was to make the book available, and not to provide exegesis, no attempt was made to explain medical terms, either those persisting or long since outdated. The spellings of the time are retained wherever they would not be misleading (typical examples are: headach, shew, Shakspere). Occasional obvious typos and errata have been corrected (e. g. where the book has a "humour the size of a walnut" pressing on the brain, the correction was made to "tumour").

Wigan also made unusually copious use of commas and dashes, to the point of distraction for a modern reader, some have therefore been deleted. A typical Wigan page is illustrated in the following example from page 130, toward the end of Chapter XI, in which Wigan is describing his conversation with a "naval gentleman" who had been institutionalized and was explaining to Wigan how it happened:

> I will explain it to you. You are of course aware that houses describe a cycloidal curve; they are not in the same place in the evening in which they were in the morning. At least you will allow that the chimneys move and you cannot suppose they move without the houses they are

> built on. Now I was proceeding to give a demonstration of this to these men but found they had such a mere smattering of mathematics that they could not follow it; so, to conceal their ignorance, they broke off the conversation and consigned me to a madhouse. A pretty country of liberty this, where men cannot dispute on a point of science but, if they happen to be in a minority, they are called mad and placed in confinement!"

In this reprinting we have deleted the commas before the words "but" and "and" in the final sentence of the above passage; similar changes are numerous but without effect on Wigan's meaning.

Some modern medical readers may be surprised to learn that for Wigan (as for Bouillaud) the lobes of the cerebral hemisphere were only three in number. And he was, of course, completely mistaken in his view that "whenever disease spreads from one cerebrum to the other, it is through the meninges, and never through the corpus callosum." But as he himself insisted in various ways in several places, however wrong he may have been in lesser respects, he was presciently correct in the essence.

As additional information continues to accumulate suggesting that the split-brain results are of significance far beyond their values as a treatment of epilepsy,[14] Wigan's book takes on additional interest, not only because it is a pleasure to read but because it shows us both the insights and concerns of a man whose prophetic vision was over 100 years ahead of the evidence which has ultimately sustained him.

REFERENCES

1. Benton, A. L. (1977). Historical notes on hemispheric dominance. *Arch. Neurol. 34:* 127–129.

2. Bogen, J. E. (1969). The other side of the brain II: An appositional mind. *Bull. Los Angeles Neurol. Soc. 34:* 135–162.

3. Bogen, J. E. (1972). Neowiganism (Concluding Statement) in *Drugs, Development and Cerebral Function*, W. L. Smith (ed.) C. C. Thomas, Springfield.

4. Bogen, J. E. (1985a). The Callosal Syndromes, in K. M. Heilman and E. Valenstein (eds.) *Clinical Neuropsychology, 2nd Edition.* Oxford University Press, New York.

5. Clarke, B. (Unpublished manuscript on the life and significance of Wigan.)

6. Efron, R. (1963). Temporal perception, aphasia and déja vu. *Brain 86:* 403–424.

7. Efron, R.; Bogen, J. E. and Yund, E. W. (1977). Perception of dichotic chords by normal and commissurotimized human subjects. *Cortex 13:* 137–149.

8. Goldstein, K. (1953). Hugo Karl Liepmann. In *The founders of Neurology* (W. Haymaker, ed.) Springfield, Ill., C. C. Thomas.

9. Harms, E. (1961). Predecessors of Morton Prince's dissociation concept. *American Journal of Psychiatry. 117:* 941–2.

10. Hunter, R. and MacAlpine, I. (1963) *Three hundred years of psychiatry.* London: Oxford University Press.

11. Isler, H. and Regard, M. (Unpublished manuscript on A. L. Wigan.)

12. Maudsley, H. (1889). The Double Brain. *Mind 4:* 161–187.

13. Ornstein, R. E. (1973). *The Nature of Human Consciousness.* San Francisco: Freeman & Co: 101–125

14. Reeves, A. (1985). *Epilepsy and the Corpus Callosum.* Plenum, N. Y.

15. Sperry, R. (1982). Some effects of disconnecting the cerebral hemispheres. *Science 217:* 1223–1226.

16. Sperry, R. W.; Gazzaniga, M. S. and Bogen, J. E. (1969). Interhemispheric relationships: The neocortical commissures; syndromes of hemisphere disconnection. *Handbook Clin. Neurol. 4:* 273–290.

17. Zaidel, E. (in press). Right hemisphere language, D. F. Benson and E. Zaidel (eds.) *The Dual Brain: Hemispheric Specialization in Humans.* Guilford, N. Y.

Preface

In looking over the following pages for the purpose of making an index to their contents, I am struck with the conviction, that (were it now to be commenced) it would be easy to execute the task much better. There are occasional negligences which ought to have been avoided, and tautology that in offending the ear is not compensated by additional force and clearness. there are also some errors in the succession of the paragraphs and chapters, and repetitions of inferences which had been already drawn and established.

The last fault, however, is not always unintentional; whenever the facts, arguments, and illustrations, seemed to lead naturally to the conclusion, I have not hesitated to proceed to it at once, although aware that, in other chapters of the book, I had already drawn the same inferences, perhaps in the same terms, from dissimilar facts, imparallel arguments, and totally different illustrations.

I know, by experience, that works of this kind are rarely read consecutively, and therefore do not trust to the desultory reader the task of drawing the conclusion from the whole collocation of evidence. The few men of science who may carefully peruse the book from title-page to colophon, will, I hope, see enough to convince them that the defects arise rather from an unpracticed pen, than from ignorance of the subject, or of the proper mode of treating it, did time and leisure admit of recasting the whole. Should the public be sufficiently interested by the novelty and importance of the theory to call for a second edition, I will endeavour to remove them.

The eminent geometricians who were employed on the trigonometrical survey of the country some years ago, did on one occasion lose their way, and were set right by a ploughman. I do not fancy myself capable of making a trigonometrical survey even of the department I have selected, but shall be satisfied with the concession of the ploughman's degree of merit, if it be found that I have liberated investigators from the quagmires and obscurities of the jungle, and pointed out a clear and practicable road to the object of their hitherto confessedly futile pursuit.

Lest however the possession of this degree of modesty be denied me, I will use another and a different illustration.

If to the rope by which the animal is tethered to the spot we make an addition equal only to one-half of its original length, we have more than doubled the space to which he was previously confined. In like manner if I have added but a few links to the short and galling chain that binds us to the earth, I shall have largely increased the field of discovery, and paved the way, I hope, for better workmen. The only limit to our researches on the nature of the mind, will ultimately be the boundary fixed by the Almighty to the powers of the human intellect—a point from which we are yet immeasurably distant. When we shall have cultivated all the faculties which He has bestowed upon us, to their full extent and perfection, then indeed will come the Millennium—an issue towards which we are steadily and rapidly advancing.

> God never meant that man should scale the heavens
> By strides of human wisdom.

Even should it be found that two or three persons have *slightly* indicated a *slight* guess at a *slight* portion of the theory I am attempting to establish, my ideas are not the less original, for no suggestion reached me till more than twenty years after I had completely arranged the whole in my own mind. The previous hints may diminish the *merit*, but not the *value* of my demonstration. If I can firmly fix the latter in the convictions of the public, it is all I desire to accomplish.—The originality may be denied without giving me the slightest pain.

He who just indicates or asserts that a certain block of marble contains a beautiful statue is not, however, placed exactly on the same level with the sculptor who clears away the rubbish and gives it form and expression. The simple fact of the vaccine disease being a preservative from small-pox was known a century before the birth of Dr. Jenner, but it was he who elaborated the proofs and established the practice. If my theory be proved beyond cavil, I may surely claim some portion of similar merit; for (if there be no defect in the mental telescope) it involves distant consequences of much greater importance than vaccination.

"It is with theories as with wells," says Swift, "you may see to the bottom of the deepest, *if there be any water there*, while another shall pass for wondrous profound, when 'tis merely shallow, dark, and empty."

The single point on which I am inclined to modify my assertions is the structure and office of the corpus callosum, respecting which, some new views have been opened to me by very recent dissection—they do not, however, in any respect interfere with the notions I have expressed as to the nature of the mind; and as the candidates for the college prize of the current year (the distribution of the cerebral fibres) will probably throw considerable light on this obscure subject, I do not, on the present occasion, put forth my own as yet crude and imperfect opinions.

I will only add, in anticipation and deprecation of critical censure, that a man cannot well be accused of precipitation or presumption who waits till his sixtieth year to promulgate opinions he has held during half his life with daily increasing conviction; which he believes to be of the greatest importance in medicine, morals, and jurisprudence—in the management of the insane—in the treatment of criminals—the education of youth—and, above all, in the discipline of *imperfect, defective*, and *distorted* minds.

ARTHUR LADBROKE WIGAN

Croydon, November, 1844

TO

A PROFOUND THINKER AND ABLE PHYSICIAN,

A SCHOLAR, A PHILOSOPHER, AND A GENTLEMAN

TO

DR. HENRY HOLLAND, F. R. S.

PHYSICIAN TO THE QUEEN

THIS BOOK IS RESPECTFULLY INSCRIBED

BY THE AUTHOR

THE
Duality of the Mind

CHAPTER I: *Introduction; Unsettled State of Mental Philosophy; A New Instrument for its Investigation; Mind and Soul*

The spot of earth on which he stands seems to every man the centre of the world, as the highest point of the heavens is always immediately over his head. This feeling is one of the modifications of self-love, a principle which, like the law of gravitation, keeps each group of particles in its place, and the whole of the groups in harmonious combination and unity. It is through the influence of this universal sentiment that each single point in the wilderness of knowledge seems, to him who sets himself to its investigation, more important than all others, and thus excites an interest disproportioned perhaps to its intrinsic value. Without this extrinsic interest, however, few men would give themselves the continuous labour of examination and consideration; life indeed is not long enough to allow any individual to benefit mankind by the results of diffused researches into various departments of knowledge. By confining himself to a single topic, and pursuing it with zeal and perseverance, any man of ordinary capacity and acquirements may elicit new and useful truths, more or less important according to the subject he has selected, and his own powers of investigation. Whatever we thus place under the mental microscope is found to possess forms and qualities which the cursory view of ordinary vision passes by unnoticed; and it is no wonder then that those who have not subjected it to a similar rigid examination, should hesitate or refuse to acquiesce in the importance of the pretended discovery. Making every allowance for this source of erroneous estimation of the relative value of our own researches and those of others, I cannot but think that the subjects treated of in the following pages are amongst the most important which can occupy the attention of a rational being. Researches into the nature and modes of manifestation of the august faculty of Reason seem to be the very foundation of all positive knowledge; and when these researches can be pursued by means of physical evidence, it is clearly an imperative duty to exhaust, as far as possible, all such testimony, before we enter on the wild region of metaphysics.

The unsettled state of mental philosophy in the present day is such as to justify any man in the endeavour to throw light on a subject so dark and intricate, more especially if the discovery of a new instrument seem to give new and extraordinary facilities for the investigation. Physiological reasoning could advance but a little way till the circulation of the blood was ascertained; and whatever may be the degree of merit awarded to myself on the present occasion, I cannot but think that I bring to the investigation of the mental phenomena in health and disease a new power, of at least equal importance, and capable of equally satisfactory demonstration.

Mr. George Combe remarks as follows: "Dr. Reid overturned the philosophy of Locke and Hume. Stewart, while he illustrated Reid, differed from him in many important particulars; and recently, Dr. Thomas Brown has attacked with powerful eloquence and philosophical profundity the fabric of Newton, which already totters to its fall. The very existence of the most common and familiar faculties of the mind is debated among these philosophers. Mr. Stewart maintains attention to be a faculty, but this is denied by Dr. Brown. Others again state imagination to be a primitive power of the mind; whilst Mr. Stewart informs us that 'what we call the power of imagination is not *the gift of nature*, but the result of acquired habits, aided by favourable circumstances.' Common observation informs us that musical talent, and a genius for poetry and painting, are gifts of nature bestowed only on a few; but Mr. Stewart, by dint of his philosophy, has discovered that these powers, and also a genius for mathematics, 'are gradually formed by particular habits of study or of business.' On the other hand, he treats of perception, conception, and memory, as original powers; while Dr. Thomas Brown denies their title to that appellation. Reid, Stewart, and Brown, admit the existence of moral emotions; but Hobbes, Mandeville, Paley, and many others, resolve the sentiment of right and wrong into a regard to our own good, perception of utility, and obedience to human laws or the Divine command. Thus, after the lapse and labour of more than two thousand years, philosophers are not yet agreed concerning the existence of many of the most important principles of action and intellectual powers of man. While the philosophy of mind shall remain in this uncertain condition, it will be impossible to give to morals and natural religion a scientific foundation; and, until these shall assume the stableness and precision of science, education, political economy, and legislation, must continue defective in their principles and application."

If this be a true representation of the present state of mental philospphy, I need make no apology for putting forth a theory which may tend to reconcile the discrepancy of opinion on such important subjects. I hope, at least, to point out a path which may lead others to a more open country, than the tangled maze they have hitherto pursued in vain.

If the facts and arguments advanced in the present work, and the inferences to which they lead, be admitted, it must be allowed that they furnish ample materials for the construction of a theory at once so novel and so important, that if its truth be established it may almost aspire to the honour of being called a discovery. This may seem too bold an assumption to him who commences the investigation, but after a patient perusal of the evidence, he will, I think, feel himself compelled to yield his assent to the claim.

I have carefully examined most of the established authors on the subject of the mind, and of its manifestations through a material organ, as well as those on the anatomy and physiology of the brain, and other writers on collateral subjects, and I cannot find one, except Dr. Holland, who has advanced a single step on the road to the important truth which I hope to establish; namely, that the mind is essentially dual, like the organs by which it is exercised. Even Dr. Holland does not follow up his own ideas to their legitimate consequences, nor arrive at the logical result to which they seem inevitably to lead, as I expect to shew in the course of my examination of the opinions he has promulgated in his essay *On the Brain as a Double Organ*, contained in his profound and instructive work called *Medical Notes and Reflections*.

A double organ the brain is not, but *dual* it is, as I shall prove beyond a shadow of doubt.

The word *Mind* is employed in so many different senses in ordinary discourse, that it will be necessary, on the present occasion, strictly to define its meaning before we can advance into the discussion on which I propose to enter; it is used so vaguely and so variously in different places by the same writer, that it is often difficult to understand the drift of his argument. By some it is held to be synonymous with soul, and by others considered as equivalent to the *Principle of Vitality* of animal life. According to Cruden, the word is used in the Holy Scriptures in nine different senses, and the word *Soul*, in five. With these varieties of signification we have nothing to do in the present disquisition, and I confine myself to the single object of shewing the absolute distinction between *Mind* and *Soul*. It seems to me that the use of these two words as convertible terms, is a serious obstacle to the freedom of investigation of the mental phenomenà, and is at the root of all the difficulties which occur in the discussion of the intellectual faculties.

When I speak of *Mind*, then, I wish to be understood to signify the aggregate of the mental powers and faculties, whether exercised by one brain or two; and when I have occasion to allude to the GREAT, IMMORTAL, IMMATERIAL PRINCIPLE, connected for a time with the material world by means of our physical organization—I shall call it by its proper name, THE SOUL.

The soul, however, is not in question on the present occasion; it lies in the domain of theology, into which I do not presume to enter. Of it we can know absolutely nothing through our own unaided faculties. Revelation alone can enable us even to conceive its nature, still more its destiny.

To attempt to form a conception of the abstract nature of *the Mind*, in the sense in which it is usually employed, or even of the vital principle, or of the essence of matter, is a pure misemployment of our time, and leads only to confusion; these things are beyond our comprehension, absolutely out of the reach of our faculties, and were probably so intended by the

Creator. On these subjects the gigantic intellect of a Newton is as impotent as that of the uneducated peasant, or the child.

In contemplating my own mental powers, it seems to me that such investigations are as futile as the endeavour to ascertain what kind of structure it is which fits the inhabitants of the planet Mercury for their position so near the sun. We are wandering beyond the bounds assigned to human understanding. With the manifestations of these essences in their phenomena we are familiar, and can pursue the examination of them to a satisfactory result. The prospect beyond is covered with clouds and darkness, and our limited vision can penetrate no further.

I have listened to the reasonings of our greatest modern philosopher, on the essential nature of matter, with wonder, admiration, and alarm:—wonder, at the exibition of mental powers, so vastly beyond the average of humanity; admiration, of the energy and perseverance with which they have been cultivated; and alarm, lest the physical structure of the material organ should be spoiled by such excessive exertion of its faculties.

"To see ourselves," says Lord Bacon, "we must look down." Let us humbly exercise within their proper bounds, the glorious faculties which it has pleased the Almighty to bestow upon us; and when we have finished our worldly task, and spun, like the silkworm, our allotted cocoon, let us wait till a more genial atmosphere shall call us to a higher destiny. When the chrysalis bursts from his torpor and his prison, and is furnished with wings, he has a wider horizon, a more extended view, and increased faculties for the enjoyment of happiness.

CHAPTER II: *Origin of the Work; Rev. J. Barlow, on Man's Power over Himself to Prevent and Control Insanity; High Intellectual Cultivation of the Clergy; There Can Be No Discrepancy between the Word and the Works of God*

The opinions here expressed on the nature of insanity, of the exercise of sound mind, and of the structure and functions of the brain, which give rise to these different states, are not of recent growth; they have occupied my attention for at least thirty years, and have appeared to me so clear, so well founded, and so obvious, that I have constantly wished to place them before the public, and have only been withheld from it by two considerations. The first, that inferences, apparently so irresistible, from facts so thoroughly established, must necessarily have been drawn by others, and that I should be contending for opinions already familiar to thinkers. Secondly, that my theory of the mental functions in health and disease was accompanied by moral corollaries, extremely perplexing and unsatisfactory; which latter reason I naturally thought might have operated with others as well as myself, and would perhaps account for the silence of so many writers on a subject of such great interest and importance.

Longer consideration, and more extensive reading and experience, have convinced me that such fears were quite unfounded, and that, in seeking during so many years for objections to my theory, instead of confirmation of it, I have neglected a duty incumbent on every man, of promulgating a *new* and important *truth*.

This mode of proceeding has, however, had one advantage; it has enabled me to anticipate or to refute, I believe, all the objections to the new doctrine. I have tried them in every way that my degree of intellect would permit, and believe them to be utterly unfounded.

It is not likely, however, that I should have put pen to paper on the subject, but for the perusal of a highly interesting little work, *On Man's Power over Himself to prevent or control Insanity*, by the Rev. J. Barlow, the Secretary of the Royal Institution. I have read it with great interest and attention. The acute and able writer goes so near the *truth*, that to use the children's phrase, "he burns;" and I can only attribute the tangent he describes, on approaching the very verge of the discovery, to an influence which has misled many other men —an error in nomenclature; vitiating the ratiocination of some of the strongest minds which have been directed to the subject.

It is from no feeling of arrogance that I use this language respecting my superiors in mental power and acquirements. The idea *has* persented itself to *my* mind, and I have dwelt on it for more than a quarter of a century, without being able to find a single valid, or even plausible objection. It explains innumerable difficulties and contradictions; it is founded on anatomical evidence, capable of demonstration, and is in strict harmony with all we know, or can infer, of the designs of Providence in a world of progressive education.

"We must not say what good shall this thing do, for the use of every thing shall be found in its season, but we dare not disguise the truth."

In reading Mr. Barlow's work, I was struck with the candid and fearless spirit in which the subject was pursued. It is evident that the object of the writer was *truth*, and truth alone, and that he was not a man to be deterred from following up a process of rigid induction, by any apprehension of the logical inferences to which it might lead, and which might seem, perhaps, to clash with received opinions, deemed essential to the welfare and happiness of mankind. In the true and honest spirit of a Christian philosopher, he seems to have felt that God intended us to execise all the reasoning faculties he has bestowed upon us, and that whatever truth was logically proved, must, in the end, be useful to man.

It was a great satisfaction to find, that in a book written by a clergyman, on natural science, there was no admixture of controversial theology. The clergy, as a body, are, beyond question, the best educated men in the kingdom, and the men who have most successfully cultivated the art of making efficient use of the reasoning faculties,—they are, therefore, admirable auxiliaries in the investigation of natural phenomena, when they will be contented to put aside, for the moment, their own peculiar science, which depends on proofs of a totally different nature. Moral evidence may be as cogent, conclusive, and satisfactory as physical evidence, but it must not be admitted as alone sufficient in the exact sciences, It has always appeared to me a desecration of theology, to mix it up with investigations of the physical laws of nature.

Whenever, by the aid of anatomy, physiology, and pathology, we have clearly established, on irrefragable evidence, certain natural facts, we may rest entirely satisfied that, however they may at first appear opposed to the doctrines of theology, they will ultimately be explained and harmonized by theologians, so as to calm the apprehensions, and convey consolation and conviction to every devout Christian. To cite only two instances out of many:

The doctrines of Galileo excited the sincere indignation of the clergy of his day, who most conscientiously persecuted him, and compelled him to disavow tenets believed to be in opposition to the Word of God. Time passed on, his discoveries were universally received as truths, and now the clergy themselves teach the astronomical facts which were at first supposed to be blasphemous falsehoods.

In like manner, the new science of geology was opposed on its first introduction; not merely by clergymen, who naturally take alarm at any apparent attack on the system it is the object of their lives to explain and defend, but by great numbers of the laity, who also believed the discoveries of geologists to be opposed to the doctrines of the Church, and dangerous to the welfare of mankind. These discoveries, however, are now universally adopted, and taught by clergymen, who even declare that the immense duration of the earth, apparently established by this new and wonderful science, is in perfect harmony with the cosmogony of Moses.

All this is a great encouragement to persevere in physical investigations. It is indeed obvious that the *works of God* can never be really opposed to the *word of God*, and that, as it has been ingeniously and reverently expressed, "whenever there is an apparent discrepancy between them, it must necessarily arise from an erroneous interpretation of the latter"—an assertion to which every man will assent, who can recollect the opposite and contradictory explanations given by different sects, of certain passages of Scripture which, to him, appear to have no ambiguity whatever.

In fact, when in this country alone, a body of more than twenty-five thousand men in succession, whose intellectual faculties have been cultivated to the highest degree that our institutions will allow, are set to explain apparent discrepancies between natural science and theology, aided by the accumulated arguments of their predecessors, recorded during so many centuries, and instigated by every motive that can influence the mind; when such a body of men are, by the institutions of society, supplied with all possible inducements to persevere in the struggle, and labour for the final triumph of religion; when honour, wealth, high station, and other worldly rewards are profusely offered to the successful controversialist, and when he is still further excited by an approving conscience, and an entire conviction that he is promoting the temporal and eternal happiness of his fellow-creatures; when this combination of selfish and of generous motives is found in so large, so intelligent, so enlightened, and so moral a body of men, the mere physician—and I use the word in its original sense, which is still retained in every modern language of Europe, except our own,—the mere *physician* must, indeed, be presumptuous, should he expect that his feeble efforts and limited discoveries can endanger a system so solid and so long established.

Let us then proceed without fear, pursue our investigations with patience and caution, make good every step before we advance to the next, and take care that each in succession be established beyond the possibility of failure; we may then, with a safe conscience, discard all consideration of consequences, in the conviction that all positive truths will, in the end, be found consistent with true religion, and useful to society. Let us accept with cheerfulness the assistance of every clergyman who will descend from his vantage-ground, and aid us in the cultivation of natural science, without apprehensions for the issue, laying down the precaution of party politicians, who hardly dare to give utterance to that which they know to be true, till they have ascertained whether it be likely to benefit or injure "THE CAUSE."

CHAPTER III: *Description of the Brain, Adapted to Non-Medical Readers; Functions of the Brain*

It is not likely that many persons will read this work who are not already acquainted with the structure of the brain; but as some may be interested in my speculations on the nature of the mind, who do not possess that knowledge, I give a short description of that organ, sufficient, perhaps, to enable them to comprehend the scope of the arguments. Should they once enter on the investigation, it possesses such strong attractions as will no doubt induce them to pursue the study of at least this portion of anatomy, for which there are in the present day such great facilities, without going through the labour of dissection. There is no part of the body of which a man of sense and spirit would less willingly be ignorant. If the great distinction between ourselves and the beasts that perish, be as I have stated, *the power of thinking of our own thoughts*, surely the organ by which alone this Godlike faculty is exercised must be an object of the greatest interest, and its structure well worthy of attention. A very slight knowledge of the manifestations of mind by a material organ would prevent a man from falling into the silly metaphysical notions which pervade the ignorant, and form one of the most formidable impediments to the acquisition of real information; would dissipate prejudices as gross as those we ridicule respecting witches and apparitions; and would give a precision to our language, the want of which is a constant source of dispute and dissension. It would enable him often to test the stories which are told to him, and prevent him from retailing as truths, things which are self-contradictory and impossible. There are some narratives of death-beds, for example, put forth with the best intentions no doubt, but which a man, with a moderate knowledge of the structure and functions of the brain would know to be false, and to have been invented by a person in perfect health, who was entirely ignorant of the physical and moral state of the moribund.

On removing the bony roof of the skull, we observe the brain, or cerebrum, lying covered by a thick membrane or skin; on cutting through this skin, we see a mass of tortuous folds like intestines, huddled together irregularly; these are called the *convolutions* of the brain. The thick membrane which covers them is attached to the skull along its central line, from front to back, and dipping down between these convolutions, divides them into two equal and similar parts, called the *hemispheres* of the brain.

Let the reader imagine a hollow frill, containing a solid substance about the consistence of new cheese; suppose the frill thus filled, to be sewed on the edge of a band, and puckered very closely, it will then form what may be compared to a sausage, which, when thus drawn together at the bottom, becomes twisted and turned in irregular serpentine folds at the upper rounded edge. Suppose a similar frill sewed on the other edge of the band, and the whole compressed into an oval box. This will very fairly represent the brain. The small space into which these convolutions are packed, pushes them all together into a mass, and the two halves would be undistinguishable, but for the strong skin or membrane, which dips down between them to the band, where the two portions are fastened.

This band is a white substance, in appearance something like the white ligament which is seen in a neck of veal; it is, however, by no means of equal consistence, being so soft as to be easily broken through with the fingers. It is called the *corpus callosum*, or great *commissure*, and forms the bond of union between the two halves of the brain, or the two brains, as it is more correct to call them. There are other small fibrous bands, which stretch across from one brain to the other, but they need not be taken into consideration on the present occasion.

Now the whole of the human body is in the beginning composed of two absolutely distinct halves, which ultimately grow together, and unite; so also with the brain; but the fibres from each half of the latter only go to the middle line, and do not pass over to the other side; and when there is a great accumulation of water under the corpus callosum from disease, its splits asunder along this line, and each half is retracted to its own side.

The covering of these convolutions, which I have compared to intestines, is of considerable thickness, is of a granular texture, and of a grey ashy colour, and the interior substance, pure white; the former is supposed to be the essential nervous matter which gives sensation, and the other functions of the brain, and the white is composed of very minute fibres, running up into it, which convey the volitions to the extreme parts and sensations from extreme parts to the mind. The object of all these convolutions would seem to be to furnish a larger surface of grey matter, than could have existed had the brain been in one uniform mass; for it would appear that the powers of the brain are created by an action of some kind between these two substances. Some have supposed it to be of the nature of galvanism. All we know is that the contact of the two is necessary to produce any of the faculties, and that the energy of these faculties is in proportion to the extent of surface of grey matter.

I have thus described the convolutions, in order to give a clear idea of their position; in point of fact, however, they do not extend down to the edge of the band, but only to a certain depth in the white mass of fibres which forms the body and substance of the brain. If we could suppose the skin of the lower edge of each convolution to be obliterated at the surfaces in contact, and the white substance to coalesce into one uniform mass, we should form a tolerably correct notion of the real state of the brain.

The membrane which I have described as dividing the convolutions into two symmetrical hemispheres, resembles a scythe or sickle, and hence called the *falx*, of which the point is towards the forehead; at the broad end it rests on another similar membrane, stretching tight across from one side of the skull to the other at right angles with the former; this is named the *tentorium*. The object of these membranes, which are as tightly stretched as the skin of a drum, seems to be to prevent the mischievous consequences of the concussion of the brain in sudden movements; as jumping, for example—the elastic membrane gives way to the impulse, and thus diminishes the shock. The falx is also of great utility in preventing the pressure of one brain on the other in lying down; and the transverse membrane, called the tentorium, performs a similar office; it forms a kind of tent (whence its name), and covers a deep hollow in the back part of the skull, which contains the cerebellum, and thus preserves it from the pressure of the superincumbent mass of cerebrum.

The cerebellum (or *little brain*) has some slight resemblance to the real *brain of thought*, but is of a much firmer consistence: like the other, it is composed of two different textures. Philosophers are not quite decided as to the use it fulfils in the animal economy. Numerous cruel experiments have been performed on living animals, with the object of ascertaining its functions, but the results are unsatisfactory and indeed contradictory. One thing, however, seems conclusively established, that it is not the organ of the reasoning faculties; it is unnecessary, therefore, to dwell upon it in a disquisition on the nature of the mind.

At the basis of the brain there are a number of little protuberances called, according to their shape, *corpora mammillaria* (mammillary bodies), from their resemblance to the form of the breast (mamma), corpora olivaria (olives), corpora albicantia, restiformia, pyramidalia, striata, quadrigemina, and many others. There is also a prolongation of the brain, called the *medulla oblongata*, forming the bulbous head of the spinal marrow, etc. etc.

From the basis of the brain pass off a number of white cords, called nerves, supplying the special senses, and also volition and sensation; and from the prolongation of the medulla oblongata (the spinal marrow) pass off nerves to all parts of the body with similar functions.

At that part at the basis of the brain, or medulla oblongata, called the *corpora pyramidalia*, the minute fibres which descend from the upper surface of the convolutions, *decussate*, or cross over from one side to the other; so that it is the right brain which supplies its influence to the left side of the body, and *vice versa*. And this division of functions is so absolute, that whatever may be the extent of the injury of one brain, it is the opposite side of the body which alone suffers, and the other is entirely unaffected. The object of this arrangement is at present incomprehensible; no doubt, in the further progress of science, it will be discovered, and be found to be quite in harmony with the whole scheme of our economy—every part of which appears to be contrived with such surpassing skill, that the more we investigate the more are we lost in admiration, wonder, and reverence.

One of the most inconceivable things in the nature of the brain is, that the organ of sensation should itself be insensible. To cut the brain gives no pain, yet in the brain alone resides the power of feeling pain in any other part of the body. If the nerve which leads to it from the injured part be divided, we become instantly unconscious of suffering. It is only by communication with the brain that any kind of sensation is produced, yet the organ itself is insensible!

But there is a circumstance more wonderful still. The brain itself may be removed—may be cut away, down to the corpus callosum, without destroying life! The animal lives, and performs all those functions which are necessary to simple vitality, but has no longer a *mind*—it cannot *think* or feel—it requires that the food should be pushed into its stomach; once there, it is digested, and the animal will even thrive and grow fat. We infer, therefore, that the part of the brain called the convolutions is simply intended for the exercise of the intellectual faculties, whether of the low degree called *Instinct*, or of that exalted kind bestowed on man, *the gift of Reason.*

The whole mass of each brain is divided into three lobes, called the anterior, middle, and posterior. The division is but just indicated by a greater depth of the convolutions, and is by no means distinct throughout. Many phrenologists deny the existence of a division into three lobes, which on their parts seems a strange contradiction, since they demand assent to their assertions, that the convolutions are divided into separate organs, which manifest different functions, faculties, affections, instincts, or propensities; and this, although it is not even pretended that, anatomically speaking, there is any distinction or separation between them. Most phrenologists go much further, and contend that these arbitrary divisions are manifested on the surface of the skull, and form an indication of the character of the individual. This is quite a different affair; and if a sufficient number of coincidences between conformation and character were established, on clear and satisfactory evidence, we could not refuse assent to the simple doctrine of Cranioscopy, whether we did or did not believe that such differences depended on the division of the brain into organs, capable of being distinctly located and recognised.

I have treated this subject elsewhere. What has been said above, as to the structure of the brain, is sufficient to give a general idea of it. If, however, the reader be not acquainted with its anatomy, he may *acquiesce* in my facts and my reasonings, but cannot in strictness be said to *judge* of them.

According to Flourens, whose opinions are founded partly on the discoveries of Sir Charles Bell, and partly on his own (and which opinions seem to meet general acquiescence and approbation), there are in the nervous system three properties or functions, essentially distinct, which I thus condense into the shortest space—that is to say:

1. That of the power of perceiving sensations, or being conscious of impressions, and the power of willing or volition—*Intelligence.*

2. That of receiving and transmitting impressions—*Sensibility.*

3. That of immediately exciting muscular contraction—*Excitability.*

But according to this writer (and his sentiments on this subject also are now generally adopted), there is, in addition to all these, a property residing exclusively in the cerebellum, or supplementary brain, and only recently discovered, which consists in the power of *co-ordinating the movements willed* by certain parts of the nervous system, and *excited* by others.

The *nerve* directly excites the contraction of the muscle.

The *spinal cord* unites the separate contractions into regular movements.

The *cerebellum* co-ordinates these movements into the forms of locomotion: walking, running, flying, etc.; while by the cerebral lobes, or two cerebra, the animal *perceives* and *wills*.

Those who are unacquainted with the perfection which the microscope has attained in this country, and the marvellous results which have been obtained from its new powers, will be startled at the assertion that a bundle of nervous fibres from the brain contains more than one hundred millions in the square inch; indeed, in some parts of the brain, these fibres may be accurately counted to the extent of fourteen thousand in the space of an inch, which would give to the *square* inch the inconceivable amount of more than three thousand millions: these numbers cannot even be comprehended by the mind; they are, however, objects of measurement and calculation, as certain as the number of cubic inches in a block of wood.

It is further stated that each of these hollow fibres contains a fluid during life, which is coagulated after death, and that this can be distinctly seen in its two states. I give this on the authority of the celebrated microscopical anatomist Erasmus Wilson, and there is none higher.

Now, if the nervous fibres be used as I have supposed, either singly, or in regular fasciculi, in the different mental processes, it is easy to conceive that physical causes may derange so delicate a machinery, and that, acting in erroneous combination, they may give rise to the phenomena of insanity, and other delusions of the mind; and this quite independent of the innumerable changes which may take place in the nervous fluid itself, and the various modifications of its circulation by disorder and disease.

I think that I have placed the statement in so clear a light as to convey to the general reader a correct idea of the nature of the nervous functions; and that, added to the description of the brain previously given, he will be at no loss to comprehend as much of the physical machinery of the mind, as is required in social metaphysics.

It is with no expectation of enabling the public to judge of the medical view of mental organization, that I thus endeavour to make the doctrine understood by the non-medical world—this would be a vain attempt. I would merely furnish means of appreciating, and motives for aiding, the researches of scientific men—to make the rules which such men lay down as the result of their investigations, comprehended and obeyed—and their recommendations adopted and enforced on others less enlightened.

CHAPTER IV: *The Duality of the Mind; Propositions to be Proved; Results if Proved*

In entering on the subject of the duality of the mind and its organs, I must begin by demanding a temporary assent to certain propositions, of which I am hereafter to furnish the proofs. If the chain of reasoning founded upon the graduated collocation of evidence be defective, the dogmas must be denied and discarded. On the concession of them for the moment, however, depends the facility of the inquiry; and this mode is the shortest for arriving at the truth.

I believe it then to be entirely unphilosophical, and tending to important errors, to speak of the cerebrum as one organ. The term *two hemispheres of the brain* is, indeed, strictly a misnomer, since the two together form very little more than one-half of a sphere.

This, however, would be of trifling importance, were it not for the deceptive effect it produces. The two hemispheres of the brain are really and in fact two distinct and entire organs, and each respectively as complete (indeed more complete), and as fully perfect in all its parts, for the purposes it is intended to perform, as are the two eyes. The corpus callosum, and the other commissures between them, can with no more justice be said to constitute the two hemispheres into one organ, than the optic commissure can be called an union of the *two eyes* into one organ; and it would be just as reasonable to talk of the two lobes or globes of the eye, as of the two hemispheres of the brain. The decussation of the fibres in the corpora pyramidalia is not merely visible, but proved by innumerable consequences necessarily resulting from it, as Hemiplegia and Paralysis. Each set of fibres retains its separate functions in passing to the opposite side, and to the opposite columns of the spinal marrow. That some of the powers and functions may be combined in the medulla oblongata, or in the protuberances which occupy the cavities at the base of the bony cranium, is no greater objection to the absolute completeness and individuality of each hemisphere of the brain, or evidence of their forming but one organ, than the fact of our seeing only one object with two eyes proves that the two eyes are not distinct, complete, and separate organs, each capable of acting alone, when its fellow is injured or destroyed.

In drawing up the following propositions, it is by no means my intention to claim for them the merit of strict sequence and logical precision, but merely to give a facility of reference in the arrangement of proofs. Entertaining no doubt whatever that every candid man, after reading these remarks, will at least adopt my nomenclature, I shall in future speak of the two cerebra instead of the two hemispheres; being certain that I shall prove the propriety and utility, nay, the absolute necessity, of using the former term instead of the latter, which has led (as I shall shew) to false inferences, and has no advantage whatever to counterbalance the mischief.

I believe myself then able to prove:

1. That each cerebrum is a distinct and perfect whole, as an organ of thought.
2. That a separate and distinct process of thinking or ratiocination may be carried on in each cerebrum simultaneously.
3. That each cerebrum is capable of a distinct and separate volition, and that these are very often opposing volitions.
4. That, in the healthy brain, one of the cerebra is almost always superior in power to the other, and capable of exercising control over the volitions of its fellow, and of preventing them from passing into acts, or from being manifested to others.
5. That when one of these cerebra becomes the subject of functional disorder, or of positive change of structure, of such a kind as to vitiate mind or induce insanity, the

healthy organ can still, up to a certain point, control the morbid volitions of its fellow.

6. That this point depends partly on the extent of the disease or disorder, and partly on the degree of cultivation of the general brain in the art of self-government.
7. That when the disease or disorder of one cerebrum becomes sufficiently aggravated to defy the control of the other, the case is then one of the commonest forms of mental derangement or insanity; and that a lesser degree of discrepancy between the functions of the two cerebra constitutes the state of conscious delusion.
8. That in the insane, it is almost always possible to trace the intermixture of two synchronous trains of thought, and that it is the irregularly alternate utterance of portions of these two trains of thought which constitutes incoherence.
9. That of the two distinct simultaneous trains of thought, one may be rational and the other irrational, or both may be irrational; but that, in either case, the effect is the same, to deprive the discourse of coherence or congruity.

Even in furious mania, this double process may be generally perceived; often it takes the form of a colloquy between the diseased mind and the healthy one, and sometimes even resembles the steady continuous argument or narrative of a sane man, more or less frequently interrupted by a madman; but persevering with tenacity of purpose in the endeavour to overpower the intruder.

10. That when both cerebra are the subjects of disease, which is not of remittent periodicity, there are no lucid intervals, no attempt at self-control, and no means of promoting the cure; and that a spontaneous cure is rarely to be expected in such cases.
11. That, however, where such mental derangement depends on inflammation, fever, gout, impoverished or diseased blood, or manifest bodily disease, it may often be cured by curing the malady which gave rise to it.
12. That in cases of insanity, not depending on structural injury, in which the patients retain the partial use of reason (from one of the cerebra remaining healthy or only slightly

affected), the only mode in which the medical art can promote the cure beyond the means alluded to is by presenting motives of encouragement to the sound brain to exercise and strengthen its control over the unsound brain.

13. That the power of the higher organs of the intellect to coerce the mere instincts and propensities, as well as the power of one cerebrum to control the volitions of the other, may be indefinitely increased by exercise and moral cultivation; may be partially or wholly lost by desuetude or neglect; or, from depraved habits and criminal indulgence in childhood, and a general vicious education in a polluted moral atmosphere, may never have been acquired.
14. That one cerebrum may be entirely destroyed by disease, cancer, softening, atrophy, or absorption; may be *annihilated*, and in its place a yawning chasm; yet the mind remain complete and capable of exercising its functions in the same manner and to the same extent that one eye is capable of exercising the faculty of vision when its fellow is injured or destroyed; although there are some exercises of the brain, as of the eye, which are better performed with two organs than one. In the case of vision, the power of measuring distances for example, and in the case of the brain, the power of concentrating the thoughts upon one subject, deep consideration, hard study; but in this latter case, it is difficult to decide how far the diminished power depends on diminution of general vigour from formidable and necessarily fatal disease.
15. That a lesion or injury of both cerebra is incompatible with such an exercise of the intellectual functions, as the common sense of mankind would designate *sound mind*.
16. That from the apparent division of each cerebum into three lobes, it is a natural and reasonable presumption that the three portions have distinct offices, and highly probable that the three great divisions of the mental functions laid down by phrenologists, are founded in nature; whether these distinctions correspond with the natural

divisions is a different question, but the fact of different portions of the brain executing different functions, is too well established to admit of denial from any physiologist.

17. That it is an error to suppose the two sides of the cranium to be always alike, that on the contrary, it is rarely found that the two halves of the exterior surface exactly correspond; that indeed, in the insane, there is often a notable difference—still more frequent in idiots, and especially in congenital idiots.

18. That the object and effect of a well-managed education are to establish and confirm the power of concentrating the energies of both brains on the same subject at the same time; that is, to make both cerebra carry on the same train of thought together, as the object of moral discipline is to strengthen the power of self-control; not merely the power of both intellectual organs to govern the animal propensities and passions, but the intellectual antagonism of the two brains, each (so to speak) a sentinel and security for the other while both are healthy; and the healthy one to correct and control the erroneous judgments of its fellow when disordered.

19. That it is the exercise of this power of compeling the combined attention of both brains to the same object, till it becomes easy and habitual, that constitutes the great superiority of the disciplined scholar over the self-educated man; the latter may perhaps possess a greater stock of useful knowledge, but set him to study a new subject, and he is soon outstripped by the other, who has acquired the very difficult accomplishment of *thinking of only one thing at a time*; that is, of concentrating the action of both brains on the same subject.

20. That every man is, in his own person, conscious of two volitions, and very often conflicting volitions, quite distinct from the government of the passions by the intellect; a consciousness so universal, that it enters into all figurative language on the moral feelings and sentiments, has been enlisted into the service of every religion, and forms the basis of some of them, as the Manichaean.

While the structure of the brain is considered as the structure of one organ only, there is not much hope of any improvement in our physiology. We know so little of the respective uses of parts in so complicated an organization, that we can form opinions of its functions only by observing the consequences of morbid changes of structure, and the connexion between changes of partial organs and changes of function; but while we consider the integrity of the whole mass of both cerebra as essential to the performance of offices which are proper to each, it is vain to expect that we shall make advance in the knowledge of the separate uses of separate parts. Had we treated the eye in the same manner, we should have contended that opacity of the crystalline lens could not impede vision, because we saw that vision remained when one lobe or hemisphere (or whatever we might call it) of THE EYE was obliterated. How much stronger would have been this illustration had the organs of vision (the two lobes of the eye, we will suppose) been concealed from our view by a bony covering, their axes directed to one aperture, and cataract only to be recognised on dissection, after other morbid changes had taken place tending to mystify and obscure the judgment. I can fancy some teacher of anatomy holding up to ridicule the doctrine that transparency of the lens was necessary to vision, and shewing, in refutation of so absurd an assertion, one *lobe* of the eye completely opaque, yet the vision perfect to the last, when every one knew that the integrity of both lobes was essential to the performance of that function, and consequently no impediment to vision. *q. e. d.*

If it be objected that my theory, as deduced from the anatomy of the brain and it functions, is mere matter of inference, I reply that the division of the spinal cord into sensory and motory columns is also a mere matter of inference; for the best minute anatomist of the present day cannot demonstrate such division; yet, the origin of the spinal nerves from the anterior and posterior portions of the cord, their combination of two functions, the loss of the motory without the sensory power in parts to which these nerves are distributed, or (according to the modern system of holding every thing to the light in a new position, and thus making it irrecognizable by all but young students) in parts *from* which these nerves *arise*; altogether these things form a demonstration just as complete and satisfactory as that furnished by the scalpel.

CHAPTER V: *Disclaimer of Materialism; Mind in its Popular Sense Connected with the Material World by Means of Our Physical Organization; Use of the Ganglionic System*

Should any one, after reading the following pages, be inclined to suspect me of a leaning to Materialism, I protest beforehand against an erroneous inference, which must be drawn either from an inattentive perusal of my book, or from my own want of power to express my sentiments with clearness and precision. No one can entertain a greater repugnance to that cheerless and desolate doctrine than myself; if this world were the *be-all* and the *end-all*, the sterile prospect would dismay the stoutest heart.

In thus speaking of Materialism, I employ the word in its ordinary popular sense, as synonymous with Atheism; but it has a very different meaning when used by philosophers, and especially by metaphysicians who are physiologists. So far from considering materialism as a form of atheism, such men, though called materialists, have perhaps a more exalted idea of the Great Governor of the universe, and of his attributes, than is entertained by any other class whatever. The awe and veneration felt by the profound anatomist and physiologist, when he penetrates to the very adytum of the great temple of nature, and seems almost in the immediate presence of the Divinity, form a worship more profound than the most sublime ceremonies ever invented by man to express his feelings of devotion. Such men see cause of admiration, wonder, and adoration, in things which the ignorant vulgar regard with complacent indifference, their prevailing tone of mind is that of reverence for the Almighty Creator, and tranquil confidence in the Divine government of the universe.

Haeremus cuncti superis, temploque tacente
Nil facimus non sponte Dei.
Est-ne Dei sedes, nisi terra, et pontus, et aër,
Et coelum, et virtus . . . .
Et Deus est quodcunque vides, quocumque moveris.

There is no class of society more essentially devout than the investigators of nature in the medical profession, and it is not likely, in the face of such abundant evidence from social statistics, that any other class will claim a superiority over them in moral conduct. The accusation of materialism or atheism, so often preferred against them, is founded on ignorance of the exact meaning of the terms they use. Neophytes among the early Christians, taking literally the metaphorical language of their professors in theology, spoke of eating the flesh and drinking the blood of their god, and even gloried in it when accused of cannibalism. It is not surprising then that the authorities should put to death without compunction, men who apparently acknowledged themselves guilty of crimes so loathsome. We do not live in such times; but anatomists and physiologists are with no more justice now accused of attributing a self-inherent thinking faculty to matter, from the flippant conclusions of young students who are not yet sufficiently advanced to comprehend their doctrines.

Whatever be the qualities and faculties possessed by the structures of the body, they must have been *bestowed*, since the same structures exist when these functions are withdrawn by death. The Creator gives to the juice of the poppy, the power of exciting or of supressing thought, of exalting our conceptions even of himself, or of extinguishing, or retarding every mental process according to the quantity we may take of it. To endow a specific portion of the frame with the power of creating thoughts, seems not a whit more mysterious and incomprehensible, nor to imply any greater exercise of Omnipotence. Vital crystallization as it has been happily called by that admirable anatomist Erasmus Wilson, is as much a gift of the Creator as the crystallization of a salt; and if God has made the brain to think, it is but a quibble to say that thinking is not the result of organization. We have been permitted to see enough of the order of the universe to excite and reward the exercise of the faculties bestowed upon us, and enough has been involved in impenetrable mystery to check the presumption which would expect to comprehend the whole scheme of Divine government. The most strenuous advocate for the separate entity of mind will allow that its connexion with the material world is through the action of a material organ, and that when this organ is destroyed or disordered, so as to be incapable of its specific functions, the communication between mind and the material world is at an end.

The light of day, however pure and colourless, if it pass through a distorted or coloured medium, will be distorted or coloured,—through red glass it will be red, through yellow glass it will be yellow; and if it pass through several media of different densities, or be twice reflected, it will be decomposed and polarized. So with the *mind*, in the sense in which that word is generally used.

To me it seems that the provision of two distinct and perfect brains, for this object, is like the provision of two ears and two eyes. In thought, as in vision and in hearing, each organ may suffice to perform perfectly all its appropriate functions, yet the two when in health produce only one result. We have only one sound with both ears, each of them hearing it at the same time. We see only one object with both eyes, each seeing it separately at the same time. We carry on only one train of thought in both brains, each thinking it at the same time; all this however is contingent, not only on the perfect health of the organs, but on their due exercise and cultivation. In disorder or disease, brain, eye, and ear, convey separate, distinct, conflicting ideas—one, or both, necessarily erroneous.

Ratiocination is so essential to the well-being of the individual, that the possession of two organs for this purpose, each capable of carrying on the function when its fellow is impaired or annihilated, seems only one more of the superabundant examples of design and contrivance in the structure of man, as a provision against accident or disease.

If perfect mind were destroyed by injury of one brain, man would lose, under such circumstances, the guide which makes him a moral agent. Responsibility for his actions could not justly be exacted, when the organ (by the due performance of whose function he was alone enabled to judge of the morality of them) was no longer complete. Without a brain to connect the soul with the material world *perfectly*, he must be either a mere animal of instinct, a madman, or an idiot. He could not be a responsible agent.

When one brain wills what is lawful and right, consistent with the duties a man owes to himself and others, and with the form of society existing at the time in the country he lives in, and the other brain suggests a process of ratiocination to justify or palliate some vicious or criminal act, the latter is sometimes attributed to "the instigation of the devil." On the approach of insanity, the patient is often found to be holding a conversation, as it may be called, between his two brains, conversing with himself. I do not mean merely talking to himself aloud, but contending with an imaginary opponent,—sometimes uttering his own conscious sentiments, sometimes those of his adversary,—sometimes mixing them, or giving them in irregular alternation—more frequently only his own, which the listener perceives to be answers to some question the patient supposes to have been asked, or some argument he believes to have been proffered by the other. Dr. Johnson represents himself to have been much annoyed in his dreams, by the superior wit of his antagonist. "Had I been awake," says he, "I should have known that I furnished the wit on both sides."

The ganglionic, or great sympathetic system of *little brains* in the interior of the body, connected by a network of nerves (like the additional spring to a watch, to enable it to go while winding up), carries on the functions of life during sleep, while the action of the cerebral organs is suspended. Connected as it is with the real cerebral and spinal nerves, it may, from local disturbance, wake up some of the organs of the mind, and unequally. In this mysterious state of torpor, and temporary suspension of the faculties, there is no consentaneity between the two cerebra, and they are probably in different stages or degrees of somnolency. If consciousness exist in either of them, it cannot exist in both, unless both were perfectly awake; if in one only, the suggestions of the other must necessarily seem external, and this would account for the double consciousness in sleep. I do but hint at the subject in this place, but expect to throw some light on it hereafter.

The command of one brain over the other (suspended during sleep or dreaming) is what Mr. Barlow means by the expression "man's power over himself to prevent or control insanity." He who is so happily constituted as to possess two cerebra, which are not only well formed and healthy, but which have been duly cultivated by religious, moral, and educational discipline, is a wise and a good man; but he who with one brain constantly furnishing arguments to excuse criminal indulgence, has yet cultivated the power of the other till it can exercise a complete and continuous control over the bad impulses, is a better man. God, who created us such as we are, can alone judge of the absolute degree of merit. It was, no doubt, for wise and just purposes that we were thus formed; had it been otherwise indeed, the whole constitution of nature in this world must have been different.

"O God!" says the Arabian philosopher, "be kind to the wicked; to the good thou hast been already sufficiently kind in making them good."

CHAPTER VI: *Progress of My Own Convictions; Proofs that One Cerebrum may be Destroyed, Yet the Mind Remain Entire; Examples from Conolly, Johnson, Cruveilhier, Abercrombie, Ferriar, O'Halloran, and Others; Reflections; Case of Cardinal, from Dr. Bright's Work; Early Remarks of Dr. Gall*

It is obvious that a disease of the brain tending to the destruction of one cerebrum; or, according to the present nomenclature, one hemisphere of the cerebrum, can rarely pass to such an extent as to destroy life (when alone we can ascertain the facts) without spreading to the other side, although it might have arrived at a very advanced stage before such extention took place. It is therefore difficult to give examples of the fact; we have, however, on record several such cases, on authority which cannot be questioned.

My own attention to the subject was attracted in the first instance by the case I am about to describe. My knowledge of the brain was at that time exceedingly limited. The theories of Dr. Gall yet slept in his own sensorium or, if promulgated, had attracted no notice; war occupied all our attention, our exclusion from the Continent was complete. A narrow-minded and despicable jealousy stifled all mental development in the nations under the iron rule of France, lest it should attract any part of the attention due to the progress of her dominion, or we might have had the advantage of Dr. Gall's sagacious plan of dissecting the brain before it had been attached to the fantastic theories which have been since pushed to so great an excess by the more enthusiastic of his followers. Had we been able to commence the dissection of the brain on true principles five-and-thirty or forty years ago, unencumbered with his hypothesis of its functions, we should probably have admitted a large portion of his deductions; and some of the quiet, steady, well-cultivated minds of anatomists in this country might have elaborated a system which should have been free from many of the gross *non-sequiturs* contended for by him and his colleagues. This, however, by the way. The case I speak of was as follows. A boy, in climbing a high tree for a rook's nest, missed his footing and fell on the sharp edge of an iron railway, one of the very earliest laid down in this country, and on a different principle from those now in use, the wheel passing in a sort of groove, instead of on the edge of a projection. The side of the iron rail stood up and was exposed to the friction of the outer edge of the wheel, which soon wore it to a sharp edge. The boy fell head downwards on this, it entered about an inch from the falx and sliced off a large portion of brain, with nearly the whole of the parietal bone; much of the brain being torn and ragged, I pared off the projecting fragments and replaced the mass, not having the slightest hope of his recovery, and only occupying myself with the task of laying on plasters and bandages to appease the anxiety of the friends. The quantity of brain lost must have exceeded four ounces, but my recollection of the case is vague after an interval of more than thirty years.

Having always read that the integrity of both hemispheres was essential to the due exercise of *mind*, I was much astonished the next day to find the patient (a remarkably intelligent lad, of twelve or thirteen years of age) in the full possession of his faculties in as high a degree as at any former period. He did not seem to suffer pain—had no delirium—and advanced steadily towards recovery; considerable new growth took place, but of its nature I have no recollection; it was probably fungous; at the end of a few weeks he was so well, that, in spite of the remonstrances of his mother, he went into the field to play; became exceedingly heated by this, under exposure to a powerful sun, and then walked deliberately into the water to cool himself. The new blood-vessels burst, and he died of hemorrhage; never having manifested from first to last any loss or perversion of mental power.

At this period, like most young persons, I had a passion for metaphysics, and felt no little bewildered at such a disruption of my ideas on the oneness of the mind, and of its organ; of the latter I did not permit myself to doubt, and yet doubted notwithstanding.

The next was a case of absorption, but of this also my recollection is imperfect, and the circumstances would have passed away from my mind altogether but for the embarrassment I long suffered in the consideration of it. One hemisphere was entirely gone—that was evident to my senses; the patient, a man about fifty years of age, had conversed rationally and even written verses, within a few days of his death; yet I knew that, according to books, the mind could only manifest itself through a complete brain (which is true enough as I now explain it), and I was in a similar state to that of persons who cannot refuse assent to geological facts, yet cannot reconcile them to the writings of Moses, in which they have absolute faith. All the observations I made at this period are useless as arguments to convince others, and I only adduce them to shew the progress of my own convictions.

Other cases came under my notice afterwards; one at Pavia and another at Paris. Little information could be obtained as to the exact degree of mind which remained in one of these cases, and there had been long continued delirium in the other, so that I cannot use them on the present occasion.

I have, however, better evidence to offer than the testimony of an unknown writer, and hasten to produce it. Let the reader bear in mind that *one well authenticated case* is quite as conclusive as a hundred; it establishes the fact stated as my first proposition—that one hemisphere, or as I prefer to call it, one brain, is a perfect instrument of thought and ratiocination. From this root springs the whole theory which I am now endeavouring to illustrate.

Dr. Conolly mentions the case of a gentleman who, from applying St. John Long's embrocation to the cheek for some ailment in the part, established so serious a disease that it spread through the orbit into the cerebrum, and by very slow degrees destroyed his life. He was a man of family and independence, and he lodged with Mr. Gill, the tailor, now of Holles Street, Cavendish Square. On examining the skull, one brain was entirely destroyed—gone, annihilated—and in its place (in the narrator's emphatic language) "a yawning chasm." All his mental faculties were apparently quite perfect. I did not see the case, but Mrs. Gill (the only person he would permit to attend upon him) declares that his mind was clear and undisturbed to within a few hours of his death. He had a perfect idea of his own awful situation, and Mrs. Gill having been gradually accustomed to the sight of horror, was alone allowed to come near him; he would not even permit his own sister or other relatives to witness his frightful condition.

This single case is conclusive.

Dr. James Johnson mentions to me another example of a gentleman under his care, who retained the entire possession of his faculties to the last day of his existence, yet on opening the skull, one cerebrum was reduced by absorption to a thin membrane—the whole solid contents of the one-half of the cranium, above the tentorium, absolutely gone. The gentleman was subject to epileptic fits, but had no other indication of cerebral disturbance.

The above cases are more than enough to shew that one cerebrum is alone sufficient as an organ of thought, but I proceed to others. In the great work of Cruveilhier, *Anatomie Pathologique du Corps Humain*, there is an account of the complete atrophy of one cerebrum, of which he gives a plate (Livraison viii, Plate v), where the intellectual powers remained uninjured, although paralysis of the opposite side was established. It is thus related:

"Alexander Sylvain Augé, aged 42, not married, was brought to the Hotel Dieu, 13th February 1830, with all the symptoms of a disease of the heart carried to the greatest extent. He had been affected from the earliest period of childhood with an incomplete paralysis of the right side, of which he could not remember the commencement. His paralyzed members were wasted and atrophied. The second phalanges of the fingers reversed on the first. From the manner in which he replies to the questions put to him, and the mode in which he expresses his desires, his intellectual faculties appear to be entire. He enjoys the use of all his senses; and, from information collected at La Chapelle near Paris, where he resided, possessed the ordinary degree of intelligence. He walked, by the help of a stick, up to the moment of his disease of the heart compelling him to keep to his bed. He died two days after his admission to the hospital, and his body was examined twenty-four hours after his death."

It is unnecessary here to cite other appearances, besides those of the brain; it is sufficient to say, that the left ventricle of the heart was much thickened, and three or four times its natural size.

"We had great difficulty in opening the cranium, by breaking it circularly with a hammer. Its thickness on the left side was, at least, double that of the right. The brain, still enveloped in its meninges, presented, on the left side, a considerable depression. . . . The dura mater being cut, the arachnoid appeared healthy; but the convolutions of the left hemisphere were thin, flattened, more consistent, and whiter, than in their natural state, leaving large spaces between them, which were filled by the infiltrated pia mater. Fluctuation was manifest at the slightest touch . . . and, on taking the brain out of its bony case, a large quantity of serous liquid escaped from the corresponding ventricle, and the mass was reduced to one-third its former size." It was altogether about a fourth part the weight of its fellow.

No one can look at the representation in the plate, without seeing at once that an organ so extensively diseased must have been entirely incapable of performing its functions; and that, consequently, *the mind was exercised solely by the right cerebrum*, which is all that I wish to prove from the case, or it would have been worth while to extract the whole narrative: it is highly interesting in many other respects, more especially from the inferences drawn by the author as to the distinction between the causes of paralysis and idiocy. He makes the case prove too much, however, in my opinion, which is a vice more common among the continental writers than among my countrymen. To speak figuratively, having proved that, so far as they have traced the curve, it is circular, they boldly pronounce that the unknown remainder completes the circle; when, perhaps, further search would have shewn that it turns in a totally different direction, or perhaps comes back on itself to the point they set out from, and leaves the remainder to be traced by another observer, starting from a different point.

Another case related in the same work (Livraison xx, Plate III), representing the right cerebrum destroyed by apoplexy, and so thoroughly disorganized as to be utterly useless, although not absorbed like the last. The woman, says Cruveilhier, " jouissait de toute son intelligence."

The next which bears upon the subject, is that of a child four years of age, who died in consequence of a blow on the head ten months previous. The left hemisphere was converted, almost entirely, into a soft, pulpy substance, resembling *blanc mange*. Paralysis had come on very slowly, and was preceded, during four months, by excessive irritability. This child had full possession of his mental faculties (Livraison xvii, page 6).

The only further example I shall give from the work of M. Cruveilhier is that of Martin, a man thirty-two years of age, whose right cerebrum, of which a plate is given (Livraison xxxiii, Plate III), was utterly disorganized by the extension of disease from caries of the petrous portion of the temporal bone. There was also an encysted tumour in the centre, and the lateral ventricle was filled with the most horribly fetid sanious pus. The man was in full possession of his faculties, and enjoyed the use of all the organs of sense, though suffering the most dreadful tortures.

Many other examples are given of destruction by cancer, softening, tumours, etc., but no mention is made of the state of mind. Where it is alluded to, it seems to be done quite parenthetically; and it is evident that M. Cruveilhier does not attach any importance to the presence or absence of the intellectual faculties. It is therefore clear that he, at least, has not conceived the idea to which his dissections inevitably lead, namely, that each cerebrum is a perfect organ, capable of all the manifestations of mind; and that, by a necessary inference, although the two may, when in health, act in unison and give only one result, like that of vision, yet that double mind must necessarily be produced in some forms of diseased action, where, one brain being sound, the other performs its duties imperfectly and erroneously. This may not always be in those specific instances which produce great destruction of parts, in which, perhaps, there is a mere gradual cessation of the power of thought, and the functions of the mind are quietly and insensibly transferred to the other brain. A case is mentioned by Mr. O'Halloran, cited by Dr. Abercrombie, where a man received an injury of the frontal bone, on the right side; it was broken to pieces. Some of the pieces were extracted at the time, others a few days afterwards. A great opening was thus formed, and extensive suppuration took place; immense quantities of purulent matter were discharged, mixed with large pieces of brain, making a "frightful cavern," as Mr. O'Halloran describes it, not less than three ounces of brain coming away at each dressing. "The cavern was terrible;"—*yet the man preserved his intellect entire till the very moment of his death.*

In another case related by Dr. Abercrombie, it is stated that the left hemisphere was diseased throughout; some parts hardened—some softened—and presented a variety of colours, chiefly rose-colour, grey, and yellow, the more diseased portions highly vascular; in some places there were distinct insulated masses, enclosed in vascular cysts, etc. The whole left hemisphere was little else than such a mass of concentric indurations and softenings. It is clear that such a brain could not perform the functions of mind, yet his understanding remained perfect to the last, for the other brain was healthy.

A man is mentioned by Dr. Ferriar, who, dying of a disease of the brain, retained all his faculties entire till the moment of his death, which was sudden. The whole right hemisphere was found to be entirely destroyed by suppuration.

It would be easy to multiply examples from the writings of eminent men, and many narratives of cases have been offered to me by living practitioners, but the above are more than sufficient; indeed one is as conclusive as a thousand.

The strong exercise of the mind for a considerable time produces brain-ache, as every one must have felt; and as the degree of this brain-ache depends much on the general vigour of all the organs of the body (good health), so must it depend especially on the vigour of the organ itself, by which the process of thinking is carried on. It seems, then, reasonable to suppose, that the organ in which that process is most painful, will leave its duties to be performed by the other, and (if we may so phrase it) tacitly acquiesce in the vicarious exercise of functions for which it is unfit. I have elsewhere spoken of this, and here again remark, that in all the cases of extensive, or even slight disease of one cerebrum, there is observed the inability to exercise continous study, or to learn by heart; that is to say, as I have stated in the propositions, to concentrate the attention of both brains on the same subject simultaneously. As they cannot go on *pari passu*, it is clear they cannot both go on considering the subject together, although the single healthy brain may still exercise perfectly all the ordinary functions of mind, of which the preceeding cases afford ample proof.

One of two things must be: either each hemisphere or cerebrum is a perfect whole, capable of exercising all the functions which, in the aggregate, form *the mind* of the individual, or else each half must exercise some of those functions, and the other half the remainder, so as between them to make up *a mind*. There is positively no other thing possible—the mind is performed completely by each brain, or jointly by the two.

Now, the exact equality in number, form, colour, texture, and character, of the various parts or organs which compose each brain, and the almost as exact equality in size, at once negative the supposition that the two cerebra perform different offices; such a supposition would be contrary to all analogy, and opposed to all rational logic; but it needs neither logic nor analogy to disprove it; for we see, from the preceding examples, that when one brain is destroyed by disease, utterly disorganized, so as to be obviously incapable of exercising any functions whatever—nay, when it is actually absorbed and annihilated, the other hemisphere, or the other cerebrum, can carry on all the mental processes which had previously been performed by the joint action of the two; and this, in spite of the extensive destruction of the physical power of the body, by the progress of a disease necessarily fatal. Were the functions of the mind performed cumulatively by the two brains, it is clear that when one of them was destroyed, portions of the mind only would be annihilated, and not the whole; that is to say, that madness would necessarily take place, and there would be an imperfect mental result, from the imperfection and defect of the organ devoted to intellectual faculties.

Having thus established my first proposition, it seems to me to form a solid foundation, on which might be erected a much larger superstructure than that which I propose to build. In abstaining from this for the present, it is not my intention to relinquish the design, and I more especially propose to subject some of the most celebrated metaphysical and ethical writings to the test of the doctrine here laid down. If I do not greatly deceive myself, it will throw light on many subjects generally considered exceedingly abstruse and incomprehensible, but which are perfectly clear and satisfactory, when we have once established the fact, that man possesses two complete and entire thinking organs; that these act in perfect unison and *oneness* while in health, but even in this state require moral cultivation to enable them to execute their duties justly and fully. The slow progress to physical maturity of the human species, compared with that of any other animal, seems a provision for longer pupilage, and more extensive instruction. If this duty be neglected, or if the discipline be defective or erroneous, the animal grows up into the most detestable combination of intelligence and physical force that infests the earth. Here is the advantage bestowed on man alone, of being able to store up the accumulated wisdom of a long succession of ages, and thus establish systems of government which shall supply the defective sagacity of individuals. I do not think that the authority thus conferred on man by implication has yet been carried to the extent that it will bear, but this is a subject too extensive and unfit to enter on here.

The case of James Cardinal, related at page 431, vol. ii, of Dr. Bright's great work, entitled *Reports of Medical Cases* (a complete magazine of valuable information on a great number of the most important diseases); this case has been pointed out as opposed to my present theory. I cannot see in what way it bears upon it at all, except in the single instance of the annihilation of the corpus callosum, where it seems fully to confirm my opinion that it is an organ of no importance, and not necessary to the functions of the brain. In Cardinal's case there was no destruction of parts, the immense accumulation of water (about eight pints) did not even separate the fibres of the convolutions, but made its way through the corpus callosum (which it split at the medial line with a smooth edge as if cut with a knife), merely pushing aside the two cerebra, which were thus turned over, but not displaced. Neither of them was injured in any other way than by compression, and even this did not very long precede death, the complete ossification of the skull not taking place till a few years before his decease at the age of twenty-nine.

The man was an extraordinary example of hydrocephalus. "His countenance," says Dr. Bright, "was not wanting in intelligence; his mental faculties were very fair; he read and wrote pretty well; his memory was tolerable." Here is no resemblance to the state I have described; but it seems to me that the destruction of the commissural connexion between the two brains is an additional proof, if proof were needed, after the many I have collocated, that they are essentially dual. As there was no disease in either of them, there could be no discrepancy in the mental functions performed by the two; they were in unison, and their action was single, like that of two healthy eyes, which give only one object, or, as the commissures had been destroyed, the comparison would perhaps be closer with the two ears.

The circumference of this man's skull was thirty-two inches and a quarter, and when emptied of its contents would hold ten pints of water. Had not the ossification been completed, it is probable that the water might have gradually accumulated to double the extent without any further inconvenience than the additional weight. The possession of even moderate intellect (and that without the slightest disposition to derangement) under such a degree of compression as the water must have produced from its weight alone, even were there still vacant space in the skull, is an extraordinary instance of the tenacity of mental functions, and is, I believe, perfectly unexampled. The mass of cerebral matter was not diminished, and the bodily health had been uniformly good.

We lay down for nature the most perfect laws, shew where the deviations are bounded by impossibilities, make admirable scientific divisions, and give them very elegant and sonorous Greek names, and after all our trouble we are set at nought.

The impossibilities are performed, our rules are violated, our divisions obliterated, and our fine names rendered ridiculous. We see this—are vexed—and begin again.

"It has been observed that one entire hemisphere has been destroyed by suppuration without the intellectual faculties having been deranged. Might one not expect that in such a case the exercise of at least half the intellectual functions would be thereby rendered impossible?

These are the words of Dr. Gall, more than thirty years ago: "I may say that these observations are *of very doubtful authority*, but let us admit that they are absolutely exact, for I have myself seen a case of the same kind in the Theresian Institution at Vienna. A clergyman suffered a long time from an erysipelas of the forehead, which often disappeared and reappeared, at uncertain periods. His whole left side gradually became enfeebled to such a degree that he could not walk without a stick; at last, he was attacked with apoplexy and died after a few hours. Three days before his death he had preached, and had been occupied as usual in the instruction of youth. On examining the right hemisphere, it was found converted into a clotted substance of a dirty yellowish white. . . . It is certain that the intellectual faculties had continued to be exercised in an astonishing manner, in spite of this extensive destruction."

In the case of Cardinal, the corpus callosum was split, as I have said, in its medial line, and the two hemispheres absolutely divided to the base of the skull; and as he retained all his intellectual powers and affections, notwithstanding the pressure of ten pints of water in his skull, it is quite evident that the corpus callosum is not an essential commissure. Spurzheim, who saw this case, declares that the fibres of the fimbriated body and entire fornix never cross the median line, and however his cranioscopy may be opposed, no one ever doubted his consummate knowledge of the anatomy of the brain, or his perfect good faith in describing it. I think myself then justified, from all I have seen, read, and manipulated, in describing the corpus callosum as merely a mechanical bond of union between the two brains, and that it does actually oppose an obstacle to the transmission of disease from one to the other, and is consequently a wall of separation rather than a bond of union. Tiedeman relates that a man named Moser had one side of his head, or *one brain*, in a state of insanity, and that he watched it with the other. I do not know how this could be ascertained, though I have not a shadow of doubt that such cases are common, and that the extreme caution of some lunatics to conceal their mental derangement, when under examination, is in reality an absolute government for a limited period of the unhealthy brain by the sound one. Thousands of men never suspected of being insane, do habitually practise this concealment of their morbid intellectual functions. It is only when this control is completely exhausted, or the man has not a sufficient motive for its exercise, that we can pronounce the case insanity. With one man a little cerebral excitement from fermented fluid will destroy this power, with another anger, and thus on through the lower instincts; and we say of such men, with strict justice, A.B. is perfectly mad when drunk, C.D. is absolutely insane when in a passion, and so forth.

At Vienna, says Gall, a minister of state was attacked for three years with a malady which he thus described to me: On the left side he constantly heard insulting expressions, so that he was always turning his eyes in that direction, to see where they came from, although perfectly convinced in the right side of his head that it was a delusion of the left side. When attacked with fever, he no longer knew it to be illusion, but long after his cure, when he indulged in wine or fell into violent anger, he felt in the left side of his head symptoms of relapse.

Another instance he relates of a fellow student at Vienna, who often complained that he could not think with one side of his head, and indeed one side was evidently lower and narrower, and altogether smaller, than the other.

Gall also relates the cases of two ladies who had a similar inability to use one side of the head, but there is little dependence to be placed on observations drawn from that sex, because of the innumerable forms of hysteria to which they are subject, and the extreme vivacity of their imagination, which mystifies every mental process. Yet Gall declares that one of these ladies observed to him that she felt as if her head were in two halves, and that all the thoughts in one of the halves were jumbled together; yet she was entirely ignorant of the real structure of the brain, and had not the least idea that such a division existed in nature.

Strange that such words, from such a source, should have dropped unheeded into oblivion—their existence even known but to a few phrenologists, and that no one, in more than thirty years, should have drawn a single inference from such important premises. It is obvious that Gall's assertions on this subject were generally disbelieved, or they could not have failed to create general notoriety, and lead to very important results.

CHAPTER VII: *Quotation from Quarterly Review; Comparison with a Theatre; Pinel; Double Volition, from Cerebral Disturbance, caused by Great Anxiety.*

A writer in the Quarterly Review (Vol. XXVII, page 113), in a criticism on Dr. Reid's *Essays on Hypochondriasis and Nervous Affections*, endeavours to draw a distinction between temporary delusions and real insanity. He says, "'It may be said, if there is a moral as well as physical eccentricity, it is probable there is a moral as well as physical insanity.' We believe no such thing. Strange habits, by intellectual operations, may produce great eccentricity of opinion and action, but they will never produce madness in the true acceptation of the word, till they have affected physically the bodily organization." This is a complete begging of the question, unless he can shew that in hypochondriasis the bodily organization is never affected. The intellectual organs, for any thing we know to the contrary, may be as effectually disordered by reflex action from the ganglionic centres, as from disease within the cranium.

"There is," he proceeds, "a condition of mind bordering on delirium, in which the patient is delirious enough to afford an example of that state, yet collected enough to observe and reason about it, which comes nearer than any phenomenon with which we are acquainted to an experimental demonstration of the double nature of our being, of the physical and moral impulses of our thoughts, which are here brought into contact and comparison."

So far, all is clear and easily comprehended; but he goes on with an unmeaning explanation, and 'the interpreter is the harder to be understood of the two.' "In this state, the ideas are moved," says he, "one minute by the will, the next by something else; one minute we can command them, another we feel them slip out of our grasp, and *whirl across the mind*—[Has this any meaning?]—with indescribable fleetness, guided, or rather hurried on, by some impulse strange to and stronger than ourselves."

How simple and easy is the explanation of this incomprehensible description of the mental operations, if we concede the question, which it appears to me that I have already established beyond cavil—the possession of two complete and perfect organs of thought with opposing volitions. When the audience at a theatre sit impatiently waiting the drawing up of the curtain for a new piece, of the nature of which they are entirely ignorant, they cannot prevent themselves from trying to form an opinion, however limited, of the performance, from the little insignificant incidents which take place during the period of suspense. A spangled shoe makes its appearance under the curtain, and one man thinks the play will be preceded by a ballet; higher up the curtain is a projection which seems to indicate the shape of a man, or a hat and feathers are seen at the side, and another person thinks it will be a tragedy, and so forth; but he who has been behind the scenes, and especially a manager, or experienced player, knows what all these things mean. Even he who has been a regular frequenter of theatres, and has constantly observed that such and such appearances, however insignificant in themselves, are invariably followed by such and such kinds of performance, will be generally right in his conjectures.

It is thus with the speculators I have named. I *have* been a close and attentive observer, and a constant frequenter of this great theatre of the mind, and fancy myself able, in some cases, to anticipate the nature of the performance. The curtain is the bony cranium which hides the proceedings; but a close attention to your own theatre, your own little microcosm, will enable you to foretell your own performances, and to give a shrewd guess at those of others.

> . . . . learning dwells
> In heads replete with thoughts of other men;
> Knowledge in minds attentive to their own.

Hospitals for the insane, says Pinel, are never without some examples of mania, marked by acts of extravagance, or even fury, with *a kind of judgment preserved in all its integrity*, if we judge of it by the conversation: the lunatic gives the most just and precise answers to the questions of the curious. No incoherence of ideas is discernible; he reads and writes letters as if his understanding were perfectly sound, and yet he tears his clothes and bed-clothes, etc.

"Here again," says Mr. George Combe,"the difficulty occurs of reconciling such facts with the idea of only one organ exercising all the functions of the mind." I agree with him; but that which he thinks proves a plurality of organs proves much more clearly a duality of brains—one sound, and, on ordinary occasions, controlling the other, and suppressing its manifestations; but, at other times, fatigued with the effort, and leaving the disordered impulse to pass unchecked. This is the more likely to happen at night, when the healthier brain is exhausted, and the other in diseased activity.

"If (adds he) every part of the brain is concerned in every mental act, it appears strange that all the processes of thought should be manifested *with equal effect* when a great part of the brain is injured or destroyed, as when its whole structure is sound and entire."

There is, I believe, no instance on record of any considerable injury to both brains being accompanied by full possession of the mental faculties. One brain,we have seen, may be annihilated, and the mind remain entire, but injury to both is incompatible with sound mind. To exercise all the mental powers and faculties, it is absolutely necessary that there be at least one sound and perfect organ.

An intimate friend of mine, a man of education, character, and veracity, has been for many years subjected to a succession of calamities and misfortunes, such as can rarely have fallen to the lot of any other man; with strong principles of rectitude, he has been more than once placed in the position of complicated embarrassment, which gave the appearance of guilt, or at any rate, of culpable indifference to opinion; while, in fact, he has been always morbidly sensible to it, and has allowed that feeling to exercise much too great an influence over his actions. He thus describes his case, in a statement drawn up at my request:

"With an intense scorn and hatred of every thing mean or dishonourable, I had been for a long time haunted with the idea that I was looked on as a dishonoured man; and although, in moments of calm, I knew this to be a delusion, and the continued respect and kindness of friends shewed me that I had not forfeited their good opinion, yet, on any excitement or temporary overwhelming sense of proximate impending danger, I could not control a morbid conviction that I had been detected in some dreadful crime—of what kind I know not; but if my vigilance were allowed to sleep for a few minutes only, images of judge, jury, counsel, and crowded court, would come before me, and unless by a very vigorous effort I could suddenly shake off the delusion, it went on till sentence of death was pronounced, and I felt all the deadly faintness which would have been produced by the real scene itself.

"My distress was infinitely enhanced from my supposed entire inability to defend myself, in consequence of being utterly unable to discover the nature of the crime I was accused of; or it seemed to me that I could make a triumphant defence.

"When alone, and in depressed spirits from diffused gout and dyspepsia, I sank into a reverie, my mind began to plan petitions to the Sovereign—addresses to the Privy Council, and to the two Houses of Parliament, on the cruel injustice of the laws which permitted a man to be arraigned and convicted of an offence of which he was not allowed to know the nature or the name.

"The whole of this time I knew perfectly and continuously that it was an entire delusion, that I had committed no crime whatever, nor was in any such absurd predicament, but, at the same time felt like a man hanging over a precipice by a branch, which he knows to be incapable of supporting his weight. Every day I became more and more awfully convinced that, whenever I should lay down the reins but for a few hours, and allow this reverie to proceed, I should wake from my trance a madman. This feeling was accompanied by the strange conviction, that if I could throw myself on the ground and scream violently for an hour, it would afford me infinite relief, and that the effort to *hold myself together* would then be comparatively easy.

"Yet, on going into agreeable and elevated society, and taking two or three glasses of wine, I generally became not merely cheerful, but almost hilarious. All that I had seen, read, heard, or thought, during a rather eventful life and diversified career, came vividly before me, and I poured forth my ideas with a fluency that sometimes left me the sole talker; when I ceased, it was not unusual to be entreated by the company to go on with my narrative, which had gradually drawn around me a crowd of listeners. Suddenly, perhaps, I recollected my old delusion; it was as if a curtain had been instantly drawn (with a sort of flash) between me and the scenes I had been describing. I could say no more; felt as if the eyes of all the world were upon me, was wretched and miserable; every disagreeable event of my life came again before me, and I in vain tried to recall one single incident or reflection of a different character; yet at other times, in public, my self-command was so complete, that on more than one occasion I have been congratulated on my fortunate lot; it being evident, they said, from my countenance, that I had led a life of happiness, ease, and leisure, and always had the sunny side of the peach for my food.

"The idea of a double identity has been a permanent suspicion with me, and the control of one self by the other a recognised sentiment; but the effort required to exercise this control was exceedingly painful and distressing if long continued, unless some fortunate incident aided my own struggles. For a considerable time the difficulty has been gradually diminishing, and has long passed away altogether; the delusion never recurs, but as a consequence of bodily indisposition, and can always, even then, be instantly dismissed by a strong effort of the will.

"One example of the nature and extent of the efforts formerly required to overcome similar delusions is too significant to be omitted.

"A sudden combination of unfortunate events having produced great aggravation of my habitual distress from moral and physical causes, I felt myself one evening entirely unable to control the expression of my mental agony in the presence of persons from whom it was of the greatest importance to conceal it. I walked down to the sea-side; it was a bright moonlight night. I wandered along the shore, soothed by the murmur of the waves, and lost in thought gradually allowed the waters to surround me. I was not aware of my situation till the little island of sand on which I stood began to sink under my feet. This roused me from a reverie intensely profound, where the few and short periods of happiness I had enjoyed in youth came back with all the freshness of their first impression. I waded through the water, savage at the interruption, and resumed my walk. I now felt more bitterly than ever my present position, and began to be alarmed at finding that my thoughts were beyond my control. I looked on the long stream of silvery light on the water, extending itself to the dark horizon of heavy clouds which bounded the view, and said to myself, almost unconsciously, 'That shining path is the road to happiness, I will follow it.' I advanced towards a boat with the intention of launching it, although the task was evidently beyond my strength, for it lay high up out of the water; suddenly the absurdity of the idea struck me, and I ran away from it, but the impulse to return was so strong that it was barely possible to refrain from again approaching it. I made another violent effort, and vowed not to walk in that direction. The effort was however beyond my power, and again and again did I pass through similar struggles.

"Becoming gradually more and more excited, I was alarmed to find myself drawn towards the boat by some invisible power, and seemed distinctly to hear a voice repeating my own words: 'That shining path is the road to happiness, follow it.' I had a strong desire to scream, but was afraid of being heard by the coastguard, and with much difficulty refrained from it. I made violent efforts to prevent myself from going near the boat, but the same words rang in my ears: 'That shining path is the road to happiness, follow it'; and while encouraging myself in the determination to keep aloof, I was horror-struck to find myself gradually getting nearer and nearer to the boat. The tide had now risen so high that a portion of it was occasionally reached by the waves, and what was at first impracticable, became apparently easy. I was terrified lest the conviction of it being possible, should make the impulse irresistible. I said to myself aloud, 'I will not go near it; I am mad; it is delusion!' Still the voice kept saying to me, 'That shining path is the road to happiness, follow it.' I got nearer and nearer, and at last, from an impulse of despair threw myself on the ground, and then felt secure; although for some time my feet continued to imitate the action of walking. I had however sufficient self-command left to prevent myself from getting again on my legs, and lay quietly on the pebbles. Gradually I became composed, from the conviction that in a lying posture I was safe. I lay an hour, till the cold roused me to sensation and perception, and then walked home perfectly composed. The following morning the scalp was puffed, like the legs after great fatigue. Had I launched the boat, I should probably have been drowned; at any rate, the act would have passed for insanity, and the consciousness of it would for a long time have prevented the establishment of perfect self-control.

"Do as you like about mentioning what follows: it may excite a more compassionate feeling perhaps towards human beings similarly afflicted, who are often more deserving of commiseration than those who have passed the dreadful rubicon.

"Instead of soothing, or indeed comprehending my destressing state, my friends and family used remonstrances and arguments to which I could not reply; they *advised* and I *acquiesced in* things decidedly against my judgment and against my will; but as I could not give satisfactory reasons for my opposition, I was, like other men of stronger minds, talked down. I felt that to begin to give reasons would put one into a state of excitement, and my disordered brain would presently betray itself—I should be mad! So, like the bird that has entirely exhausted itself in the vain attempt to escape from his cage, I folded my wings, and lay down with a panting heart and stupified brain—not to think—not to consider—not to reason—not to complain or remonstrate, but to endure, *ipse meum cor edens*, to gnaw my own heart in silence.

"Mad I was not—mad I have never been—and, encouraged in the exercise of self-control by the issue of that great mental conflict, *mad I will never be.*"

The tendency in the case just recited seems to have been to physical violence and garrulity, especially to great muscular exertion. Had the gentleman been in a situation to tire a couple of horses under him, to play some games at tennis, or use other laborious exercise, fatigue would perhaps have brought on muscular exhaustion, and the sound brain would then have resumed its control.

How many human beings are in this lamentable situation! Yet it is one rarely pitied—the man is blamed for want of energy and exertion, when he really gives an extraordinary example of both those meritorious qualities. In the modern system of managing insanity, had this poor man gone a few steps further, he would have been subjected to a treatment founded, as I think, unconsciously on the dual theory. His brain would have been soothed by excessive kindness and tenderness of manner. His imperfect power of commanding the disordered organ by the sound one would have been encouraged and strengthened; the imperfect function would have been left for a time in abeyance, and its irregular manifestations checked and discouraged, till they gradually subsided into tranquillity and repose.

CHAPTER VIII: *False Perceptions; Errors of the Organs of Sense; Example of Delusion; My Own Delusion; Case of Nicolai and Dr. Bostock; Case of Cerebral Disturbance from Diffused Gout; Double Mind; Self-Restraint; Case of Moral Insanity*

It must be observed that it is not the greater or less degree of power of the intellectual faculties over the passions (the animal propensities) which I here speak of. This may be more or less powerful, and more or less exercised, according to the temperament, the position in life, the religious convictions, the moral atmosphere in which the individual has been brought up, and the degree of cultivation bestowed on the intellectual powers in the establishment of that which is the object and basis of all moral discipline—self-restraint. It is not of this I would now speak, because these are healthy exercises of healthy faculties; it is the control by the sane intellectual faculties of the insane faculties; the tyranny of the sound ratiocinator over the unsound ratiocinator, that is the present object of consideration.

The organs which recognise the objects of sense, may give false perceptions; but if the intellectual portion of the brain be sound, the mind resists the false evidence. I have, for example, a predominant taste of garlic on my gustatory nerves, pervading every article of food. It is only a process of reasoning which can convince me that it is a false impression, and induce me to reject the evidence of my senses. So, if the portions of both brains with which the auditory nerves communicate convey to my intellect the false impression of deep-toned bell, when I know that there is no bell of the kind within audible distance, my mind at once concludes that the whole is the result of local or general disorder, which I accordingly take measures to remove. I remember hearing a bell, at Mola di Gaeta, with a very peculiar sound; it probably was a musical note of an exact pitch which had never struck my ear before from any instrument, or it might have been something in the quality of the tone, independent of its position in the musical scale. I happened at the moment to be in the midst of a long train of painful emotions, and the two things became associated in my mind. I never heard the same bell again; but in passing Mont Cenis I encountered one of those whirlwinds called a "tourmente," and felt that I had taken cold in my ears, which began to be slightly painful, when I suddenly heard the peculiar sound of the bell of Mola di Gaeta. I was entirely convinced that I heard a bell; looked round for a campanella in vain, and tried, with as little success, to persuade my companions of the truth of my convictions. All the way from thence to Beauvoisin the same sound continued in my ears, renewing all the painful ideas associated with first hearing it; and it was not till I had sat for some time in a very hot room at Martigny that it ceased to annoy me. On resuming my journey the sound was renewed, and it was not till after a hot bath, and free injection of the ears with warm water, at Lyons, that I finally got rid of the distressing delusion.

In this case, the false information conveyed by both brains could not have been recognised as false by the direct process of reasoning, that is, comparing the separate impressions of the two brains, but gave way to the evidence of others. Had this been inaccessible, I must necessarily have remained convinced that there was a bell at Mont Cenis with exactly the same tone as that at Mola di Gaeta.

These cases are however very different from that of one intellectual organ in opposition to the other. If, for example, one brain tells me to swallow a quantity of stones, in order to revenge myself on certain persons for supposed insults, and to proportion the number of the stones to the number of the persons who have offended me, or to the number of imaginary insults (not a very uncommon delusion), my sound brain discards the reasoning as absurd and ridiculous, and for a time compels its fellow to acquiesce in a rational view of the case, or depend on the testimony of others; but when the disordered affection extends to the other brain, the absurdity is believed and acted on. A medical man of great attainments, formerly President of the College of Physicians, was under my care with this curious delusion, and had very nearly starved himself to death believing, that as the stones could not dissolve, it was useless to eat; he would not take a particle of food for seventeen days. I restored him, by convincing him that the stones would promote digestion, as in the gizzards of birds; and when thus rescued from starvation and well fed, he recovered his senses, and the stones were voided by the bowels.

The late Mr. Anderson, of Cobham, a retired medical practitioner of advanced age, and I believe the first man who professed to be an "oculist," was the subject of a controllable delusion of a curious description. When in a large party, especially in a ballroom, unless he made a strong effort to prevent it, his imagination gradually and slowly went on removing one article of clothing after another from all the persons present, then their integuments, then layer after layer of muscles, then removed the viscera and, at last, left them all bare skeletons dancing before his eyes, and he burst out into loud laughter at the ridiculous scene. He could at any time stop the morbid process at an early stage, and it was only when his mind was engaged on some other topic that these vagaries were allowed to pass unchecked. Sometimes he watched them out of pure curiosity, but if he allowed the series to be completed could not prevent laughter at the absurd exhibition. Disease of one cerebrum was discovered after death.

My explanation of this phenomenon is that one cerebrum was disordered, and from time to time in a state of temporary insanity, but that the other was perfect and capable of entirely controlling its fellow, unless its attention were occupied, and it were neglecting its duty of sentinel.

Had this disorder of mind passed on a little further—had the diseased functions become a little stronger, and the healthy functions a little weaker, this gentleman would have been justly pronounced insane, and subjected to restraint. There are thousands of such cases.

When very young I once mounted to the top of a church to view the prospect. The church stood on a high rock, and the ascent to it was by several hundred steps; on the other side, the wall of the building was almost continuous with a perpendicular face of the rock, and thus gave an immense elevation.

Plumbers who were engaged in repairing the lead work had made a fire at the base of the spire, and while watching the melting of the metal, I leaned on the balustrade which surmounted the square portion of the tower. It was old and loosened by decay, and as I rested on it gave way and fell to the bottom of the rock: for a few seconds I was balanced on one leg, or seemed to be so balanced, for in the excess of my terror, I lost my consciousness. I fell in the right direction, however, and lay for some moments insensible.

On my recovery I became gradually ill, and for a week gave considerable alarm to my friends. I now believe that it was followed by meningitis. It is not extraordinary that I dreamed of the accident for a long time afterwards, and entertained a positive horror of going to sleep. Time gradually effaced these impressions which were, however, succeeded by a strange delusion. I imagined my bed to be surrounded by little imps of the height of my knee, whose object was to pull my hair (then worn reaching to the waist), and prevent me from going to sleep. I had fears also that they might scratch my face or injure my eyes; but there was no superstitious horror respecting them—it was rather anger and indignation. At the same moment that I saw these little devils I was perfectly aware that it was a delusion and, in summer, often got up and dressed myself and set to learning my lessons for the next day; but in winter, and in darkness, I had not the power of dismissing these disagreeable companions, though equally certain that they had no real existence. I perfectly remember that (still believing it a delusion) I made myself a stout cudgel, with a noose of string to fasten round my wrist, and always took this to bed with me. Having now a conviction that I could drive away the little non-existent wretches, should they attack me, I slept with comparative tranquillity, and gradually recovered from my delusions. Yet such was, throughout, my conviction of the whole being a deceptive phantasma, that I carefully concealed my proceedings even from my own brothers, who slept in the same room. It was well no one slept in the same bed, or he might have had his brains beaten out before I could recover my consciousness.

I call this, one cerebrum in a state of disease or disorder, and one healthy, capable of watching and, in some degree, controlling its vagaries.

The case of Nicolai, the Berlin bookseller, has been often quoted, but, though familiar to medical readers, is probably little known to the public; I therefore insert it here as an established fact which bears upon my argument.

Nicolai thus describes his delusion: "At ten o'clock in the forenoon my wife and another person came to console me; I was in great perturbation of mind, owing to a series of incidents, which had altogether wounded my moral feelings, and from which I saw no possibility of relief; when suddenly I observed, at the distance of ten paces from me, a figure of a deceased person. I pointed at it, and asked my wife whether she did not see it. She saw nothing, but being much alarmed, endeavoured to compose me, and sent for a physician. The figure remained some seven or eight minutes, and at length I became a little more calm. In the afternoon, a little after four o'clock, the figure which I had seen in the morning again appeared. I was alone when this happened: a circumstance which, as may easily be conceived, was by no means agreeable. I went therefore to my wife's room and related it; but thither also the figure pursued me—sometimes present, sometimes absent, but always the same standing figure. After I had recovered from my first impression of terror, I never felt myself particularly agitated by these apparitions, as I considered them to be, what they really were, the extraordinary consequences of indisposition. On the contrary, I endeavoured as much as possible to preserve my composure of mind, that I might remain distinctly conscious of what passed within me. I observed these phantoms with great accuracy, and very often reflected on my previous thoughts, with a view to discover some law in the association of ideas, by which these or other figures might present themselves to the imagination. The figure of the deceased person never appeared to me after the first dreadful day, but several other figures shewed themselves afterwards very distinctly; sometimes such as I knew, mostly however, of persons I did not know; and among those known to me were the semblances of both living and dead persons, but mostly the former; and I made observation that acquaintances with whom I daily conversed never appeared to me as phantasms—it was always such as were at a distance.

"When these apparitions had continued for some weeks, I could regard them with the greatest composure. I afterwards endeavoured, at my own pleasure, to call forth phantoms of several acquaintance, who I, for that reason, represented to my imagination in the most lively manner, but in vain. The phantasms appeared to me in many cases involuntarily, as if they had been presented externally, like the phenomena of nature, though they certainly had their origin internally. At the same time I was always able to distinguish, with the greatest precision, phantasms from realities. I never once erred in this, as I was in general perfectly calm and self-collected on the occasion. I knew perfectly well when it only appeared to me that the door was opened and a phantom entered, and when the door really was opened and any person came in." These figures appeared to Nicolai when alone or in company, or even in the street, and continued to haunt him for about two months. At last they disappeared; sometimes returning for a time, and for the last time while he was writing an account of them.

Here, it seems to me, that the perceptive faculties in one brain were in a state of occasional disorder or disease, and took on the same kind of action that they would have done had the perceptions been the consequence of real sensations. The other brain being healthy, not merely in the parts ministering to ratiocination (comparison and judgment), but in the exercise of the perceptive faculties, knew that those perceptions of its fellow were unfounded in fact; and the difference between the perceptions produced by the real object and by the imagination were easily distinguished. One brain was, as we so often see, watching the other, and even interested and amused by its vagaries; as soon at least as comparison had been exercised a sufficient number of times (had been *cultivated*, that is), and had acquired a new sense, much in the same mode as in the operation of castle building, the sound brain watches the amusing exercise of the perceptive faculties in its fellow, which it could interrupt, but does not, because the process is agreeable.

A similar delusion was experienced by Dr. Bostock; it was as follows: "I was labouring under a fever, attended with symptoms of general debility, especially of the nervous system, and with a severe pain of the head, which was confined to a small spot situated above the right temple. After having passed a sleepless night, and been reduced to a state of considerable exhaustion, I first perceived figures presenting themselves before me, which I immediately recognised as similar to those described by Nicolai; and upon which, as I was free from delirium, and as they were visible for three days and nights with little intermission, I was able to make my observations. There were two circumstances which appeared to me very remarkable: first, that the spectral appearances always followed the motion of the eyes; and secondly, that the objects which were best defined and which remained the longest visible were such as I had no recollection of having previously seen. For about twenty-four hours I had constantly before me a human figure, the features and dress of which were as distinctly visible as that of any real existence, and of which, after an interval of many years, I still retain the most lively impression; yet neither at the time nor since have I been able to discover any person whom I had previously seen who resembled it.

"During one part of this disease, after the disappearance of the stationary phantom, I had a very singular and amusing imagery presented to me. It appeared as if a number of objects, principally human faces or figures on a small scale, were placed before me and gradually removed, like a succession of medallions. They were all of the same size, and appeared to be all at the same distance from the face."

This admits of the same explanation as the case of Nicolai; but the writer, being a better informed and more learned man, gives a clearer description of it.

How common are similar delusions in children; but their alarm and their want of judgment prevent them from recognising the objects as unreal. A child wakes up from its sleep and sees horrible phantoms before its eyes, nor does this sort of delirium subside even for some time after candles are brought in, and it is able to recognise its father and mother. It has the two sets of perceptions, each complete; but the disordered ones are most powerful, and it is only by soothing words and caresses that it can, from moment to moment, shake off for an instant the constantly recurring delusions of the disordered brain. Generally, in such cases, it has appeared to me that the disturbance was in both brains; that one became gradually re-established for some time before the other: at first, the child flies to the arms of its parents for safety, but does not recognise them; gradually, it becomes conscious of real objects, but has a *pari passu* conviction of the reality of the phantoms; after a time, the disturbance in the other brain also ceases, and composure is restored. Few parents with a numerous progeny but must have witnessed similar distressing phenomena. Whatever the state of brain in the children, and however unable we may be to describe it, or to give it a name, I conceive that during its stage of recovery, when the child begins to smile at its terrors, it is identical with that of Nicolai and Dr. Bostock. It almost always arises from indigestion.

Every medical man must have heard patients, in an incipient or subsiding delirium, express their distress at the immense multitude of faces which come out from the darkness and surround the bed. They are quite aware of the unreality of the phantoms, but cannot dismiss them from their perceptions.

Much insight is obtained into the nature and origin of mental derangement, and of the antagonism of the two brains, by careful observation of the disease as a consequence of diffused gout, and scarcely less from watching puerperal insanity. In these cases, the immediate, *direct*, *proximate* cause is known to us; in the latter instance it is obvious from the first, and in the former from the result; but while waiting this result, we may commit great and grievous mischief, by a mistake in the probable origin of the disease, of which I will give a striking example.

A gentleman of large hereditary fortune, having a very numerous family, chiefly of girls, resolved to lay down his expensive establishment, for the sake of making provision for them. He let his house, sold his carriage and his large stud of horses, gave his hounds to a friend, and retired to a house of moderate size, with one man-servant and three females, and, with a good library; he occupied himself in aiding the tutor and governess in the tuition of his daughters and younger children. His pride was much hurt on first encountering the change, for he was generally supposed to be a ruined man, and not a few stories were told of his shameless extravagance which had brought him to his present degradation, although in fact he had always lived much within his income. I mention these things to shew that he was a man with strong self-command and high principle. "I bide my time," was his consolation, and he often declared that he had never experienced real happiness till after his change of habits; yet he was morbidly sensible to slights, and had the change in his position been compulsory instead of voluntary, I do not think he could have survived the vivid sense of degradation. When it was found, however, that out of his annual savings he was regularly investing large sums in the names of his daughters, that no interruption had ever taken place in his eleemosynary benefactions, and that he was even able to purchase portions of land, for the purpose of completing the form and compactness of his estate, public opinion entirely changed, and the man who had been so largely abused as a spendthrift became as extravagantly lauded as a hero. He was simply a man of high principle and great self-command.

This gentleman came under my care, with a long list of anomalous ailments, and it was not for a considerable time that I was able to form a decided opinion of their origin. It was one of the two

> monster ills that mimic all the rest—

gout and hysteria—it was *gout*. Having always cultivated the practice of forming a medical opinion slowly, and adhering to it pertinaciously, I was not turned from my convictions by the many contradictory opinions of other advisers, in some respects superior to myself. I could not go through with them on every occasion, the logical process by which I had convinced myself; for all the reasons were not always present to me in the same order and force, but I knew that I *had* investigated thoroughly and satisfied myself absolutely, and that no other series of arguments, however consecutive, could produce a more absolute conviction. I therefore remained of the same opinion.

The gentleman gradually became bewildered in mind. He expressed occasional alarm at the excessive rapidity of his thoughts, and spoke of the difficulty of convincing himself that he had parted with his hounds; he repeatedly rang the bell for the keeper, and then, perhaps, before the servant could answer it, recollected, and was ashamed of the error. His expression was, "there always seems to be another person *thinking with my brain*, and telling me things that I know to be false, but which I have the greatest difficulty to prevent myself from uttering as my own." The slightest opposition to any absurd sentiment which he uttered under this impulse made him furious, but by affecting assent to his assertion or confused attempt at argument, and by a tone of great sympathy and compassion, I could sometimes gradually and gently lead him to explain the two trains of thought which were passing through his mind, and I very much regret not having committed them to paper. They were, however, as completely unconnected as two trains of thought passing through the minds of two distinct persons; yet, in the midst of the confusion produced by this mental disturbance, he could sometimes, as he phrased it, "suddenly pull up and throw himself on his haunches." It went on in this manner till he became entirely unable to control his morbid trains of thought, and it assumed the character of positive insanity. His friends took steps to place him under restraint; a conclave assembled at his house, keepers and a strait-waistcoat were provided, and it was only by most forcibly pleading the frightful consequences of such a proceeding to the welfare of his daughters, and shewing the obstacle it would create to their establishment in life, that I procured a little delay. Sometimes I could assign such reasons for my belief as seemed to me irresistible—more frequently I could only oppose my dogged conviction to the acute arguments of an able man, and I was *talked down*. There is something, however, so impressive on others, in an absolute faith like that which possessed me, that I succeeded for more than a week in procuring delay; at last, I was allowed four-and-twenty hours more as the very latest period they would consent to wait, at the expiration of which he was to be removed to an establishment for the insane. Happily, four-and-twenty hours were not required to prove *me* in the right (which was a matter of trifling importance), but to save *him* from a degradation which I firmly believe would have had fatal consequences. In the night he was seized with pain in the great toe, which in a few hours swelled to a great size—all his delusions vanished, and his reasoning powers became extraordinarily acute, as is, I believe, always the case under an established fit of gout, however the temper may be spoiled.

Had this man waked from his insane dream to find himself in a strait-waistcoat, and surrounded by plebeian controllers of his actions, I think it highly probable that, with a mind so susceptible and a sense of personal dignity so acute, his indignation would have produced a revulsion which might have rendered his recovery hopeless, and the belief of the friends in my ignorance would have been confirmed.

To this day, the gentleman does not know the extent of his obligation to me, for he had but a vague recollection of his former state, and it was never thought safe to make very specific allusions to it, although of the transition state he had a very vivid remembrance, and it was his narrative that mainly aided to establish in my own mind those principles, if I may so term them, which led to my present theory.

Non-medical men may perhaps think it strange that a generally diffused disease like gout should attack only one brain, and that a malady pervading the whole body, whether in the blood or not, should fix upon one organ alone; but this is universal, and a slight consideration will explain it. Whatever be the nature of the poison circulating in the veins, it will first manifest itself by disorder or change of structure in some one part, though it may afterwards extend to others; one eye will be affected alone, perhaps by a virus pervading the whole system; in scrofula, one gland, and so forth. The length of time of the state of transition may be of any duration; and while one brain is the seat of disease which gives erroneous perceptions or suggests erroneous arguments, the other may be so completely healthy that it entirely dominates the disordered one, and not only prevents its morbid volitions from being exercised, but carefully conceals them from observation, conscious that they would inspire not sympathy but contempt. In like manner, millions of human beings have criminal volitions passing through their minds, which, were the means of gratification suddenly presented, accompanied by a conviction of worldly impunity, would pass into acts; but the early and continuous cultivation of self-command, fear of punishment (the social conscience), religious principle, self-respect, risk of detection, and a hundred other motives, keep them always in the path of duty.

> . . . . thoughts impure
> May pass through mind of angel, or of man,
> And leave no stain.

Each man knows his own bad volitions, which he has been able to suppress; but he knows not which of his neighbours, whom he thinks so pure, have had the same difficulties to encounter; still less does he know those who have indulged their evil propensities undetected of all but One.

Place the individual subjected to these morbid impulses in a position of impunity, so low or so high in the social scale that he is either above shame or below it, and we see how much of the morality of society depends on positive law, and how little on virtuous self-restraint. There are only two classes of men who know how numerous are such cases. Clergymen of the Roman Catholic faith, and those medical men whose general benevolence and calmness of manner invite the confidential communications of their patients. Such men hail with delight the new system of prison discipline, which will produce a greater reformation in society than even Father Mathew.

The long course of self-restraint which has acquired the respect of our fellow-creatures may suddenly cease, and a man of high character be reduced to infamy by exposure. Where no previous misconduct can be traced, it is more charitable, and generally more just, to attribute the misdeed to mental disturbance—a sudden increase of bad volitions or diminution of power in the functions which control them, arising from positive physical disease. There is little fear of this sentiment being carried too far. I will give only one instance, for it is a dangerous subject, and as we cannot on these occasions *open the head to ascertain the truth*, it is safer for society to punish than to give extensive impunity; just as it is safer and more extensively benefical to mankind that the marriage tie should be indissoluble, although the enforcement of the bond is often accompanied by the most cruel tyranny and injustice.

The following case is more especially connected with the government of the propensities than with cerebral antagonism, but it bears on the point indirectly. The gentleman held a situation in which he had many younger persons under him. I purposely leave the designation obscure. He had risen to the head of the office by long and exemplary services. He was a widower, and had had a considerable family, all of whom however died in their youth. He exercised a paternal control over his subordinates, and was extremely respected by every one who knew him. His salary was ample, however, his excessive benevolence had kept him always poor, but as his style of living did not imply the expenditure of more than half his income, he had the reputation of wealth. Gradually, towards the age of sixty, this gentleman became garrulous and light in his conversation, and the others in the office suspected him to have been drinking. He had many rebuffs from the persons under his command, but this in no degree changed the indecorous levity of his conversation, which had formerly been remarkably dignified, and as reserved as was compatible with his excessive benevolence of disposition. Months and months passed on, his language became gradually worse, and at last was of the most depraved obscenity. This shocked and disgusted his juniors, and he was seriously threatened with exposure by them. The propensity was checked for awhile, but after repeated offences and repeated forgiveness by the young men, they made a formal complaint to his superiors. The offender was taken to task very seriously, but, as the young men had given rather a lenient representation of his conduct, he was permitted one more trial, with the assurance that his next offence would be followed by dismissal.

There was soon an opportunity of putting the threat in force, for his conduct and conversation became more and more gross and disgusting. He was dismissed.

Having made no provision, he suddenly found himself utterly destitute, but did not make known his position. He packed a bundle of necessary clothes, put in his pocket whatever money and trinkets he possessed, and wandered about the country without aim or object. Every one lost sight of him for two or three months, when he was found in a remote part of the kingdom *literally dead on a dunghill*, where it is supposed he had laid himself down for warmth; his money was gone, and from the state of the stomach and intestines, it is probable that he had died of want of food as the immediate cause, but on examining the interior of the skull, there was found extensive softening and disorganization in the left cerebrum, and the other was not free from disease. He could not have lived long, though under proper care the disease would not have been immediately fatal.

Whether it was a weakening of the intellectual powers which destroyed the control over propensities always in excess, or an increase of the propensities from disease or disorder in the parts of the brain appropriated to those functions, can be only matter of conjecture, but the change was probably owing to both causes. At what exact point of time it commenced cannot be known, but the self-command so early acquired and so long cultivated, perhaps continued in one brain, while the other was beginning to be disorganized; and we may conceive many struggles and victories before the contest was finally given up, and he gave way to the full impulses of the grosser passions.

CHAPTER IX: *Sentiment of Pre-Existence; Explanation; Princess Charlotte's Funeral; Impressions on the Senses; Phrenology; Clergyman with Opposing Convictions; Remarks of Mr. Solly; Cerebellum; Antagonism of the Two Brains*

There is a mental phenomenon of frequent occurrence, so common that I do not remember ever to have met with a person who had not experienced it more than once—yet, I believe, Walter Scott is the only writer who has made mention of it. He calls it a "sentiment of pre-existence." It is a sudden feeling, as if the scene we have just witnessed (although, from the very nature of things it could never have been seen before) had been present to our eyes on a former occasion, when the very same speakers, seated in the very same positions, uttered the same sentiments, in the same words—the postures, the expression of countenance, the gestures, the tone of voice, all seem to be *remembered*, and to be now attracting attention for the second time. *Never* is it supposed to be the third time.

Now this delusion occurs only when the mind has been exhausted by excitement, or is from indisposition or any other cause languid, and only slightly attentive to the conversation. The persuasion of the scene being a repetition, comes on when the attention has been roused by some accidental circumstance and we become, as the phrase is, wide awake.

I believe the explanation to be this: only one brain has been used in the immediately preceding part of the scene, the other brain has been asleep, or in an analogous state nearly approaching it. When the attention of both brains is roused to the topic, there is the same vague consciousness that the ideas have passed through the mind before, which takes place on reperusing the page we had read while thinking on some other subject. The ideas *have* passed through the mind before, and as there was not sufficient consciousness to fix them in the memory without a renewal, we have no means of knowing the length of time that had elapsed between the *faint* impression received by the single brain, and the *distinct* impression received by the double brain. It may seem to have been many years.

I have often noticed this in children, and believe they have sometimes been punished for the involuntary error, in the belief that they had been guilty of deliberate falsehood.

The strongest example of this delusion I ever recollect in my own person was on the occasion of the funeral of the Princess Charlotte. The circumstances connected with that event formed in every respect a most extraordinary psychological curiosity, and afforded an instructive view of the moral feelings pervading a whole nation, and shewing themselves without restraint or disguise. There is, perhaps, no example in history of so intense and so universal a sympathy, for almost every conceivable misfortune to one party is a source of joy, satisfaction, or advantage, to another. The event was attended by the strange peculiarity that it could be a subject of joy or satisfaction to no one. It is difficult to imagine another instance of calamity by which none could derive any possible benefit, for in the then state of succession to the throne no one was apparently even brought a step nearer to it. One mighty all-absorbing grief possessed the whole nation, and was aggravated in each individual by the sympathy of his neighbour, till the whole people became infected with an amiable insanity, and incapable of estimating the real extent of their loss. No one under five-and-thirty or forty years of age can form a conception of the universal paroxysm of grief which then superseded every other feeling.

I had obtained permission to be present on the occasion of the funeral, as one of the Lord Chamberlain's staff. Several disturbed nights previous to that ceremony, and the almost total privation of rest on the night immediately preceding it, had put my mind into a state of hysterical irritability, which was still further increased by grief, and by exhaustion for want of food, for between breakfast and the hour of interment at midnight, such was the confusion in the town of Windsor that no expenditure of money could procure refreshment.

I had been standing four hours, and on taking my place by the side of the coffin, in St. George's chapel, was only prevented from fainting by the interest of the scene. All that our truncated ceremonies could bestow of pomp was there, and the exquisite music produced a sort of hallucination. Suddenly, after the pathetic Miserere of Mozart, the music ceased, and there was an absolute silence. The coffin, which was placed on a kind of altar covered with black cloth (united to the black cloth which covered the pavement), sank down so slowly through the floor, that it was only in measuring its progress by some brilliant object beyond it that any motion could be perceived. I had fallen into a sort of torpid reverie, when I was recalled to consciousness by a paroxysm of violent grief on the part of the bereaved husband, as his eye suddenly caught the coffin sinking into its black grave, formed by the inverted covering of the altar. In an instant I felt not merely an *impression*, but a *conviction*, that I had seen the whole scene before on some former occasion, and had heard even the very words addressed to myself by Sir George Naylor.

Often did I discuss this matter with my talented friend, the late Dr. Gooch, who always took great interest in subjects occupying the debateable region between physics and metaphysics; but we could never devise an explanation satisfactory to either of us. I cannot but think that the theory of two brains, as above stated, affords a sufficient solution of the otherwise inexplicable phenomenon. It is probable that some of the examples of religious mysticism, which we generally set down as imposture, may have their origin in similar hallucinations, and that in the uneducated mind these apparent recollections of past scenes, similar to the present, may give to an enthusiast the idea of inspiration, especially where one brain has a decided tendency to insanity, as is so often the case with such persons.

Almost every man who starts a new theory is held responsible for all the extravagant opinions and arguments of those who adopt it, and thus discredit is thrown on the original idea. I am quite prepared to expect the accusation of having asserted madness to be a disturbance, disorder, or disease of one brain only. Let me expend a few words in anticipation of this mistake.

I believe that real madness resides in both brains, or in parts of both brains. It is only conscious delusion that is confined to one of them. An erroneous conviction, affecting any of the special senses, no doubt is a disturbance of the organs of both brains devoted to that sense, quite independent of the intellect. Were it otherwise, there would be contradictory evidence, the patient would be conscious of the discrepancy, and discard it on the same evidence which leads us to discard the belief in the sound of a bell when we have a cold in the ears.

We may conceive, for example, that the olfactory ganglia of one side may be disturbed without the other being affected, yet still the disgusting odour resulting from the perversion would be the only sensation of which the sufferer was conscious, because the healthy ganglion would *only not perceive*, it would not *contradict* the testimony; so with the portions of the brain which give sensation to the ears and the eyes—if one side perceive, and the other simply does not perceive, the error must be believed; but if, at the time that an offensive odour is smelt, the individual is still capable of appreciating the perfume of a rose; or if the eye seeing a ghost, sees at the same time a real person in his proper shape and colour, it seems quite evident that such affection is of one brain only; the two contradictory sensations give rise to incompatible perceptions, and the intellect then recognises the delusion.

In like manner of the moral sentiments, the degree to which the disturbance may extend to both brains is the measure of the delusion or insanity. It can scarcely be called complete, while the patient laments his own loss of the qualities on which he had, perhaps, formerly prided himself. He will say I detest myself for these propensities—for my cruelty to my wife or my children; it is causeless, yet I cannot help it. He will shed tears while lamenting the malignant pleasure he takes in tormenting his dependents, and say, as I have more than once heard, "Surely it is the devil who puts these cruelties and abominations into my head; it is not my natural disposition, and I hate myself all the while I am doing these things." Here *both* the *real* reasoning organs of the *intellect* appear to be in their natural state, for the judgment formed is correct, though the impulses are no longer under the control of the will.

The phrenologist (in the full extent of the term, as used in popular language) justly holds these facts as proofs of the existence of separate cerebral organs for different functions. It is when he passes on to the arbitrary appropriation of parts, and to the assumption that such parts may be identified on the surface of the skull, that we hesitate to follow him on the vague and scanty authority of observations necessarily fallible in every case but our own, since the real mind cannot be known to others. The best and most virtuous of mankind *may be* only a hypocrite of extraordinary skill and perseverance. I have heard from Catholic priests of high character and exalted understanding, narratives of death-bed confessions by persons of immaculate reputation,which throw a frightful light on the mass of wickedness sometimes concealed by a halo of piety and good deeds. Such cases of partial moral and sensuous perversion are widely different from the intellectual disturbance of which the following is an example:

A clergyman, of middle age, called on one of the most eminent of the physicians devoted to the treatment of insanity, whose reputation is spread over the whole civilized world, and addressed him to the following effect: "I am come to consult you in my embarrassment, and hope you will give me a candid opinion. I have been for some time engaged in a speculation into which I have unfortunately drawn one of my intimate friends, and totally ruined him. It is a dreadful thing that a man of my station, and at my time of life, should have engaged in so wicked a scheme, but there is no truth in it. I know that I have not done any such thing—that I have not entered on any speculation, or made attempts to induce any one to join me—still it is so, and I am overwhelmed with my guilt." After a pause he added, "I believe I must ask my friend to write me a letter to say there is no truth in the matter, and then, by always reading it, I shall perhaps be able to convince myself."

Similar delusions are familiar to every medical man conversant with insanity. Two contradictory and incompatible convictions. Here is no defective government of moral or sensual propensities, but two distinct acts of the thinking powers destructive of each other. It seems to me absolutely impossible to conceive any other explanation than the possession of two distinct minds—results of two distinct organs of thought. The individual could not tell which of the convictions were true, had he not the means of comparing them with those of other persons. It is not strange that in days of superstition and ignorance this state of brain should have been attributed to *possession by an evil spirit*, and if the disease progressed so as to give rise to epilepsy, the presence of such evil spirit was *proved*, for indeed the syllogism was complete in all the forms of logic. Above all, if it passed on to the madness of volition, and the unhappy being uttered two contradictory trains of thought; if one brain remained sufficiently complete to conceive and lament the wickedness of the other, and the want of power to control it—we need not wonder at the prevalence of the belief, and that the clergyman was resorted to for relief instead of the physician. It is a strong proof of the general intellectual progress of the nation, that in the later editions of the Prayer Book the "Form for the Exorcism of Evil Spirits," is omitted; it has been quietly and unostentatiously suppressed—a wise proceeding, whether with or without authority. Railroads will abolish the absurdity universally.

This state has but a very slight resemblance to the perversion of the moral sentiments, or of the senses, to the ungovernable state of the animal instincts, to the permanent delusions of the madman, or to the diseased idea of the monomaniac; but it may gradually change into any of them. I believe there is no form of cerebral disturbance which may not pass by slow transition into any other form of mental "unhealth," or indeed scarcely a disease of the body which may not be the cause of mental aberration, although it appears that little more than one individual in a thousand is thus liable to the terrible calamity.

I repeat, then, that the possession of two minds does not imply that disorder or disease of only one will produce insanity, although we have no example of disease of both being compatible with a full possession of the mental faculties.

Mr. Solly, in the chapter of his work on the brain, entitled *Physiological Inferences from Pathological States*, after giving many cases of extensive injury to one brain, with the perfect possession of the intellectual faculties, makes the following remarks. It is inconceivable how he could have marshaled such an array of evidence, and then stopped short of the inevitable inference:

"In considering these extraordinary cases the question naturally arises how it is, if the brain be the organ of the mind, that the mind occasionally remains perfect though the brain itself suffers severe injury, and even sustains the loss of a portion of its substance. Without pretending to be able positively to solve the question [He is perfectly capable of solving the question, were he not deterred by that fatal error in nomenclature, *the brain*, instead of the *two brains*], I cannot help venturing on the following explanation. The intellectual faculties in different individuals of the human race differ from one another as much as the human mind itself differs from that of the brute creation. The intellectual powers of a Newton are as much raised above those of the common hewer of wood and drawer of water, as the mental faculties of the labourer are raised above those of the dog which follows him to the field. Now this difference of intellectual power, though no doubt arising partly from the original conformation of the brain [who can doubt it?], must proceed mainly from the circumstance of the faculties of the mind in the one case being highly cultivated and constantly exercised; while in the other case, they have always remained dormant, and never being called into action their loss is scarcely to be perceived. When the brain has been injured, and the faculties of the individual have not appeared to suffer, it is likely the ideas of the individual have never been sufficiently abundant to attract notice to the loss of such of them as depended on that part of the instrument of intellect which has been injured."

In the whole of this paragraph there is too much of metaphysical language, but it may be thus stated in harmony with my theory.

When two brains, originally well formed, have been highly cultivated, one alone is sufficient, not merely to carry on all the functions of mind, but to overcome the tendency of the diseased or injured organ to vitiate the faculties of its fellow, which is a very natural and reasonable presumption (*à priori*). I have said that the power of one brain to control the morbid volitions of its fellow may be indefinitely increased by exercise and cultivation, may be lost by desuetude, or may never have been acquired, as in the case of the "hewer of wood and drawer of water," supposed by Mr. Solly.

How incomprehensible it seems, that he who wrote the preceding should append to it the following words, and yet not make them the basis of a theory which at once explains all the facts. Like almost all other writers whom I have consulted, he just stops short of the logical conclusion, and makes it a stumbling block instead of a bridge.

"The circumstance has also been accounted for by the phrenologists upon the principle that the mental organs are double, and that the loss of one is not therefore easily perceived; and this opinion is certainly supported by the fact, that *there are no cases on record in which the mental faculties have remained undisturbed when the disorganization has extended to both sides of the brain.*"

Quite true; one brain may be injured, mutilated, absorbed, lost, gone, and a hollow cavern left in its place, and yet all the faculties of the mind continue to be exercised in their ordinary degree of perfection; but it is essential to sound mind that the other brain remain perfect. If disease or injury extend to that, there is an end of the true functions of mind, not merely of that faculty which the phrenologists have located in the spot now occupied by disease, for there is not a shadow of proof to connect the locality of the disease with the *nature* of the mental disturbance. The mind is disordered or destroyed, and there is an end.

"It is clear," as Mr. Solly remarks, "that if, in accordance with the derangement or obliteration of individual functions during life, morbid alterations of individual portions of the nervous system were met with after death, no surer evidence of the connexion between function and organic structure could be desired." This, however, is by no means the case; and although I do not cite the fact for the purpose of opposing it to the doctrines of phrenologists (when separate from cranioscopy); it is not even contended by the professors of that science, that any correspondence has been detected between the destruction of a faculty (as memory, for example) during life, and disease discovered by dissection in the part assigned by them as the seat of the faculty.

This certainly is only negative presumption, and by no means a proof of the fallacy of the doctrine of phrenology, since the disease must have advanced much beyond such lesion as might annihilate a faculty before it would endanger life. The strongest fact against that popular theory is, however, as above stated, that no instance has been shewn of injury of corresponding parts of the two cerebra, after the loss of a faculty hitherto considered to be exercised in its integrity only be consentaneous action of both. In so far then as my doctrine shews that one brain (and consequently, one phrenological organ) is sufficient for the full manifestation of the phenomena of mind, it partly removes that objection.

Phrenology, however, whether true or false, is in no way connected with these doctrines, and does not come within the scope of my plan. I do not profess to understand the subject. It has advocates and opponents respectively among the ablest men of the age; and till phrenologists themselves approach unanimity in their minute divisions and localisations, it would be useless to attempt its discussion. I confine myself to the topic I have studied, and as Sir Charles Bell says, "I write what I have seen and what I know."

If it be true, notwithstanding the denial of some anatomists and the consent of others, that each brain is divided into three lobes, it is probable that the three great divisions of the intellectual organs described by phrenologists are correct. It is certain that the intellectual portion of the brain does really exercise a control over the propensities, as there is clearly some degree of self-command exercised by those who have lost one cerebrum from disease. It is, however, necessarily very difficult to ascertain the exact degree of this self-control in such cases, because the helpless state of the patient places him in a false position, and like the animal mutilated by experimental physiologists, the inferences to be drawn from his actions are not what might reasonably be drawn from the same actions in the perfect and healthy being.

The cerebellum also makes a part of the *exterior form*, from which character is inferred by these philosophers, yet if there be one fact more clear than another as to the functions of this mysterious organ, it is that it has no connexion with the reproductive faculty, but is chiefly a co-ordinator of muscular actions. All the symptoms arising from inflammation, or other lesion of the part, may be attributed to the inevitable disturbance of the medulla oblongata in its vicinity, the great centre of vitality. If we are to put faith in the experiments of Flourens (and I know not how we are to withhold assent from that which appeared conclusive and satisfactory to Berthollet, Portal, Pinel, Dumeril, and Cuvier), the whole of the cerebellum has been removed without destroying that faculty or its impulses; but the entire subject is still involved in obscurity, and we can infer but little as to the human brain from experiments on the lower animals.

Cruveilhier gives a plate with an accompanying narrative of a girl of eleven years of age, born absoutely without a cerebellum, and who would probably have lived to maturity but for defective nourishment and neglect. She died scrofulous and atrophied, in the Orphan Hospital at Paris, where she had gradually sunk during the fifteen months since her admission, being indeed at that time in a state of hopeless disease. There is one inference he draws from the case, in opposition to Gall and Spurzheim, which it is no disparagement of his veracity to say that I do not believe. He could only have his information from persons in the hospital unworthy of trust on such a topic. I know by experience how ready those persons are to lend themselves to prurient curiosity, and that they can easily perceive on which side the inquirer wishes for evidence. There is no presiding judge to prevent *leading questions*; and if decency would permit, I could give some striking examples of this want of veracity on the part of the attendants in Italian, French, Swiss, and German hospitals, and even in our own, where, however, the manifestation of this sort of curiosity is held to be as degrading as it is unnecessary.

The cerebellum has been taken away in slices, without interfering with the *mental* functions of the animal, or even with its propensities. The cerebrum itself has been entirely removed, and the animal has lived and grown for ten months without a mind. These extraordinary and cruel mutilations have hitherto produced no result to be depended on, and they are attended with so deadening an effect on the moral feelings of the operator and his pupils, that one can hardly wish them to be continued unless they presented a greater probability of benefit.

If the character of the individual depended not on a thing admitting of demonstration, as the antagonism of the two brains, but on certain organs assumed to exist (destructiveness, for example), balanced by other organs (benevolence), I cannot understand why the brain so formed should not act during health with uniformity on all occasions. Can we suppose it possible that whenever the organ of destructiveness of the right cerebrum is in a state of inflammation or of excitement, the organ of destructiveness of the left cerebrum is in a similar state of inflammation or excitement? This would be one of the most arbitrary assumptions to be met with in medical reasoning, and contrary to all analogy. It would require an immense number of the clearest facts to establish it, which certainly are yet wanting. The "organ of veneration," for instance, is separated from its fellow by the septum of the falx. It can have no communication with it but by a long circuit of membranes; for even in the corpus callosum I expect to prove that neither fibres nor arteries pass across from one side to the other. Either we must give up all attempt at reasoning in physiology, and resolve every thing into "it is because it is," or we must reject an inference so utterly improbable. Can it be conceived that disease should spread from one to another of organs so insulated, and so situated, without involving other organs (or parts) in contact therewith, and thus changing the character of the influence which the original malady or disorder might have upon mental impulse, and therefore upon action?

But with the demonstrated antagonism of two unequal brains an explanation is easy. The diseased action which produces one mode of mind in the right cerebrum may be balanced or neutralized or controlled by another mode of mind produced by the healthy action of the left cerebrum, which, having thus the possession of reason, can call to its aid external circumstances, to assist in the government of the disordered right cerebrum, as in the cases alluded to. A healthy organ must be, *caeteris paribus*, more than equal in power to a diseased one; and the whole set of mental functions acting in harmony and order like a regular army, must on ordinary occasions overpower a tumultuous mob of impulses in its fellow. When the opposing forces are in great disproportion, and the healthy brain can no longer control the unhealthy brain, the case becomes one of partial insanity or conscious delusion, or else it is absolute mania, when all self-government is lost. Either the disordered brain now keeps down the manifestations of the healthy one, which only gives occasional and transient glimpses of reason, or the disease has spread to both sides—both are disordered, and there is little hope of restoration.

The gradations by which this fatal result is brought about are of unlimited variety. We see one person perfectly conscious of his ungovernable impulse, and when exhausted by the physical exertion excited by his cerebral disturbance, he can reason upon and lament his extravagance; another is continuously conscious that he is acting wrongly, even during his most violent paroxysms of rage laments and bewails his wicked impulse, and feels remorse while he is giving way to it. One man is capable of watching the vagaries of his other self, and even finds amusement in the process—another is distressed and alarmed at the contemplation. One can overpower his diseased propensities when in the presence of a person greatly his superior in station or age, or even in size; another is withheld from giving way to his delusions by the dread of ridicule. One will be deterred from a maniacal act by a sense of religion; another by fear of worldly consequences. All these seem to me modifications and degrees of disorder in one brain, more or less under the influence of the other, just in proportion as that other partakes or does not partake of the disease which disturbs the functions, the perceptive or affective faculties, or the reasoning powers, of its fellow.

CHAPTER X: *Examination of the Opinions of Dr. Holland; Comparison of the Theory with a New Railway; the Brain as a Double Organ; Examples of the Double Mind; Inferences; Mode in Which Alone They Can be Drawn from Examination After Death of the Insane*

There is not, I believe, one of the propositions in this work which has not passed through my mind, and produced the impression of its absolute truth many times during the last twenty-five or thirty years. Nevertheless, I should scarcely have ventured to put them forth so boldly, but for the confirmation they receive, up to a certain point, by the argument of Dr. Holland.

The great learning and experience of that gentleman, the remarkably sober and cautious character of his mind, his rigidly inductive spirit, and his reticence in pronouncing positive opinions while there remains a shadow of doubt on his mind—these things stamp a value on every thing he promulgates. When I find then, that by a separate process of reasoning, and without any knowledge of his arguments and illustrations till long after I had completed my theory, I arrive at a result *including* that which he has pronounced, I cannot but feel confirmed in my opinions, and must consider the whole as firmly established, if I can shew that my further progress in the same direction is a logical consequence and inevitable inference from the premises.

In examining his very interesting work, *Medical Notes and Reflections*, I wish to express myself with the respect and deference due to an accomplished scholar and able physician. This feeling must not, however, prevent me from discussing with freedom the opinions he has published—for if they contain error, that error becomes doubly important in its effect on others, through the influence it derives from the large experience and high character of the writer.

Most men, I think, will regret that, with his just claims to the possession of copious learning, varied information, exact knowledge, abundant experience, and great natural sagacity, his style of writing should be rather suggestive than dogmatic—that, when he especially is one of the men best qualified to speak *ex cathedra* and pronounce his opinions oracularly, he should, from his continual mental comparison of the vast *unknown* with the limited *known* (as I conceive it), so often express his *belief* instead of his *absolute conviction.* Young readers, who should be spared the torment of doubt on points of cardinal importance, may be inclined to think even those which he has established to be in their very nature incapable of proof, and may well consider as yet undecided, things on which even Dr. Holland will not pronounce without reserve.

Not having the same claims to confidence, I, for my own part, cannot *afford*, if I may so express myself, to state my opinions so modestly; and at the risk of being charged with presumption I shall, in cases where I have no doubt whatever, venture to say "it is," where Dr. Holland would probably say "may it not be."

Were I writing on a recent subject of temporary interest and of minor importance, I might hesitate to dogmatize; but after thirty years reflection, I think myself justified in speaking with boldness and decision. Believing that my theory will form a great trunk of railway to an important truth, and that innumerable branches will hereafter diverge from it, it certainly behoves me to be convinced that the main line is in a right direction; of which indeed I do not entertain an atom of doubt. To carry on the metaphor, I believe that the value of this original line will not be fully appreciated till the branches are formed and are found to connect together in one harmonious whole a large portion of the vast country of moral physiology.

I hope, therefore, to be pardoned by Dr. Holland, if in the examination of his opinions and suggestions, I should inadvertently express myself without sufficient deference to his speculations. It seems to me that he has reasoned most acutely and correctly in a line *parallel to the truth*, and which, therefore, could not arrive at it; but that a very slight alteration of the point of departure would have inevitably led him through exactly the same train of reasoning to the same result as myself; and even his error, if it be error, I attribute to his deference for the opinions of others. No one can admire more than I do the clear ratiocination of his mind and the legitimacy of his conclusions, wherever he will permit himself to express his sentiments without reserve. On topics strictly medical he writes so lucidly, so candidly, and with such a thorough knowledge of the subject he treats, that it is quite impossible to withhold assent. Still I must presume to say that, on subjects partly metaphysical his deference for the opinions of others detracts from the value of his own. He never distinctly advances an opinion of which he has not thoroughly investigated the foundation; but he often expresses doubtfully that which, if he would entirely discard the sentiments of other men, and trust exclusively to his own experience and reflection, he might put forth as *certain*, and thus save much embarrassment to the reader of his lucubrations. Dr. Holland opens his chapter "On the Brain as a Double Organ" in the following words: "I am not sure that this subject of the relation of the two hemispheres of the brain has yet been followed into all the consequences which more or less directly result from it. Symmetry of arrangement on the two sides of the body is common indeed to all the organs of animal life. But the doubleness of the brain, like all besides pertaining to this great nervous centre, offers much more of curious speculation than the same constitution of other parts. That unity of consciousness in perception, volition, memory, thought, and passion, which characterizes the mind in its healthy state, *illud quod sentit, quod sapit, quod vult, quod viget*, is singularly contrasted with the division into two equal portions of the material organ which more immediately ministers to these high functions. Yet, on the other hand, in the almost exact symmetry of form and composition of each hemisphere, in their relation precisely similar to the organs of sense and voluntary motion on each side of the body, and in the structure of the nervous connexions subsisting between them; we find argument not merely for the correspondence of functions, but even for that unity or individuality, of which consciousness is the interpreter to all. This unity, indeed, as it actually exists, is of necessity compatible with the conformation of the brain as a double organ, even had we no such presumption to refer to.

"Here it must be admitted, we are close upon that line, hardly to be defined by the human understanding, which separates material organization and actions from the proper attributes of *mind*; the structure which ministers to perception from the percipient; the instruments of voluntary power from the will itself. Our existence may be said to lie on each side this boundary; yet with a chasm between them so profound and obscure, that though perpetually traversing it in all the functions of life, we have no eye to penetrate its depths."

There is, in the passage just quoted, a much deeper process of thinking than will be obvious to a common observer. I recommend the reader to peruse it attentively at least twice (for I myself certainly did not comprehend its full meaning till after a second deliberate perusal), and when he fully understands its object, I will ask him whether the idea of the *oneness* of the mind be not here the sole obstacle to the acknowledgment of the perfect duality of the cerebral organs *and their functions?* To me it seems that Dr. Holland's fixed notion on that subject is like the fixed notion of the opponents of Galileo, that the earth was stationary in the centre of the system; and that had his mind been free from prepossession on this subject, he could not have resisted the influence of such evidence as he has himself accumulated.

All the facts Dr. Holland has stated from his own experience, and many more which he subsequently cites, seem to me to range themselves so easily, so naturally, and so satisfactorily, on my theory, that I cannot but feel entire confidence that he will adopt it; and certainly he cannot deny that it would satisfactorily explain a vast number of the phenomena of disease which do not seem to admit of any other solution.

Dr. Holland does not give entire credit to the statement of Cruveilhier, which I have cited, that the mental faculties remained perfect when one hemisphere or one cerebrum was destroyed by atrophy; but after the mass of evidence I have marshaled on the subject, he cannot, I think, any longer refuse his assent. As one case well attested settles the question, I have limited myself in the number of examples; but it would have been easy to enlarge the list from sources of unquestionable authority.

"Mental derangement," says Dr. Holland, "however the name may be used, is not *one thing*, nor can it be treated as such. It differs in kind not less than in degree; and in each of its varieties we may trace, through different cases, all the gradations between a sound and an unsound understanding. . . . These singular phenomena, while connected on the one side with dreaming, delirium, and insanity, are related on the other by a series of gradations with the most natural and healthy functions of the mind."

That is to say, as I explain it, there is every gradation of disease or disorder in one brain, and every degree of control by the other; from that absolute tyranny I have spoken of, to the fading away into acquiescence, or till the same power is lost and the case has passed into absolute insanity or dementia.

"It is not difficult to understand how some of the most singular incongruities of madness may arise from this coinage of the brain, this struggle between spectral illusions and actual impressions on the senses, each severally credited, and each brought to bear upon action. The combination of these conditions may be so various, the changes among them so rapid, as to expain every degree of such mental aberration, as well as the diversity of forms under which it occurs; from the simple reverie of the absent man, to the wildest incongruities of the maniac."

How simple is the explanation of these diversities if my theory be accepted as a guide.

"A familiar example of what may be termed the first stage of insubordination to the will" [*a happy term, I wonder that its very adoption did not lead him further*] "is that of certain musical sounds coming unsought for upon the mind, and even tormenting it by their persistence, despite every effort to put them aside."

The healthy, or comparatively healthy, brain recognises them as erroneous impressions, because not perceived by both brains; but the wrong action is either too powerful to be controlled, or the right action too weak to control it.

Dr. Holland relates a case of a gentleman of advanced age, who struck his head against the corner of a sofa with violence; an hour or two afterwards, there came on a failure in the memory and articulation of words; the sounds he uttered were unintelligible, and he was conscious of it. The following day the memory and speech returned, and continued free from disorder. Two days afterwards, while driving out in his carriage, he heard two voices close to his ear, in rapid dialogue, almost without meaning. He was conscious of the fallacy, but unable to check or withdraw the perception of them, or to change the phrases. When reading, similar voices seemed to accompany him, sometimes getting a few words in advance, *but not beyond what the eye might have reached.*" [I call this one brain reading faster than the other.]

"In another case, a gentleman who had believed and acted on similar delusions, where there was no obvious disease, passed by a well-marked passage, from this state to one in which, having still similar sensations, he recognised and treated them as delusions." That is, both brains having been disordered at first, he had no means of knowing the fallacy of the impressions; but when one of them recovered he could judge correctly. "I inquired from him," says Dr. Holland, "how, when the articulate sounds seemed still present, he had learned to regard them as illusions? He told me it was by his never discovering any person in the places whence the voices had come; chiefly by finding himself able on trial to suggest the words seemingly uttered by some one external to himself."

"This fact," adds Dr. Holland, "abounds in curious inferences; it appears to make a breach for the time in the identity of the rational being. We have the strange phenomenon before us of thoughts and emotions rising within the mind, and arranged in the phraseology of words; which words, however, by some morbid perversion of the functions of the brain, are received and believed by the consciousness as coming from persons without. It is, if such expression be allowed, *a sort of duplicity of the mind in its dealings with itself.*"

Strange, that Dr. Holland does not go a single step further, and view this disordered process as a proof of the duality of the individual; of two brains, each carrying on a distinct and separate train of thought, one sane and the other morbid; a thing which is shewn by innumerable exemplifications in health and disease.

In speaking of instances of moral derangement and gradual change of habits, passing from under the control of the will, Dr. Holland remarks that the understanding "is really perverted or enfeebled in most of these cases, and no longer gives that direction and balance which is essential to the healthy state of mind." That is, as I should state it, the disorder has gradually spread from one brain to the other, and self-control is destroyed.

"The existence of more doubtful cases, such as graduate between reason and insanity . . . is attested by the actual difficulty often experienced in dealing, both legally and morally, with these cases, and by the observation of their progress, as well when first passing the limit of reason as when re-entering it in the course of recovery." Is not this the inevitable result of causes such as I have described? The disorder or disease of one brain extends to the other, and correct judgment is not to be expected till, not merely one brain be re-established (which gives consciousness of the error), but till the other brain has made considerable progress towards recovery.

Dr. Holland further observes: "It has been a familiar remark, that in certain states of mental derangement, as well as in some cases of hysteria, which border closely upon it, there appear, as it were, *two minds*; one tending to *correct* by more just perceptions, feelings, and volitions, *the aberrations of the other*, and the relative power of the two influences varying at different times."

At this point I concluded that the author had arrived at the same result as myself; his previous arguments having so logically led to it; when to my great surprise he suddenly turns away from the direct path, and proceeds as follows:

"Admitting the general truth of this description, as attested by many and curious examples, the fact may be explained in some cases by the co-existence before the mind—[*the mind!* when he has just shewn that there are two] of real and unreal objects of sense, each successively the object of belief, a phenomenon possibly itself depending on the doubleness of the brain, and of the parts ministering to perception, though we cannot obtain any certain proof that such is the case. But this explanation will not adequately apply to the instances where complete trains of thought are perverted or deranged, while others are preserved in sufficiently natural course to become *a sort of watch on the former.*"

This "double consciousness" Dr. Holland calls a rapid fluctuation of mind from one train of thought to another ". . . where the mind passes by alternation from one state to the other, each having the perception of external impressions and appropriate trains of thought, but not linked together by the ordinary gradations, or by mutual memory."

How can memory be consistent with two simultaneous trains of erroneous thought, each confusing and mystifying the other? We know that each brain *can* act as a separate whole, when its fellow is destroyed. We know that *it does so act;* and we know by a superfluous abundance of evidence that the two are capable of acting synchronously and erroneously in disease, thus confounding two distinct trains of thought; double *mind* from disease, as double *vision* from disease.

The whole of his chapter "on the brain as a double organ" is well deserving of repeated perusal. It is still further in harmony with the present theory, and would almost seem to be intended to illustrate it, but that towards the end the writer uses the following expression: "without referring to the several parts of this complicated structure, or to the effects of morbid changes upon these respectively, in altering the relation of the two sides, *and the functions which are perfect* ONLY FROM THEIR ENTIRE CORRESPONDENCE."

This assumption seems the grand source of error in every work I have read on the subject of the mind. It is the undoubting faith in this dogma that has made the deepest thinkers resist conviction, just as the absolute reliance on the fact of the earth being stationary made the men of the time of Galileo reject his doctrines. We have seen that although the two brains (for here lies the error, the belief in the *oneness* of the thinking organ), perform but one function in the perfectly healthy and properly cultivated voluntary exercise of their energies, each is capable of acting singly for all the modes of mind; and it is not then true that for this exercise of mind there is required the entire correspondence between the two sides of the cerebrum, or the two cerebra. Were it true that such a perfect correspondence were essential to the exercise of the intellectual powers, common sense would be as rare a possession as the faculties of Newton, Shakspere, and Walter Scott.

"Here indeed we may still seek for an explanation in *supposing* the two states to be never strictly coincident in time; and this view is sanctioned by what observation tells us of the inconceivable rapidity with which the mind shifts its state from one brain of thought or feeling to another—a fluctuation and rapidity much greater in reality than we recognise by language, or in common contemplation of the subject. Articulate speech, in fact, is often unable to keep pace with such changes, nor have we any means of measuring by time these momentary passages of mental existence crowding upon each other, and withal so interwoven into one chain that consciousness, while it makes us aware of unceasing change, tells of no breach of continuity. If the latter explanation be admitted, then these cases come under the description of what has been termed *double consciousness*, [How nearly has the writer approached the full discovery: it requires but one more step, and the whole is lucidly plain.] where the mind passes by alternation from one state to another, each having the perception of external impressions (not always) and appropriate trains of thought, but not linked together by ordinary gradations or by mutual memory (one of the trains of thought, however, generally rests in the memory). I have seen one or two singular cases of this kind, but none so extraordinary as have been related elsewhere. Their relations to the phenomena of sleep, of somnambulism, reverie, and insanity, abound in conclusions of the deepest interest to every part of the mental history of man."

Which then is most probable? That the mind considered as a whole—the homogeneous brain, the double brain—should exercise false and correct perceptions alternately, at intervals of less than a second of time—should be in healthy and disordered action in this rapid alternation—should perform its functions truly and falsely, in varying succession—should appreciate justly and absurdly, without a perceptible pause between the two processes. Which, I say, is most probable—that these contradictions, repugnant to all analogy, should take place, or that the two minds of two complete brains (which I have proved to exist) should be acting in synchronous discordance? And as there is only one instrument by which the two can manifest their ideas to others, the tongue should be guided to its utterance sometimes by one brain and sometimes by the other, in irregular alternation? I can anticipate no answer but assent to my original proposition: that in disease there are *two minds*, however single may be the result of the *healthy* and harmonious action of the cerebra.

"Even admitting, however, that these curiously contrasted states of mind are never strictly simultaneous [Why admit a fact contrary to all experience and all analogy, and which renders a clear and simple subject unintelligible], it is still a question whence their close concurrence is derived; and in the absence of any certainty on this obscure subject, we may reasonably look to that part of our constitution in which manifest provision is made for unity of result from parts double in structure and function. This provision, we know, in many cases, to be disturbed by accident, disease, or other less obvious cause; and though we cannot so well shew this in regard to the higher faculties of the mind (I think we shew it clearly) as in the instance of the senses, and voluntary power, yet it is conceivable that there may be cases where the two sides of the brain (this unhappy expression—"two brains," would have deprived the subject of all ambiguity)—the two sides of the brain minister differently to these functions, so as to produce incongruity where there ought to be identity or individuality or result.

"It is not easy to carry this argument beyond the form of a mere question, etc. etc."

Should the writer of the above passages read these speculations, I feel entirely satisfied that he will be of a different opinion. I can only account for his thus stopping short, as I account for the fact that small-pox had ravaged this country for generations before it entered into the head of any one to suppose it contagious—a thing of which we now seem to have a superabundant proof. There were in those days physicians as acute minded as Dr. Holland, but they had been taught that the miasmata floated in the atmosphere, and this answered the purpose of explaining the phenomena of its propagation as effectually as that we now adopt—like the two doctrines of electricity.

Had Dr. Holland depended solely on the evidence presented to his own senses, and weighed in his own mind, and had he gone on with the investigation to its natural result, the theory I now propound would have come before the world with an authority which would have insured its reception, and it would not have remained for so humble an individual as myself to make up for the deficiency. I am ashamed to say that I had not read Dr. Holland's work till my own was nearly completed. The only excuse is that, having relinquished practice, I was no longer seeking to keep myself "*au niveau des connoissances actuelles.*"

"By no quality (says Dr. Holland, page 253) is one man better distinguished from another, than by the mastery acquired over the subject and course of his thoughts, by the power of discarding what is desultory, frivolous, or degrading, and of adhering singly and steadily to that which it enlarges and invigorates the mind to pursue."

Should the duality of the mind be conceded by the author, this elegant passage will stand thus: By no quality is one man better distinguished from another than by the power of compelling and continuous attention and obedience of the feebler brain to the volitions of the stronger, and of concentrating the energies of both organs on the same subject, thus mastering difficulties insuperable to the weaker instrument of thought, or indeed to the stronger, while its attention is disturbed by the feeble and imperfect exercise of mind by its fellow. This wonderful faculty, improved by cultivation till its exercise becomes easy and habitual, gives the power of discarding what is desultory, frivolous, or degrading, and of adhering singly and steadily to that which it enlarges and invigorates the mind to pursue.

Whether we may hope to see the subject taken up by this enlightened philosopher in the track I have pointed out, I cannot anticipate; but should my examples and inferences produce in him the same entire conviction of the truth of the doctrine that possesses my own mind, he is of all men best calculated to follow it out to its ligitimate consequences, and throw light on one of the most difficult and embarrassing subjects of human contemplation. It cannot be denied that I have proved the completeness and sufficiency of each brain; because I have shewn that it can even exercise its functions in spite of the general disturbance which accompanies the destruction of the other.

If either brain, then, be a perfect instrument of thought, the consentaneity of the two, when acting together, must always necessarily depend on the due performance of conjoint functions by each of them, were such consentaneity essential to the exercise of mind as is generally supposed. In shewing that such complete concurrence is not essential to effect this object, it seems to me that future investigators of the structure, functions, and diseases of the brain, are liberated from a very embarrassing clog. Had all the cases of death during insanity been anatomically examined, without the impediment presented by a conviction of the oneness of the brain, we should have had a mass of facts collected from which some great mind would have been enabled to draw very important inferences.

How complete this separation—this perfect individuality of the two brains—is shewn by the extent to which disease may progress in one of them, absolutely in contact with the sound one, and yet the latter remain in all its essential functions unaffected. The great commissure forms at once a bond of union and a wall of separation, and, as far as my experience goes, it is absolutely incapable of transmitting inflammation or malignant disease from one organ to another. Both indeed may be liable to the same disease, because both may have been supplied with unhealthy blood, or subjected to the same moral or physical causes of disturbance and disorder; but I believe, though I do not assert, that whenever disease spreads from one cerebrum to the other, it is through the meninges, and never through the corpus callosum. Those who are attached to a great establishment, or engaged in the office of teaching anatomy, and who have consequently dissected more extensively than myself, will be able to decide on the degree of truth and importance in this remark.

It is only a few of the cases of death from accident, or suicide during insanity, that can be available for this purpose. Hanging and drowning produce apoplexy, and make it impossible to judge of the previous state of the brain. Cutting the throat may, from the extensive hemorrhage, remove all traces of previous inflammation. It is the occurrence of pure accidents, as falls, and poisoning, and death by gunshot alone among the modes of suicide, that would enable us to judge of the living state by post-mortem appearances. These are necessarily rare, but if carefully examined may yet throw great light on this obscure subject. The common examinations of persons who have died from insanity can give us very little insight into the curable stage of the disease or diseases, since extensive subsequent disorganization must have taken place before it passed on to the destruction of life.

I may mention here (*par parenthèse*) an extraordinary case of a gentleman under the care of Sir Charles Bell in the year 1807, who, in a paroxysm of maniacal delirium, shot himself through the head. The ball passed in a little above one ear and came out nearly at the same point on the other side, wounding, one would suppose, many parts essential to life. The gentleman was the next moment perfectly sane, and lived several days. I cannot remember how long, but believe it was nearly a week, neither do I know the appearances on dissection, but no doubt the case was recorded.

CHAPTER XI: *Power of Resting One Brain; Castle Building; Case of Delusion From Pride; Another From Reverse of Fortune; Equivocal Hallucination; Case of a Painter; Gentleman Who Saw His Own Self; Lady Who Thought Herself Mary Queen of Scots.*

Apparently the power of *resting* one brain is almost as absolute with some persons who have acquired a command over irregular volitions, as of covering up one eye when diseased, and making use of the other alone. In the latter case a sudden flash of light, or a shower of stars, seen by the disordered organ, will occasionally interrupt and confuse the perfect vision of the other; and in the mental phenomena, we see a steady consecutive train of thought interrupted for an instant by a remnant of mental delusion—this is not unfrequent in the progress of recovery from deranged mind. It is in the exercise of the imagination chiefly that we rest one of the intellectual instruments, as it appears to me—a placid acquiescence of the torpid brain leaves the other free to follow its own vagaries; but should any casual circumstance, a sudden noise, the entrance of another person, a shock of any kind, or even an accidental concussion—if I may so call it—of two thoughts from the two brains occur, it instantly excites attention, or the concurrent action of both of them—this leads to *judgment*, the romantic or extravagant ideas in which we had been indulging are immediately perceived to be erroneous or absurd, and we resume our usual habit of discrimination, and that degree of ratiocination with which we are respectively endowed by nature.

The well-known process called castle-building—in which some persons can indulge till the false impression shall influence their actions—seems to me explicable in the same manner. One brain is allowed to go on with a train of thought which produces pleasurable sensations, unchecked by the conscious other, till the effort required to stop the disordered process becomes difficult or impossible. While the volition remains omnipotent, the case is merely the power of dwelling exclusively on pleasurable ideas—of which hope is one of the forms. The further indulgence of the habit produces almost the effect of truth, and the dull realities of life become insipid. In this state the person is fanciful and capricious, sometimes acting in harmony with the real position in society, sometimes putting forth absurd claims to respect and homage from equals. This degree of delusion is often produced or aggravated by the reading of novels and romances, where the painful effort of stern self-command necessary to the prosaic details of obtaining a livelihood are scarcely touched on, and the actors and actresses, either by fortune or station, are represented as possessed of umlimited power of locomotion, and have leisure for the indulgence of their own thoughts and the furtherance of their own plans; for no writer of judgment—no successful writer—will minutely describe the sordid details of life, or works which are only read for the pleasurable sensations they create would be soon cast aside and neglected.

I have known many individuals who have indulged—perhaps I might say cultivated—this passion to such an extent that they cannot on ordinary occasions control it, and are only capable of the necessary effort when alarmed at the idea of its being mistaken for insanity. I know more than one example of a person in the very lowest station in life, who has felt to the day of her death a conviction that she should be ultimately discovered to be the daughter of some great person, or should inherit some great fortune; although there was no more rational probability of such an event than that she should inherit the throne.

The extraordinary changes which accompany those overturnings of the social structure produced by revolutions—the sudden alternations of fortune witnessed in a nation rapidly rising in prosperity—the progress of new inventions like printing, steam power, and rail-roads, which derange all combinations, and make foresight useless—the general prevalence of gambling, or the predominance of some temporary delusion, as the Mississippi scheme of law, the South-Sea bubble, lotteries, speculations in the funds, and a hundred analogous causes of excitement—all tend to promote the indulgence of this habit of castle-building. Let it pass a little further, and it becomes a monomania; still further, and it degenerates into positive mental derangement. The power of self-control is lost—the person is insane. He thinks himself king, emperor, conqueror, Christ, or the Deity, and assumes the authority which he believes to be befitting the character.

Yet, in almost all these cases, there is a remnant of doubt in one of the brains at least, that he is neither king, emperor, nor Deity, but plain John Smith. He submits to the orders of a menial, eats coarse food, and gives way to needs which are incompatible with his supposed important character.

I give a few examples of these delusions, not for the sake of proof, for proof is unnecessary, as every person of common sense and observation must have noticed instances of them; but rather for the sake of shewing the gradual transition from perfect mind (so far indeed as we can properly use the term perfect mind in speaking of created being) to positive insanity.

A lady of birth so exceedingly humble and low that it would be held degrading in every form of society, was in early youth raised to a respectable position through the accidental success of some very equivocal speculations in trade by one of her relations. She received a reasonably sound and moral education, and was by temperament exceedingly religious. Remaining in a state of celibacy, partly from fastidious delicacy as to the station of the men she might have married, she lived alone, and, with an adroit servant to flatter her prejudices and promote her own interest, by ministering to the morbid passions of her mistress, indulged in novels and castle-building during a long series of years. I knew her when the passion was recent, and she would bear a jest on her assumption of dignity as contrasted with her position in childhood; it gradually passed on, till accident gave her a taste for heraldry. A cousin, whom she patronised and provided for, was apprenticed to an undertaker, and in his occasional visits of gratitude to his benefactress gave her a little insight into a science calculated to minister to her taste. She studied it with avidity, found persons of her own name among the highest ranks of the peerage, and gradually persuaded herself that she was of illustrious descent.

With those who did not know her origin, she was always supposed to be a lady of high hereditary dignity, whom events, to which she obscurely hinted, prevented from occupying the station to which she was born. With myself, and with all who had known her from childhood, or who knew any of her relations, she never entered on the subject; though, no doubt, when enjoying the homage of the low people who supposed her a person of birth, she was as fully conscious of the delusion as when she was conversing with the original acquaintances of her family.

Notwithstanding this preposterous passion for imaginary aggrandisement, and, virtually, the *lies* she was compelled to utter or sanction, she was really, in all other respects, a person of strict veracity and high principle, with a very vivid sense of religious responsibility; but when her sound convictions were unaided by her consciousness of the presence of some one who knew her assertions to be unfounded, it was not in her power to control the propensity.

As time went on, she became herself alarmed at the hold that this and similar delusions had obtained over her mind, and she made vain efforts to shake them off. The lapse of years, aided by the disturbance occasioned by the changes of the constitution at about fifty had, however, established these delusions till they became perfectly ungovernable, and she at last firmly believed herself to be a person of high rank, compelled to conceal her position for political reasons. She died in this conviction, strictly speaking *mad*; but as she spent her moderate income judiciously, and had no impatient heir to sue out a writ *de lunatico inquirendo*, she remained only a *whimsical lady* to the last, and her will has been very properly acted on as valid.

I know not at what point of this long case it would have been possible to draw the line between sound and disordered mind, but it would not have been so difficult to decide the point at which restaint should be enforced had her property been capital instead of a life annuity, and she had been induced to dissipate it absurdly in an attempt to imitate the style of living of her supposed rank.

Another case is that of a gentleman of respectable birth, excellent education and ample fortune, engaged in one of the highest departments of trade, or rather commerce. He was a kind-hearted, generous being, who never turned away a deserving (scarcely an undeserving) petitioner, yet so judicious a manager of his income, and so moderate in his self-indulgence that his fortune, for a long time, sustained no material injury from the many successful appeals to his benevolent feelings. He went on, beloved and respected, yet always inspiring his true friends with fears that his excessive tenderness and humanity would ultimately lead him to distress; this, indeed, gradually took place, and no longer being able to indulge in his wonted generosity he looked about for means to increase his income.

In one of those national paroxysms of gambling delusion of which I have spoken, he was induced to embark in one of the plausible speculations of the day, and not merely lost the whole sum he had ventured, but, from the establishment by law of the fact of copartnership, became responsible for all the defalcations of the company he had joined. He was utterly ruined.

Like other men, he could bear a sudden overwhelming reverse better than a long succession of petty misfortunes, and the way in which he conducted himself on the occasion met with unbounded admiration from his friends. He withdrew however into rigid seclusion, and, being no longer able to exercise the generosity and indulge the benevolent feelings which had formed the happiness of his life, made himself a substitute for them by day-dreams, gradually fell into a state of irritable despondency, from which he only gradually recovered with the loss of reason. He now fancied himself possessed of immense wealth, and gave without stint his imaginary riches. He has ever since been under gentle restraint, and leads a life not merely of happiness, but of bliss; converses rationally, reads the newspapers, where every tale of distress attracts his notice, and being furnished with an abundant supply of blank checks, he fills up one of them with a munificent sum, sends it off to the sufferer, and sits down to his dinner with a happy conviction that he has earned the right to a little indulgence in the pleasures of the table; and yet, on a serious conversation with one of his old friends, he is quite conscious of his real position, but the conviction is so exquisitely painful that *he will not let himself believe it.*

A very affecting example of the power of imagination and the danger of indulging it, is well known to me. Men of seventy years of age familiar with London will recognise the individual, but I will not give his name lest it should hurt the feelings of his respectable family.

A painter who succeeded to a large portion of the practice, and, as he thought, to more than all the talent of Sir Joshua Reynolds, was so extensively employed, that he informed me he had once painted (large and small) three hundred portraits in one year. This would seem physically impossible, but the secret of his rapidity and of his astonishing success was this: He required but one sitting, and painted with miraculous facility. I myself saw him execute a kit-cat portrait of a gentleman well known to me, in little more than eight hours; it was minutely finished, and a most striking likeness.

On asking him to explain it, he said, "When a sitter came, I looked at him attentively for half-an-hour, sketching from time to time on the canvass. I wanted no more, I put away my canvass, and took another sitter. When I wished to resume my first portrait, *I took the man and set him in the chair,* where I saw him as distinctly as if he had been before me in his own proper person—I may almost say more vividly. I looked from time to time at the imaginary figure, then worked with my pencil, then referred to the countenance, and so on, just as I should have done had the sitter been there—*when I looked at the chair I saw the man!* This made me very popular; and as I always succeeded in the likeness, people were very glad to be spared the tedious sittings of other painters. I gained a great deal of money, and was very careful of it; well for me and my children that it was so. Gradually I began to lose the distinction between the imaginary figure and the real person, and sometimes disputed with sitters that they had been with me the day before. At last I was sure of it; and then—and then—all is confusion. I suppose they took alarm. I recollect nothing more; I lost my senses; was thirty years in an asylum: the whole period, except the last six months of my confinement, is a dead blank in my memory, though sometimes when people describe their visits, I have a sort of imperfect remembrance of them; but I must not dwell on these subjects."

It is an extraordinary fact, that when this gentleman resumed his pencil, after a lapse of thirty years, he painted nearly as well as when insanity compelled him to discontinue it. His imagination was still exceedingly vivid, as was proved by the portrait I saw him execute, for he had only two sittings of half-an-hour each; the latter solely for the dress and for the *eye-brows*, which he could not fix in his memory.

It was found that the excitement threatened danger, and he was persuaded to discontinue the exercise of his art. He lived but a short time afterwards.

It was exceedingly affecting to listen to his conversation. He would say, "These fellows know nothing of the principles of their art, but they are so conceited that they will not be taught. I was talking to Sir Joshua the other day, and he remarked—"No, no, no—" and he would put his hand to his forehead, and say in a low tone, "that was before my misfortune."

At another time he would talk of George the Third, and observe that we might now expect some improvement: "The king told me last week that he expected great things from his Academy of Fine Arts. No, no, no, that was before my misfortune."

Now, had this gentleman been a person without a profession he might have remained under his own self-control to the end of his life; he would have exercised the faculty rarely, and only for his own amusement. I have known numerous examples of the power he possessed, but in more moderate degree, and have often heard persons declare that if they could draw, they could take a portrait of one not present, or of a past scene; but they were always able to lay down the delusion at will. Suppose this faculty a little more powerful, add a little superstition, and you have ghosts and other phantasma. Suppose the faculty indulged to excess (we can most of us remember amatory delusions of equal intensity) till it is no longer under the control of the will; or, as I should state it, suppose one brain indulging in these gambols, and the other looking on and watching it—we call it a mere play of the imagination, but let it spread to the other brain and produce confusion of identity, and we have insanity.

I knew a very intelligent and amiable man, who had the power of thus placing before his eyes *himself*, and often laughed heartily at *his double*, who always seemed to laugh in turn. This was long a subject of amusement and joke, but the ultimate result was lamentable. He became gradually convinced that he was haunted by himself, or (to violate grammar for the sake of clearly expressing his idea) by his *self*. This other self would argue with him pertinaciously, and to his great mortification sometimes refute him, which, as he was very proud of his logical powers, humiliated him exceedingly. He was eccentric, but was never placed in confinement or subjected to the slightest restraint. At length, worn out by the annoyance, he deliberately resolved not to enter on another year of existence—paid all his debts—wrapped up in separate papers the amount of the weekly demands—waited, pistol in hand, the night of the 31st of December, and as the clock struck twelve fired it into his mouth.

I remember very well some of the conversations he related as taking place between himself and his other self; and though at the time they merely furnished amusement, and did not suggest the idea of a state of which I should now be glad to witness an example, yet, if such conversations were given piecemeal by a madman, they would form exactly the sort of incoherence we notice in the insane, especially if there were intervals when the thoughts being too rapid for utterance a number of links in the chain were dropped, the whole would then resolve into nonsense. In sitting by his side, reading to myself, I sometimes heard him exclaim, "Well, that takes me quite aback; I must consider a little for an answer," and then laugh heartily at the idea of his imaginary argument with himself. It seems indeed quite as easy to conceive that a man might place before himself the image of himself, which he had seen in a glass, as the image of an absent acquaintance.

I know not what effect such an example might produce on others, but to me it seems only to be explained on the hypothesis of two brains with distinct and contradictory trains of thought at the same time. The inference seems irresistible that, with conflicting volitions and conflicting trains of thought, there are in the disordered cerebrum two perfect and complete organs of the understanding in habitual antagonism, and that uniformity of *will*, when consentaneity does not exist, is produced by the tyranny of one brain over the other. Firmness of character, which when we disapprove the mode of its manifestation, we call *obstinacy*, either arising from the perfection of this tyranny, or from the continuous joint-action and harmony of two organs.

There was some time ago, in a public establishment, a pauper lunatic who believed herself to be Mary Queen of Scots. She was extremely anxious to conceal the *fact*, and it required some address to induce her to speak on the subject; in every other respect she was perfectly rational. Being a woman of considerable accomplishments, she was generally occupied in giving instruction to the children of the officers of the establishment, from whom she was most anxious to conceal her claims to the throne. Indeed, if I am correctly informed, she was at such times very doubtful of their validity, and had a misgiving that it might be a delusion; but if, when only two or three persons were present, she were treated for a while with great deference and respect, the delusion then took possession of her, and if seriously asked about her rank she would confidentially confess that it was true, but must be kept a secret—that her friends in Scotland were assembling for her rescue, and that she should soon be in a position to reward her benefactors; she had no wish to punish her enemies. When reminded that she had been beheaded, she explained the matter by stating that a waxen figure had been substituted for decapitation; and when surprise was expressed that she had grown no older in the lapse of centuries, she remarked that an absolute sovereign, like her sister Elizabeth, could easily falsify history. Yet there were moments when she appeared ashamed of the delusion, and seemed to feel as if detected in a falsehood.

Now I can conceive that this lady's original state of mind, before she was subjected to restraint, had been very similar to that described of the indulgence of false ideas on the subject of high birth. The latter being independent, was enabled to continue her delusive enjoyment; but the former being incapacitated for her employment, could no longer earn her own living, and became a pauper lunatic. The more sordid and sad were her occupation and employment, the more (probably) was she tempted to indulge in the pleasures of imagination—as players take refuge from the wretched cares of their precarious life in a sort of half-belief that they are the characters they represent.

The strange delusions of madmen are sometimes very slight perversions of a natural process of reasoning; and it was the contemplation of such cases, no doubt, that induced Locke to draw his celebrated distinction between the insane and the imbecile—that the former reason right from wrong premises, and the latter reason wrong from right premises—a very unfounded and untrue representation. In all pointed sentences, says Johnson, some truth is sacrificed to brevity. There are certain forms of insanity which are scarcely exaggerations of hypochondria. Certainly, if a man believe himself to have been turned into salt, he is right not to go out in the rain; if he think his legs made of butter, he acts wisely to keep out of the sun; or if he suppose his body to be made of glass, it behoves him to be cautious of falling; but surely this cannot be called reasoning rightly from wrong premises. His premises are certainly wrong, but his reasoning is wrong also; it wants the great basis of all reasoning—*comparison*, without which there is no judgment.

As a specimen of the slight variation in the mode of reasoning, which makes the difference between sanity and insanity in a discourse, I cite the following:

A naval gentleman who had been the subject of a verdict of lunacy from a writ *di lunatico inquirendo*, spoke to me thus: "Do you know Dr.——and Dr.——?"

"Slightly," I replied.

"Then," said he,"you know the two most obstinate fools in London. It is on their evidence I am here; it is they who are mad, not I. I defeated them in argument, and they have put me in confinement out of revenge. I will explain it to you. You are of course aware that houses describe a cycloidal curve; they are not in the same place in the evening in which they were in the morning. At least you will allow that the chimneys move, and you cannot suppose they move without the houses they are built on. Now I was proceeding to give a demonstration of this to these men, but found they had such a mere smattering of mathematics that they could not follow it; so, to conceal their ignorance, they broke off the conversation, and consigned me to a madhouse. A pretty country of liberty this, where men cannot dispute on a point of science but, if they happen to be in a minority, they are called mad and placed in confinement!"

On all other subjects, during a very long conversation, this gentleman evinced no sign of disturbed reason; narrated to me all the events of his life, during the eighteen years that I had lost sight of him, with perfect correctness; and discussed a variety of political and light literary topics with as much composure as ever. I took advantage of a pause at a moment when he was peculiarly tranquil, and asked him to explain to me what he meant by chimneys making a cycloidal curve, when he very composedly began to describe the earth's course round the sun and revolution on its axis, and I saw that his morbid idea of the cycloidal curve was nothing more than a vague recollection of the nature of the cycloidal curve which a point on the earth's surface does really describe in space, from these two combined motions; but that, in the disordered state of his mind, he had confounded this with an actual change of position, from day to day, of objects on the earth's surface. He believed that a summer-house seen from his window in a certain position in the morning, was invisible in the afternoon, though before his eyes; and when I declared it to be visible, he endeavoured to make me understand that, although strictly speaking visible, it was so only from the effect of refraction, and that the summer-house had changed its place at the rate of four minutes to a degree. By-and-by, becoming excited, he contended that the parterres in the garden had also changed their relative position while we had been talking; and then went on to the most extravagant and absurd assertions about cycloidal curves, till all power of ratiocination was lost in confusion.

Now, if we consider this case attentively, we shall find it to be so very slight a deviation from correct conception, that we can all recollect examples of vain persons assuming acquaintance with subjects on which they are profoundly ignorant, and making mistakes of equal absurdity. If we could suppose them to persevere obstinately and permanently in their erroneous opinions, we should merely set them down as conceited fools; and if we found them incapable of comprehending the absurdity when explained, we should justly call them insane; but we should not be justified in depriving them of liberty, unless we found that their collateral vagaries were injurious to others or to their own safety, which was the case with this gentleman.

I do not give this as bearing on the duality of the mind, but as one of *modes* of erroneous reasoning, in the hope of aiding in the effort now making by so many able writers to familiarize the public with the manifestations of mental disturbance, and thus diminish the superstitious terror with which insanity is regarded. It is seen that there is as little resemblance between the cerebral disturbance which thus distorts an established idea, and the cerebral disturbance which leads to suicide or murder, as there is between the scarlatina which merely gives a temporary headach, and the scarlatina which in a couple of days leads to delirium and to the putrefaction of all the fluids of the body, and causes death more rapidly than the plague.

CHAPTER XII: *Dr. Abercrombie's Treatise on the Mental Powers; Cases of Hallucination; Cerebral Disturbance Without Disease; Morbid Appearances on Dissection; Hallucination Confined to a Single Point; Nature and Causes of Insanity; Circumstances in Which Argument May Be Addressed to the Insane*

Dr. Abercrombie, in his Treatise on the Mental Powers, after citing various cases of mental impressions spontaneously arising in the brain, without the causes which in the perfectly healthy state would give rise to them, states the following instances of conscious delusion: "A lady under his care, in a slight feverish disorder, saw distinctly a party of ladies and gentlemen sitting round her bedchamber, and a servant handing them something on a tray. The scene continued in a greater or less degree for several days, and was varied by spectacles of castles and churches of a very brilliant appearance, as if they had been built of finely cut crystal. The whole was in this case entirely a visual phantom, for there was no hallucination of the mind. On the contrary, the patient had from the first a full impression that it was a morbid affection of vision, connected with the fever, and she amused herself and her attendants by watching and descibing the changes in the scenery. Now I suspect that in this case there occurred what I have very often seen with weak-minded persons of strong imaginations, a little attempt at mystification. The false impressions are at first real, but if the patient be conscious of the delusion, they are a subject rather of alarm than curiosity. When the narration of them, however, is found to excite interest in the bystanders, the invalid is very apt to go on drawing on her imagination for future facts, and making up a false narrative, with no more sense of defective veracity than Walter Scott in writing his romances. How often we see this in children. The attention paid to these delusions by patients of this class is widely different from the philosophical examination of a man who understands the structure and functions of the brain, and exercises an enlightened curiosity in the investigation of an unusual and interesting phenomenon.

Another case, related by Dr. Abercrombie, is of a gentleman, also his patient, of irritable habit and liable to a variety of uneasy sensations in his head, who was sitting alone in his dining-room in the twilight, the door being a little open. He distinctly saw a female figure enter, wrapped in a mantle, and the face concealed by a large black bonnet. She seemed to advance a few steps towards him and then stop. He had a full conviction that the figure was an illusion of vision, and amused himself for some time by watching it, at the same time observing that he could see through the figure so as to perceive the lock of the door and other objects behind it. At length, when he moved his body a little forward, it disappeared.

The appearances in these two cases were entirely visual illusions, and probably consisted of the renewal of real scenes or figures in a manner somewhat analogous to those in Dr. Ferriar's case, though the renewal took place after a longer interval. When there is any degree of hallucination of mind, so that the phantasm is believed to have a real existence, the affection is of an entirely different nature, as will be more particularly mentioned under another part of our subject.

So far Dr. Abercrombie—I explain these matters very differently. Whatever may be the effect on the fibres of the brain of certain real impressions on the organs of special sense, we know that these fibres have the power of taking on similar actions (vibrations, undulations, or whatever be the name we give to these mysterious and incomprehensible movements or states) when the external cause does not exist. We see this in madness, intoxication, dreaming, somnambulism, the delirium of fever, and hysterical excitement. If both brains be subjected to this pseudal action, we can have no means of judging of the truth of the facts—we are compelled to believe the evidence of our senses; but if one brain only be subjected to the erroneous action, the other is still capable of entertaining true ideas on the subject and, perceiving that the evidence afforded is not harmonious, rejects it as a delusion.

It is widely different when the same disturbed and abnormal action extends to both brains, and it then depends entirely on its degree of permanence whether we give it the name of transient delirium or insanity. Every medical man must have seen cases of painful dismenorrhoea, accompanied by delirium; the patient is for the time insane, but no one would call this *insanity*, because he knows that it arises from a temporary cause, and that it is certain to subside in a short time. It is, however, while it lasts, as purely mental aberration as any case that was ever subjected to the strait waistcoat.

In the early stage of this affection I have known a young lady stretch out her hand to an imaginary relation to whom she was attached, and be perfectly miserable at the want of cordiality of her friend in not reciprocating the offer. She would address to her vehement remonstrances on her cruelty, but was quite satisfied if any other person would perform the office vicariously, and was entirely unconscious of the substitution. In an earlier or later stage of the disturbance of the mental functions, she would be conscious of this and similar delusions; it was in that stage then not hallucination, but affecting only one brain in the commencement, gradually extending to the other, or in the latter stage of subsidence leaving one brain in its normal position, and forming the *status* I have called conscious delusion.

Among the examples of temporary disease which shew how very imperfect is our knowledge of the cerebral functions, the following is one of the most remarkable. It is related by Dr. Abercrombie—case 151, page 428.

A young lady, after a variety of attacks resembling St. Vitus's dance, which were always relieved by cupping on the temples, was affected at the end of two or three years of occasional suffering by violent convulsive movements of the legs and arms, and indeed of the whole body; these convulsions were much increased by touching her, or approaching her with the apparent intention of touching her. There was occasional difficulty in swallowing, resembling hydrophobia. After lying for an instant she would throw herself, by a strange convulsive spring, entirely out of bed, and being on the floor, a similar spring would throw her into bed, or to the top of a chest of drawers five feet high! Her mind remained entire, and she could give no other explanation than that the impulse was irresistible.

After a time this was succeeded by a rotatory motion of the head, continuing without interruption night and day for several weeks together; and, if the head or neck were touched, the motion increased to a most extraordinary degree of rapidity. During the attacks she could only sleep in the sitting posture, and the motion continued during sleep, though in a more moderate degree; but if she happened to slip down, so that her head touched the pillow, it was instantly increased to a frightful degree of rapidity. These paroxysms were relieved by nothing but cupping on the temple to the extent of ten or twelve ounces, when the affection ceased in an instant, with a general convulsive start of the whole body. At the expiration of about four years it was decided to leave the next attack to nature, and attend only to peculiar functions which were in a state of abeyance. In the midst of a violent paroxysm, which had lasted three weeks without any intermission, night or day, of the motion of the head, the whole ceased (as from cupping) with a sudden start—other natural functions were restored, and she became perfectly well.

I quote this extreme case to shew how extensive may be the disturbance of the brain, and how formidable its influence on the bodily actions, without any actual disease of the organ. Let us suppose a similar state of the cerebral mass affecting only one side, and in a very slight degree, and it is easy to conceive that the most extravagant insanity might be produced, leading to motiveless murder or suicide, and yet no traces be left, on examining the brain, to shew the nature of the cause which gave rise to it. In the present case the disorder was entirely sympathetic. Had it been a married woman it might have led to the destruction of her children, as we so often see in the insanity of the inferior animals: pigs, horses, cows, and sheep. Those who know nothing of the diseases of animals will perhaps be surprised to learn that idiopathic insanity is as common with them as with human beings. It does not exist so long, for they are cured by the knife or bullet.

A boy, aged eleven, had a sudden attack of dimness of sight, amounting to blindness. It went off in a few minutes, but from that time vision was gradually impaired, and lost altogether in a year. He then had an affection resembling chorea; and, after a short time, suffered an attack in which he lay speechless for three days—this was followed by hemiplegia of the right side. He complained much of his head, which appeared to his friends to enlarge, and he sometimes lost his speech for two or three days. *His intellect was not affected, but at times was extremely acute.* He died after coma of five weeks continuance, about a year after the attack of hemiplegia, and two years from the commencement of the disease.

On dissection, it was found that the membranes adhered firmly to the surface of the middle lobe of the left hemisphere of the cerebrum. On raising them, fluid escaped in great quantity from a cyst contained within the lateral ventricle, and which had advanced nearly to the circumference of the brain; it contained about sixteen ounces of limpid fluid, and besides this, there were several ounces in the proper cavity of the ventricle. It is worthy of remark, as shewing the little importance attached to the connexion between lesion of brain and lesion of intellect, that in the work of Dr. Abercrombie (from which I have taken the above case), *Pathological Researches on Diseases of the Brain and Spinal Cord*, in forty-six examples of disease destroying life, narrated in the Appendix alone, besides those in the body of the work, and many more alluded to, the state of the intellect is only spoken of in this one case, and in two more of tumour growing from the *cerebellum*. In one case, descending within the dura mater into the spinal canal, as low as the sixth spinal nerve, Dr. A. only remarks, "senses entire to the last;" but whether the senses of sight, smell, etc., or the intellectual faculties, he leaves uncertain.

The other case is of a medical man, in the meridian of life, who had for a year been subject to attacks of dyspepsia with headach. "In October 1815, he had severe headach with fever, which was relieved by blood-letting; then complete want of digestion, headach, general emaciation, and frequent vomiting, which occurred chiefly in a morning. He had various uneasy feelings, which he referred to his liver; and his complaints were ascribed to this source by the most eminent practitioners whom he consulted. In August 1816, he had severe headach, and nothing agreed with his stomach, almost every thing being vomited. After some time the pain was relieved, but the morning sickness and vomiting continued, with increasing emaciation, torpid bowels, frequent eructations, and hiccup. At the end of September he had twice a slight convulsion. *Mind entire*—but conversation induced headach, and sometimes convulsion. October 9th, died suddenly in convulsions.

"There were four ounces of fluid in the ventricles. On the inferior part of the left lobe of the *cerebellum* there was an encysted tumour, the size of a French walnut. [How very carelessly are such descriptions drawn up; if it were of any importance to name the size, it makes a difference of more than double, whether the walnut has its outer shell or not], besides a vesicular portion connected with it containing yellow serum," etc.

I cite these two cases of disease in the cerebellum, not as being strictly within the scope of my investigation, but to shew how very little attention has been paid to the subject by anatomists, and therefore that it is probable the theory here propounded may lead to useful results, by pointing out a field of discovery yet uninvestigated.

"Among the most singular phenomena connected with insanity, we must reckon those cases in which the hallucination is confined to a single point, while on every other subject the patient speaks and acts like a rational man, and he often shews the most astonishing power of avoiding the subject of his disordered impression when circumstances make it advisable for him to do so."

The mental process is simple enough, if my theory be admitted—the man has a disordered sentiment or conviction in one brain, of the absurdity of which he is perfectly convinced in the other; he will say, for example, "I know that I am dead, and yet I know that the idea is absurd;" or " I am very ill, and it is strange I cannot believe it." He may, however, have this diseased idea in one brain, and be *not quite* convinced on the other that it is entirely false and unfounded, but merely that it is so completely in opposition to the general belief of mankind, that he would make himself ridiculous by stating it. Is there any man who has never had a crotchet of which he is perfectly assured, yet which he abstains from uttering, because he knows it would be impossible to convince others of it? Men in general suppose that a notion is positively either *right* or *wrong*, and that there is no medium, whereas the gradations are infinite, and that which is *right* to one man is *not quite right* to another, *wrong* to a third, and *monstrous* to a fourth. In the case of positive insanity of one brain, the trouble of controlling it by the other may be, and most frequently is, a painful effort, only to be undertaken through the influence of some strong motive as, for example, that of obtaining liberty. Such a man can for a time *wind himself up*, as it were, and determine that the notions of the disordered brain shall not be manifested. Many instances are on record similar to that told by Pinel, where an inmate of the Bicêtre, having stood a long cross-examination, and given every mark of restored reason, signed his name to the paper authorizing his discharge, *Jesus Christ*, and then went off into all the vagaries connected with that delusion. In the phraseology of the gentleman whose case is related in an early part of this work, he had "held himself tight" during the examination, in order to attain his object; this once accomplished, he "let himself down" again, and, if even *conscious* of his delusion, could not control it. I have observed with such persons that it requires a considerable time to wind themselves up to the pitch of complete self-control, and that the effort is a painful tension of the mind.

When thrown off their guard by any accidental remark, or worn out by the length of the examination, they *let themselves go*, and cannot gather themselves up again without preparation. Lord Erskine relates the story of a man who brought an action against Dr. Munro for confining him without cause. He underwent the most rigid examination by the counsel for the defendant, without discovering any appearance of insanity, till a gentleman asked him about a princess with whom he corresponded in cherry juice, and he became instantly insane. This was in Westminster; and by the strange anomalies of law he was enabled to bring another action in the city of London, when he had so completely wound himself up to the "sticking-place," that it was quite impossible to elicit the slightest evidence of insanity, and the cause of justice was only obtained by permission to record the evidence taken in Westminster. Another similar case is related by Lord Erskine, which was detected by addressing the patient as the Saviour of the World; till he heard which he had given perfectly rational answers during many hours of cross-examination. Another case occurred at Edinburgh, where a gentleman, under a process similar to our writ of lunacy, was about to be dismissed for lack of proof, when a witness, who had been detained till the last moment by an accident, came into court and asked him what news from the planet Saturn, he instantly relapsed into incoherence, and gave evident proofs of insanity.

Such cases are common. No one attempts an explanation of them, yet once admit two perfect instruments of thought, one of them out of order (which I have proved till there cannot rest a doubt, I think, on the mind of any one), and these cases are as simple and as easily explained as dropsy or jaundice. This is a subject on which I have thought so long and so deeply, that I cannot admit the possibility of error. If the evidence here collected be not sufficient to establish the fact, then we must for ever remain in darkness.

I would not speak presumptuously on the subject, or affect to place myself on a level with some of the great writers I have quoted, but when such a man as Dr. Abercrombie, whose reasoning powers are so acute and whose opportunities of investigation so unlimited, makes use of an expression like the following, I cannot but think that he, like others, does not allow himself the full use of his faculties, but that certain prepossessions incapacitate him for a thoroughly unbiased judgment:

"Of the nature and cause of that remarkable condition of the mental faculties, which gives rise to the phenomena of insanity, we know nothing."

Certainly not, if we are to regard "faculties" as the soul, or even the vital principle; but if we look at them as the physician is alone entitled to regard them, as functions dependent on organization, then there is no difficulty in the matter whatever. I have elsewhere alluded to the fact, that the pressure of a finger at the aperture in the cranium made by the trephine shall extinguish the senses of taste, smell, hearing, and sight; a slight increase of the pressure extinguishes memory, imagination, perception, volition, judgment, and all the faculties which in their aggregate compose the mind. The body remains a mere lump of organized matter, dependent on the ganglionic system for its vitality, and possessing only a sort of vegetable life, without consciousness. Take away the finger, and all these faculties are restored, without even a consciousness that they have been temporarily interrupted. These are mysteries which reason would vainly try to unravel. He who makes the attempt would be as mad as he who should attempt to explain the physical structure of the body by Revelation. Whatever is attainable by our own faculties is left by the Creator to our own researches, and there seems a satisfactory reason for the gradual acquisition of knowledge in a world of progression. No doubt the Almighty could, had he so pleased, have given us the knowledge at once, of all we shall ever be permitted to know; but that was obviously incompatible with the scheme laid down for the government of this world; and in working out our own knowledge we have a succession of acquisitions, each of which is a source of pleasure, but in the knowledge of the soul and its destiny, reason cannot take us onwards a single step—it is to Revelation alone that man can look for an explanation of the mighty mystery.

"Of the nature and cause of that condition of the mental faculties" seems to me as void of meaning as the words "of the nature and cause of that condition of the motion of a watch," etc. We know absolutely nothing of either but of the machinery. The abstract nature of momentum, elasticity, motion, or matter, are mysteries quite as inscrutable as the nature of mind. If we mean the phenomena of either, then it is not true that we are ignorant of them; we are as well acquainted with the derangements of the brain as of the watch, though we cannot rectify them so easily, and over many of the causes of derangement we have no control whatever. Let us not be deterred from advancing to the end of our tether, and examining every thing in the little circle to which it bounds us, because there is an unlimited space beyond it which we are not permitted to traverse, and the nature of which we are utterly unable to conceive.

It is not, then, the condition of the mental faculties which gives rise to insanity; it is the condition of the mental faculties which *constitutes* insanity; and, except in so far as the tracing the particular chain of ideas may lead us to an accessible organ, whose derangement gave rise to them, there seems no object whatever in making a distinction between the different forms of mental derangement. It is not one specific form of bodily disorder or disease which gives rise to one specific form of mental disturbance. The corporeal disorder disturbs the reason, and the form of the hallucination is an object of only futile curiosity; it does not in the least guide us in the treatment, except in so far as it indicates the nature of the bodily disease, or the organ specially affected.

If the nature of the hallucination decided the nature of the cause—the moral cause, then the proper treatment of some of the forms of insanity would be by reasoning with the patient, and convincing him of his delusion by arguments shewing its wickedness or absurdity. No one, I should think, ever adopted this mode twice; yet it seems, at the first glance, so natural and so consistent with common sense, that any man without experience of insanity would be excusable for trying it once. A very little reflection would shew the incongruity of attempting to rectify the disordered state of an organ by the disordered exercise of that organ. *You appeal to pure reason, because pure reason does not exist to appeal to.* The absurdity is evident. If the arguments you use be good and effectual, then they are unnecessary, since, if the patient be capable of understanding, comprehending, and acting upon them, the patient is *not* mad.

It is difficult, however, for those who are unfamiliar with mental derangement to abstain from attempts to convince the insane of their errors; and I have seen very wise persons occupied in thus *pushing against the side of the boat they are sitting in, in order to push it on;* and this, after they have listened with apparent conviction to the arguments above stated. Those who are experienced in the matter see the absurdity and know the futility of the attempt, and are inclined to affect acquiescence in the vagaries of the lunatic, rather than reason with him.

There is, however, one form, or I should rather say, one degree or stage of insanity, where argument avails something; and that is where the healthy brain is just beginning to waver in its convictions as to the reality of the delusions of its brother; where there is yet self-command when a motive is presented, and the sound organ requires to have its convictions confirmed by something external; where, for example, the state of conscious delusion is slowly passing into that of unconscious delusion, or the disorder of one brain beginning to pass into the other; a strong appeal made to the reasoning powers of the sound brain will, in such cases, sometimes induce and enable it to resume the reins it was just laying down in despair. The endeavour to overcome the delusions by which we are persecuted (and which we know to be delusions), is among the most heroic of human efforts, and it is rare that the attempt is successful, unless aided by a feeling of piety and submission.

In this case, as in that of young ladies, to which I have alluded, it is of importance to keep away all books of controversial divinity; indeed, all religious books which touch on dogmas or articles of faith; for, if some point of mystery happen to catch the attention of the unsound brain, it is like a spark among gun-powder, and all self-control is at once destroyed. Piety cannot be too much cultivated, or religion too carefully avoided. I use the word *piety* in the sense of quiet reverence for the Deity, acting as a ruling principle of moral conduct, and *religion* as a set of observances, ceremonies, and dogmas, for the guidance of the world, under a body of men set apart to inculcate piety and submission to the will of God. It is the *result (piety)* which should be impressed on a man in this position of equivocal intellect, the *means (religion)* is for the guidance of the healthy minded. I therefore urge conversation with a person judiciously pious, and careful avoidance of religious books. The omission of this distinction produces incalculable mischief, as every physician familiar with the insane must have witnessed.

I have, however, entered more fully into this subject elsewhere, and perhaps have indulged in too close a repetition of the arguments. The subject deserves to be dwelt on.

CHAPTER XIII: *Two Processes Carried on Together; Counting Steps; Objections to the Explanation; The Animal is Created Dual at First; Gradually Joined; Moral Responsibility; Considerations on Phrenology; Differences in Form and Texture at the Base of the Brain*

If we attentively observe any person engaged in a mechanical employment, as spinning, sewing, or other occupation requiring but little attention, from the habit having been so long and thoroughly acquired, we shall find perhaps that they are at the same time singing or talking to an acquaintance. It is not till the art has become perfectly familiar, that this is possible; in the beginning it requires the attention of both brains—that is, *study*; but we know that, however rapid the process of spinning or sewing, each separate step of it is accompanied by a separate volition. If I write my name, it is true I do it so rapidly, and with so little mental effort, that the act seems to be purely mechanical, and to require no aid from the mind; but any one who will consider the matter, must see that in the formation of the capital letter L, for example, I have to bear in mind that I must carry my pen upwards sloping to the right, must lean but lightly on the paper—must, on arriving at a certain height, turn to the left and form an arch—then, bring the line down at a different angle, with heavier pressure, must produce a peculiar curve to the right, till I arrive at a certain point, then direct my pen to the left again, taking care not to make an acute angle at the spot where the curves are reversed, and so on. All this before I have got half through a single letter, although the whole signature occupies only a few seconds. George IV, and many persons whom I have known, could go on making a succession of signatures with great rapidity, all the while conversing on a subject of importance, or telling a story of deep interest; but suppose a knot in the thread with the spinner or sewer, or a hair in the pen of the writer, anything to require even the momentary attention of the two brains, and one process or the other, the singing or the spinning, the narrative or the signing, instantly stops. I have noticed this in innumerable instances, and can explain it no otherwise than on the supposition that the two brains are occupied on the two distinct subjects. One is calling to mind the words and tune of the song, and guiding the numerous organs of the voice in their execution of them, while the other is directing the process of spinning or sewing; but the moment a difficulty occurs, either in the mechanical operation or in the memory of the words, attention is required: the two thinking organs must employ themselves on the same subject, and the two synchronous acts become incompatible till that difficulty is removed. I fancy—but this I put forth as pure hypothesis, and ask no assent, although convinced of it myself—I fancy that, when the occupation is resumed, the two brains transpose their labour, and that this is one of the reasons of the relief found from slight occasional interruptions. The power of directing two trains of thought at the same time has been often attributed to great men. Conquerors, kings, and high ministers, dictating to two secretaries at once, metaphysicians explain by rapid alternation: this would be satisfactory had we nothing better to assign, but the testimony is not of a kind to be depended on. Whether true or not in those cases, I have myself more than once witnessed a banker's clerk casting up a long column of figures, which practice had rendered easy, while not merely conversing with another, but telling an amusing tale, with great rapidity; and this without an interval of even a second of time in the narrative. If from defective light, or any other cause, more attention was required (that is, the attention of *both* cerebra), his narrative ceased instantly, till the obstacle being removed, the two trains of thought were resumed with the same fluency and facility as before. There is no banking house in London that will not afford an example of this faculty. I confess myself unable to conceive any other explanation of it, than the possession of two brains, each carrying on its process simultaneously, as we have seen in the former examples cited.

Among the many trivial examples of this dual process, I may mention one perhaps peculiar to myself, although analogous phenomena are observed in others:

When my list of patients was very large, or cases of peculiar severity or difficulty kept me in a state of anxiety, or my rest had been disturbed, I found it impossible to prevent myself from counting my steps, more especially in ascending stairs. I attempted by incessant conversation with the person who was accompanying me to prevent this annoyance, but in vain. On arriving at the top, I always knew the number of stairs, however numerous. The same when walking arm-in-arm with a friend along a frequented street; I went on to a thousand steps, vexed and worried, yet quite unable to stop the process, although I had been at the same time keeping up an animated conversation the whole distance. Often did I set out with the determined resolution not to allow such a ridiculous propensity to master me, but in vain: the firmer my resolves against it, the more accurate my calculation. Yet, when perfectly well, and with the feeling of freshness and health, I had not the power to perform the same process; and, indeed, whenever I did overcome the propensity, it was by *trying* to act upon it—that is to say, *study* with both brains.

I cannot devise any other explanation of this *disease*, if I may so call it, than the discordant exercise of two brains, and the inability to stop the involuntary process of that which was disturbed. The mere form of what Dr. Holland calls *insubordination* is of no importance—it might have been the rapid flow of thought of pervigilium. The character of the process is that of being uncontrollable—the mode in which it is manifested is nothing.

It has been objected to this explanation, that in some manufactures and mechanical processes there are a great number of movements performed by the same person at once, which, according to this doctrine, would each of them require a brain to attend to it—that, if two brains be necessary for two synchronous acts, five brains would be necessary for five concurrent acts, as each would require a separate volition.

After an attentive consideration of this objection, and an examination of every example offered to me, I still retain my opinion, for the following reasons:

1. The acts spoken of are only continuous muscular movements of the greatest simplicity.

2. That such acts become perfectly automatic, and so far from needing a continuous volition, they do, when once established, really go on spontaneously, and require a distinct act of volition to stop them, or they would continue till fatigue produced pain, when they would equally cease from an act of volition. Every one, I think, must be conscious of this.

3. That, in the cases where this explanation does not suffice, the combination of several movements requiring intellect is produced by rapid alternations of thought, but that only two steady continuous movements are possible where each of them requires a continuous exercise of skill and judgment.

Every instance I have known admits of this interpretation, and I cannot but think that, if the reader will set himself attentively to examine the cases in which numerous concurrent actions take place, he will find that not more than two are really the result of synchronous volition; and that the slightest difficulty or impediment which necessitates consideration, or an exercise of the two brains conjointly, at once reduces them to one single act of the mind. Should his examination not be satisfactory, he will discard this from my list of proofs.

When the want of consentaneity between the two brains, of which I have spoken, is the effect of sympathy with visceral disturbance, or excessive mental application, and not of positive disease of structure or function in the brain itself, it may often be removed by a moderate excitement from wine and stimulating food. It is a dangerous advice to give to those whose self-control has not been properly cultivated, but to men of a different stamp I have never hesitated to recommend it, and with the most satisfactory results. The want of harmony in the action of the two brains produces a feeling of intense distress, of which pervigilium is only an aggravated degree. Short of incipient madness, which in excess it very much resembles, there is no malady which excites a more acute misery. It is this feeling which so often leads to habitual excess in drinking; the relief experienced from moderate excitement has the unfortunate effect of increasing the desire for vinous stimuli, and the habit thus acquired is, as we see, the great curse of society. The positively pleasurable sensation which the early stages of intoxication produce, leads to a repetition of the indulgence when not required by the discrepant action of the two brains; but this degree of enjoyment is much beyond that which is necessary to reestablish the union of the thinking organs, and the practice, by exhausting their energy (and especially that of the feebler of them), lays the foundation of increasing disorder. We do not, however, forbid the use of opium because of the mischiefs it produces in excess; nor are we to be deterred from the use of a moderate quantity of wine, because of the danger that we may acquire the habit of drinking.

I conceive that, in the case of the gentleman who tried to push off the boat, it was the discrepancy between the action of the two brains which caused his unhappy delusions, and the temporary restoration of their union which produced the tranquillity of which he speaks, from going into agreeable society and taking a few glasses of wine. That gentleman is habitually abstemious, and the two or three glasses of wine would with him produce the effect of a bottle on those who drink their pint daily at their dinner.

However regular and uniform may be the employment of the two arms, the two legs, or the two eyes, we always find that one of them becomes fatigued and exhausted before the other; it is not likely indeed that any two limbs should be so exactly parallel in structure and power as to be capable of exactly similar exertion with exactly the same amount of fatigue. Independent of the difference to which I have before alluded, as arising from the superior power of the left cerebrum, which gives the greater control over the right hand and the right foot as instruments of volition, there must necessarily be a variation, however slight,between the energies of the two halves of the body, formed as they are separately, and only gradually united. Nay, in the laborious continued exercise of vision, it is always one eye which becomes fatigued and inflamed before the other, although these organs are connected by a real commissure, and are much better entitled to the name of "a double organ" than the brain.

Is it at all extraordinary then that the two brains should be unequally exhausted by the joint exercise of their common powers? and that, as each is proved to be a perfect instrument of thought, and all other mental operations, they should sometimes give discrepant results, similar to the state of the whole brain from excessive mental exertion.

Richeraud remarks that, in tracing the scale of animals from the fish to the ape, the brain gradually becomes more and more complex—the same advance is observed in the foetus as it progresses to the perfect animal in the class of mammifers, at the head of which is man; the brain of the human foetus is at first simple, and exactly resembling that of fishes, next advances to the form of the brain of reptiles, rises by degrees to that of the bird, and at last attains that oneness and proportion which constitute the human animal. In this gradual and successive development and addition, we always see the organization advance from the circumference to the centre—that is, the sides or halves first appear; the nerves which are to give sensation and volition *take their rise in the organs*, to which in common language we say they are distributed; they at last insert themselves into the great nervous mass of the brain and spinal marrow, called the cerebro-spinal axis, from which they are to derive their functions, the right half and the left half unite and adhere—sometimes by a simple union, sometimes by commissures or interlacement and decussation of fibres.

All seems then to prove that man is strictly made up of two complete and perfect halves, and that no more central and common machinery is given than is just sufficient to unite the two into one sentient being, and provide for the due synchronous action of the two animals.

To ask *why* this strange organization should have been established is futile. That it is for a wise and beneficent purpose the whole constitution of nature seems to prove; but when the philosopher attempts to search deeply into the cause, he is compelled to acquiesce at last in the reason that satisfies the simple peasant without the trouble of inquiry—*it is because it is.*

This fact of man being composed of two halves, gradually united together, being clearly established, there will seem less objection to the theory here laid down, since it is obviously in harmony with the known laws of nature. We may even shew that such a combination of two distinct animals into one is not only the invariable practice, but that, little as we know of its objects, it possesses some advantages, inasmuch, for example, as that the slightest accident would otherwise disturb the whole system. There will be little difficulty in conceding that the thinking organ more especially should partake of the same duality, since, but for such a precaution, the guide which is to direct all our voluntary actions would be dethroned when most needed.

If the consciousness be single, which it always is in health, and even in sickness—for the exceptions in this country are not one in seven or eight hundred individuals—if the consciousness be single, it suffices to establish the individuality of the being.

It is a mysterious subject—but what part of the animal structure is not mysterious? Enough is accessible to us to excite and reward rational curiosity, enough impenetrably concealed to check presumption. Perhaps in some other of the myriads of worlds these apparent discrepancies do not exist; and in those imagined abodes the inhabitants may be endowed with organs capable of conceiving and appreciating mysteries beyond the comprehension of *our* humble faculties.

If it were permitted to argue a physiological and pathological question with reference to the presumed designs of Providence, we might ask, "Is it likely that, when each of the comparatively unimportant functions of sight and hearing is provided with two distinct organs, perfect and complete—each capable of performing its duties during the indisposition, disturbance, disease, or destruction of the other—is it probable that so pre-eminently important a function as ratiocination (a function essential to the well-being, and almost to the existence of the individual)—that this would have been entrusted to a single organ, so that the slightest injury would annihilate its completeness as an instrument of thought, or, as it is usually termed, a medium of communication between mind and the material world? It seems to me that all who believe in the responsibility of man must at one acquiesce in at least the strong probability of my theory; for if a slight injury or disease could destroy the completeness of the mind, how could there be room for those struggles which constitute the merit of a responsible agent, when the means by which he had to judge of the morality of his own actions had been annihilated?—he had no longer a complete mind, and was, necessarily, no longer responsible.

The more deeply we contemplate the structure and functions of man, as adapted to the world in which he is destined to live, the more are we struck with wonder at the simplicity of the means by which such mighty results are produced. *A slight inequality in the two brains is sufficient to produce all the varieties of character which are to be found in the world.* The doctrines of some ultra-phrenologists seem incompatible with free-will; yet every sane man feels a conviction beyond all reasoning that he has, while in mental health, the power *to do* or *to abstain*. If the two brains were exactly equal in form, energy, and function, must not the individuals always act alike from inevitable instinct? If so, the present scheme of society would be at an end. Even conceding that the propensities are exercised by separate organs—as combativeness, amativeness, etc., it is past comprehension how the strictly intellectual faculties can be exerted singly: it seems more logical to consider them as modes of the mind (temporary combinations in action of single cerebral fibres, or of established fasciculi), than distinct organs. We see that there are three lobes—we see that there are a pair of brains and millions of fibres; but the division in the convolutions which forms them into distinct organs, still more their appropriation, is not proved, although the number of striking coincidences collected by phrenological philosophers is too startling to permit us entirely to deny the existence of these divisions.

To believe that one part of the intellectual organ exercises the power of ideality, another of comparison, another of memory, seems as illogical as to suppose that one part of the eye judges of form, another of magnitude, and a third of colour; or that one part of the ear takes cognizance of the loudness, another of the quality, and another of the musical tone. It seems more reasonable to suppose that the intellectual organ is employed upon the whole process of thinking; this, however, I leave to the phrenologists, whose doctrines I cannot quite understand. Their minute divisions, where they can shew no anatomical distinction, seem gratuituous and unnecessary, while all the phenomena which these minute divisions are invented to explain are quite in harmony with the grand division into two perfect brains, each composed of three lobes and myriads of fibres, added to the various bodies at the base of the cranium—all these acting together, or separately, or in opposition, or in varied combination. To this extent the anatomical structure can be demonstrated without assuming arbitrary divisions, which cannot be demonstrated. The number and variety of parts distinguishable by our senses are quite sufficient to account for every discrepancy of action, and every difficulty

How is it that the two organs of the same faculty, on the two sides of the head, should be so perfectly consentaneous, when the faculty is defective or disordered? It seems almost contradictory to common sense to imagine that disease in a certain arbitrarily defined portion of a convolution should be accompanied by exactly similar disease in the same portion of convolution or organ on the opposite side, having no connexion with it but at the base of the brain—so entirely separated indeed, that, as I have shewn, the organs, or congeries of organs, in one half of the cranium, are capable of carrying on the intellectual functions alone and perfectly, when the corresponding congeries of organs in the other half of the cranium have been annihilated.

The fact that so many great minds, great anatomists and great physiologists, are satisfied with the evidence the phrenologists offer, and the arguments they found upon it, cannot be allowed much weight, since there are a still greater number of great minds, anatomists and physiologists, who do not merely dissent but openly oppose the doctrines. We must wait still longer for the universal adoption of the system. That it will be greatly modified by successive investigators there can be no doubt; in the mean time, the number of extraordinary coincidences which have been collected between the shape of the head and the "shape" of the mind will ensure the permanence of the discussion, and ultimately lead to the adoption of a doctrine satisfactory to all.

That the intellectual organization of the individual is in some way connected with the shape of his head, is a fact proved beyond question, although single cases may appear to contradict the inferences, and numerous cases defy cognition; nevertheless, it is not easy to acquiesce in the correctness of the arbitrary division of the understanding. Of the propensities, the sentiments, the perceptive and reflective faculties, the grand division seems logical and reasonable; although the location of the three divisions leaves room for much more evidence before it be satisfactory; but the minute sub-divisions of the cranioscopists are by far too fantastic and arbitrary to deserve attention.

In this, as in other sciences, discredit is thrown on the real discoveries of the learned, and the sagacious inductions of the wise, by the flippant remarks and superficial examinations of the ill-informed and the silly, who *will* jump up and ride behind wherever the wise man turns his steed. As alchemy led to chemistry, so will phrenology perhaps lead in time to a correct knowledge of the brain and the intellectual faculties. I am old enough to remember the dissections of that organ forty years ago, and the advance from the mode of slicing the brain and reasoning upon its functions—which was then thought philosophical and satisfactory, to the present state of the science—seems to me much greater than the space from our present degree of knowledge to absolute certainty. I hope phrenologists will be satisfied with *proving up to a certain point*, and not be so anxious to complete a system for which the materials are not yet sufficiently abundant, nor the inductions uniformly correct, even from those facts which are entitled to entire confidence.

No one, I think, who looks at the great variety of form and texture of the organs below the corpus callosum, can hesitate to acknowledge that they must be intended for different functions and purposes. The corpora olivaria, the mammary bodies, the pituitary, the pineal glands, and the medulla oblongata, for example, must be intended, like all other parts of the body, to serve some specific purpose.

According to Foville, the external shape of the skull depends mainly on the shape of the ventricles!—but all these things are purely speculation. We want still a large examination of morbid appearances on dissection, as connected with previously recognised disturbance of intellectual functions during life, before we can be in a position even to argue the question. To shew how much this has been hitherto neglected and entirely overlooked, I may mention that in a synopsis of forty-six cases of cerebral disease by Dr. Abercrombie, the state of the intellectual functions is only alluded to in one single instance. If a man of such acquirements, of so much sagacity, and of such great experience in these diseases, can have overlooked or disregarded the connexion between organs and faculties, it is not likely that others should have been more attentive to it. I cannot but hope that even I may be instrumental in drawing attention to a subject of great interest and importance by the present theory of duality, of which the investigation can only be successfully pursued by those who cultivate the large field of experience afforded by a public establishment.

If it be true that the multitudinous cerebral fibres act always in the same specific fasciculi, or in the same combination of specific fasciculi, in order to produce the same faculty on the same process of ratiocination, then phrenology is so far true; and if the action of these fasciculi has the effect of elongating them so as to produce pressure on the corresponding internal surface of the cranium, and if the bony case make a corresponding concession of space to the elongation of these specific fasciculi, then cranioscopy is true also; but there are so many arbitrary assumptions in arriving at such a result, that a vastly greater mass of evidence must be brought forward before phrenologists and cranioscopists have a right to claim general assent to their doctrines. Hitherto the proofs accepted have been so exceedingly lax and uncertain, that phrenology has suffered much more from its friends than its enemies. If my assent be absolutely required, for instance, to the allocation of faculties around the eye as essential to the science, then I unhesitatingly reject the whole, nor think it even worthy of examination.

CHAPTER XIV: *Phrenology Continued; Case of Spectral Illusions, and Commencement of Moral Insanity, Cured by Bleeding; Other Cases; Mental Pictures by an Artist; Inability to Remember Faces; Inability to Distinguish Dreams From Realities; Robert Hall and Cowper*

If each brain be a perfect instrument of mind, then it is not a very extravagant hypothesis to suppose that one brain may be courageous and the other cowardly, and be the cause of various other modifications of character. May not this give rise to the strange discrepancy between the actions of the same person at different times? If under the influence of suppurative fever, a man of the undaunted courage of Charles the Twelfth of Sweden became timid and irresolute, may we not suppose that some other malady shall sometimes produce in one brain only the modification of mind which the suppurative fever produced in both? and if fermented liquors can excite both brains, habitually timid, into a state of enthusiastic courage, why may not other stimulants produce an equal change in one of the brains only, when from the nature or modification of the stimulant its influence is confined to one of them? The two brains may not be equally susceptible to the influence even of a general cause, any more than a gouty or other disorder of the whole system shall affect both eyes with disease—it is almost always confined to one of them.

I can conceive, but do not assert, that the strange contradictions we sometimes notice in men who have raised themselves into notoriety by practising on the religious credulity of their fellow-creatures, may arise in a great measure from this cause—that with one brain a man is a hypocritical knave, and with the other a fanatical enthusiast. One of the most extraordinary men which the last half-century—so prolific in extraordinary men—has produced, was the late William Huntingdon, the preacher. That man contained moral gunpowder enough to split the world asunder, had it been placed under compression. Happily, being left open, it made little noise and did no mischief. I have listened to that man with the greatest psychological curiosity, and have often said to myself long before it occurred to me to take up the question physiologically, "That man has two brains in one skull—sometimes one has the command, and sometimes the other." That he was equally sincere as knave and fanatic, I firmly believe; and his voluminous writings—twenty thick octavo volumes—shew the double mind at every page.

A gentleman who had been under treatment about six months before for a severe attack of phrenitis, and had only been restored by the aid of very active remedies administered by a very judicious practitioner, I afterwards saw in a state which was called perfect recovery. He had for some time resumed his active habits of business; but, although considering himself perfectly well, complained confidentially to me that for some time he had been constantly arguing with himself on an increasing apathy towards his wife—not physical apathy, quite the contrary—it was a strange disinclination to be in her society; he found himself frequenting the haunts of his former bachelor state, against his intention and almost against his will, yet received no gratification from any indulgences they afforded, and was constantly harassed by a feeling of remorse for neglecting the society of his wife, whom he had married from choice, whom he respected and thoroughly loved, and who was exceedingly tolerant of his indifference, from a belief that it was caused by pecuniary anxiety. I endeavoured to convince him that it was a moral change produced by a physical change, and that it would pass away with the consolidation of his health. He remained some time in this state, when he gradually began to see faces in the dark—afterwards in the day-light; groups of faces, constantly changing their shape; sometimes a portion of one face would join itself to a portion of another face; sometimes parts of faces—eyes, noses, mouths, cheeks, and forehead, would float about in vast numbers before him, and from time to time unite themselves in the most fantastic combinations. The whole occupied his mind, and rendered him incapable of continuous attention to any subject of importance requiring deep consideration. A large bleeding and a blister to the nape of the neck immediately restored him to vigorous health, and all his original delight in the society of his amiable and affectionate wife. Such cases are very instructive, and should make us "slow to judge."

Most writers class the annoyance of spectral illusions along with forms of genuine mental derangement, but they have really no more connexion than delirium and fever; the two things may chance to concur, but neither of them is a necessary consequence of the other, and it seems a strange mystification to represent them as modifications or forms of insanity. In many cases it seems only as if the eye, or at least the optic nerve, took on spontaneously the same action that it would naturally have done had the object been really before it; an action, vibration, undulation, or whatever name may be given to the process, exactly similar to that presented by the voluntary act of the painter already spoken of, of which we often see examples in children, who many of them possess the power of conjuring up a vivid image of whatever they wish to see. In other cases the figures represented are not objects which have been seen, but objects conceived by the imagination; and as, in what may be called *healthy dreams, we never renew a mental image*, but only those which have really passed before our eyes, so it is only in the disturbed or deranged state of one brain that these fanciful figures are presented as spectral illusions. However vivid they may be, the other brain recognises them as unreal, and is able to contemplate them with composure; this was the case with Dr. Bostock and with Nicolai, already cited. When once this explanation is admitted, all mystery is at an end. The many cases related by Dr. Abercrombie are all illustrative of this fact; but it is rare that such things make any but a very transient impression, unless by a strange coincidence some event or misfortune become connected with them.

The following story I know to be true. It is a striking example of past impressions assuming the character of reality, and producing almost an equal effect on the unhappy possessor of a vivid imagination. That the delusion should be manifested in three members of the same family, only shews that the three brains were similarly constituted.

A youth of eighteen, having no tendency to enthusiasm or romance, and an entire absence of superstition, was residing at Ramsgate for the benefit of his health. In a ramble to one of the neighbouring villages, he happened to go into a church towards the close of the day, and was struck aghast by the spectre of his mother, who had died some months before of a painful and lingering disease, an object of great compassion and commiseration. The figure stood between him and the wall, and remained for a considerable time without motion: almost fainting, he hastened home; and the same spectre appearing to him in his own room, for several successive evenings, he felt quite ill from the agitation, and hastened off to Paris to join his father, who was living there. At the same time, he determined to say nothing of the vision, lest he should add to the distress already weighing him down from the loss of a tender and affectionate wife, the object of his unbounded love.

Being compelled to sleep in the same room with his father, he was surprised to observe that a light was kept burning all night—a thing quite contrary to custom, and for which there had always been previously a great dislike. After several hours of watchfulness from the effect of the light, the son ventured out of bed to extinguish it. His father soon after woke up in great agitation, and commanded him to relight it, which he did; much wondering at the anger displayed, and the marks of terror on his father's countenance. On asking the reason of the alarm, he was put off by some vague excuse, and told that at some future time he would be informed of it.

A week or more had elapsed when, finding his own rest so very much disturbed by the light, he once more, when his father appeared in a sound sleep, ventured to extinguish it; but the father almost immediately jumped out of bed in the greatest trepidation, remonstrated with him on his disobedience, relighted the lamp, and told him that whenever he was left in the dark the spectre of his deceased wife appeared to him, and remained immoveable till he could again obtain a light, when it disappeared.

This made a strong impression on the boy's mind; and fearing to aggravate his father's grief should he relate the Ramsgate adventure, he soon after left Paris and went to an inland town about sixty miles off, to visit his brother who was at school there, and to whom he had not communicated what had occurred to himself, for fear of ridicule. He had scarcely entered the house and exchanged the usual salutations, when the son of the schoolmaster said to him, "Has your brother ever shewn any signs of insanity? for he has behaved very strangely lately. He came down stairs the other night in his shirt, in the greatest alarm—declared he had seen his mother's ghost, and dared not go into his room again, and then fainted away from excess of terror."

Had there been a coincidence in point of time, how would this have seemed to corroborate the superstitious belief that the spirits of the dead return to the earth. One could hardly expect them to disbelieve an evidence apparently offered to three of the family, and it would require a great deal more knowledge than the public possess, to enable them even to comprehend the nature of the mental delusion. The mother was an object of great interest and affection, and had died under circumstances so awfully distressing, that an intense impression had been made on the minds of all of them. Each of the family has the power of forming a voluntary image of any object at will on shutting the eyes, and each can draw from memory a representation of it, more or less accurate. It is not strange that all should be thinking of the being they had lost, that their affectionate regret should enhance the impression, and that thus an object should come unbidden to the mind, the presence of which they had the power to command by an act of volition. It spoils the interest and romance of the story to give this explanation, but the truth should not be withheld.

A celebrated artist of the present day, whose extraordinary fertility of imagination is a subject of wonder and admiration to every one, remarks that the preposterous figures and faces which he puts forth, always seem to him to exist already on the paper, and that his hand does nothing more than trace the outlines and fix them with the pencil. This faculty bears some resemblance to that of the unhappy painter; but in that case there was little power of *creating* images, and in his ambitious attempts at historical composition, he never was successful in inventing new faces and forms, but was always compelled to select human models for the characters he would represent. Whenever he deviated from this, he failed. I believe indeed that the artist I have spoken of above does not really *invent* the preposterous faces we so often laugh at, for in the most extravagant vagaries of his pencil, we seem to recognise them as characters we have seen. It is probable that he has stored in his memory an immense variety of countenances, and merely exaggerates the peculiar characteristics of each to produce the ludicrous effect. Such men seem very liable to mental delusion when under the influence of cerebral disorder, but a large portion of mankind are totally without the power of creating or recalling an image of what they have seen. They are as liable as others to moral insanity and to the insanity of volition, but I am not aware that we have any example of such men being the victims of the form of mental disturbance which is alluded to by Dr. Bostock, Nicolai, and others.

Among the curious defects in the functions of the brain, is one which was brought to my notice a short time ago: A gentleman of middle age, or a little past that period, lamented to me his utter inability to remember faces. He would converse with a person for an hour, but after an interval of a day could not recognise him again. Even friends, with whom he had been engaged in business transactions, he was unconscious of ever having seen. Being in an occupation in which it was essential to cultivate the good-will of the public, his life was made perfectly miserable by this unfortunate defect, and his time was passed in offending and apologizing. He was quite incapable of making a mental picture of anything, and it was not till he heard the voice, that he could recognise men with whom he had constant intercourse. He was not at all fanciful in the matter, but was always in a state of alarm lest he should lose the sense of sight, imagining that the disorder or disease lay in that organ alone. When I inquired more fully into the matter, I found that there was no defect in vision, except that his eyes were weak, and that any long continued employment of them gave him pain. There was no appearance of that morbid vanity which induces a person to affect peculiarities of constitution, but on the contrary, a strong desire to conceal his defect from the world. I endeavoured in vain to convince him that an acknowledgment of the defect would be the best means of removing the unfortunate effect it had produced in alienating friends. He was quite determined to conceal it, if possible, and it was impossible to convince him that it did not depend solely on the eyes.

One of the most distressing effects of long continued anxiety of mind, when the daily duties are incessant, and demand a continuous painful mental exertion to fulfil them, is, that imperfect conviction as to the reality of the objects which suggest ideas. For example, a man has vivid dreams—not always on the subjects of his waking thoughts, but generally excited by them through some analogy which is forgotten. He is quite unable to decide whether the friend he meets did really give him instructions to draw up a will—to make a plan of a house—to perform an operation on a diseased finger—to baptize a child—to send in a cargo of coals—or any other thing according to his profession or occupation,—or whether he only dreamt of it. When this kind of confusion comes over the mind of a solicitor or a medical man, the consequences are rapidly fatal to his reputation—the alarm is very naturally taken, and the mischief is aggravated by the well-meaning remonstrances of his friends. I have heard a man say, "Did you tell me to do so and so?" "Did you tell me to call upon you, or did I dream it?" In its aggravated form it is a frightful calamity, and can be alleviated only by the excessive kindness, indulgence, and forbearance of those around him. He has a sound brain and a disordered brain; the latter gives false information and unreal impressions so vivid as almost to baffle the judgment of the former; our remonstrances and arguments, however well intended, are felt as intense cruelty—you are aggravating the evil you wish to remove, and you run the risk of establishing positive insanity. If the man be so fortunate as to possess an affectionate and gentle wife, much may be done to restore his disordered brain; if, indeed, he have any object of *fondness*, it will do much to soothe and tranquillize his mind. Removal from business or travel avail nothing—*coelum non animam mutat;* it is the reaction of the tender propensities which alone has influence in these cases, and in pervigilium.

But, indeed, are not kindness, compassion, soothing attentions, forbearance, gentleness, indulgence, and forgiveness, the great instruments of cure in all cases of cerebral disturbance? If, reader, you have ever had the happiness to accompany Dr. Conolly round the noble establishment of Hanwell, and have witnessed the effect of his gentle and apostolic manner on the disordered minds of the poor unfortunate beings committed to his care—how the violence that would have revolted against restraint melts down under his calm and benevolent glance, while his tone of intense compassion speeds its way to the inmost recesses of the heart—if you have witnessed this, as I have, with tearful eye, you need no further argument to convince you that the Christian doctrine of forgiveness of injuries, and the exercise of persevering compassion for the perversions of the human intellect, were laid down by one who knew every secret spring and motive of humanity.

Professor Heinroth, in his "Seelenstoeringen," makes an assertion which is in harmony with the feelings of a large portion of the public (and especially of the religious public), that "moral depravity is the essential cause of madness—sin and guilt, and evil conscience, the real origin of mental derangement." The number of persons who put faith in this horrible doctrine is materially diminished of late years, but it is still a formidable and influential phalanx. Imagine a man, or several men, of this stamp, governors of a lunatic asylum, and think of the frightful consequences that may arise from their mischievous activity.

When Dr. Pritchard wrote his larger work on insanity, only seven or eight years ago, he thought it necessary to consider and refute such opinions—to contemplate seriously the arguments of those who considered that the disease was in the *motion* of the watch, and not in the watch itself, and he condescends to discuss the crude absurdities of these crazy enthusiasts. In the present day, I presume it is unnecessary to speak of them but as the delusions of the vulgar, and that no man with pretensions to science or literature will be found to take up the argument. We know that some of the best of human beings have been the victims of cerebral disease producing self-accusation, and ultimately mental derangement. Had Robert Hall lived in the present day, it is more than probable he might have been cured of the delusions which rendered so good a man miserable. Had he lived a little earlier, his aberrations might have been rectified by fire and fagot, and the other tender mercies of the day.

In the memoirs of that amiable and highly-gifted man, the poet Cowper, we have a most striking example of the influence of two opposing brains—the sound one unfortunately in this case so highly imaginative, as to be in some degree incapacitated for its office of controller, and still further unfitted for its duty by the fervour of religious enthusiasm. "The use of a Church establishment (as a high dignitary once remarked to me) is not to encourage, but to direct and control religious feeling, which will be always in excess if left without the guidance of men of sound education acting on system." Cowper had not the benefit of this kind of discipline, but fell among crazy enthusiasts who encouraged the hallucinations which should have been restrained. Instead of exercise in the open air, amusements, travel, and the study of physical science, he was induced to dwell on his deranged impressions, and made to believe that his strange visions and ecstasies were the product of inspiration, or at least direct influences from Heaven. All those motives, which would have led him to restrain by the strong volition of his comparatively sound brain, the morbid delusions of the other, were thus taken away, and he was taught to encourage feelings which common sense (had it not been mystified by religious fervour) would have shewn to be the results of disease; the natural consequence was confirmed insanity, and he remained for nearly two years a positive maniac. On his recovering from this state, he was for about ten years in a condition of comparative happiness—acquiesced entirely in the delusions of the diseased brain, and ceased to cultivate opposition to it—believing that he was now converted and received into a state of grace. He had his "experiences," his ravishing emotions—he bathed in spiritual light, and felt the most transcendent tranquillity and bliss; but this gradually changed into a conviction that he was a reprobate of heaven, and for ever cut off from salvation.

CHAPTER XV: *Diffused Disorder Affects Only One Side; Death of Dr. Wollaston; Imbecility Compatible With High Moral Qualities; Story of the Two Children; Character Changed by a Spicula of Bone; Case of Antagonist Convictions in a Clergyman*

If it be objected that a diffused disorder is not likely to produce disease in one cerebrum only, I answer that such limited effects from general causes are common—the *suffusio dimidians*, for example, where only one half of the field of vision is perceived by the mind, has been known to arise from exposure to marsh miasmata. I had under my care a young gentleman about sixteen, who, from sleeping only one night in the neighbourhood of Barking in Essex, returned to town with feelings of indescribable distress, of which he could give no other description than that he felt *very ill.* On visiting him the next morning while he was in bed, I found one half of his face and forehead in the most profuse perspiration, while the other half remained perfectly dry and harsh. On turning down the bedclothes, the same appearance was manifested throughout the body, but not quite so distinctly; the median line in the face forming an absolute boundary and demarcation. "I have known a patient," says Dr. Holland, "suffering under various symptoms of diseased brain, who frequently saw only half his face when looking in the glass; and very recently I have met with an instance where a father and daughter had each the liability of this affection. In another instance in a young lady, the occurrence was always followed by intense headach."

We are all familiar with the effect of gout, which, affecting the whole system (or rather both systems) to a violent degree, ultimately expends its malignancy perhaps on one toe. If it locate itself in onc brain, is it at all wonderful that it should produce insanity? A case of this kind I have already narrated. It is not necessary that it should produce the same effects on the cerebrum as in the toe—that it should create inflammation, pain, and swelling in the brain; it is enough if it set up a very slight disturbance in one of the cerebra in order to break up that harmonic unison of the two which is necessary for single mind. If, by a slight degree of peculiar irritation in one of these organs, it excite therein ideas of violence or murder, or a disposition to suicide, it depends entirely on the healthiness of the other organ—on its degree of cultivation, and of remaining power—whether the propensity be followed, or not followed, by corresponding action. In the great majority of cases, there is so perfect a *consciousness in the sound brain* that the sensations, perceptions, and volitions of the other, are morbid and unnatural, that if its faculties have been duly cultivated it can prevent these morbid volitions from passing into action.

If malaria can produce such effects on the *body*, we may easily conceive other causes capable of inducing similar disordered states of the *sensorium*, as we see, indeed, in the impoverished state of the blood from long suckling, from the insertion of specific poisons, and from many other causes.

It would seem that, in the optic commissure, the external fibres of each nerve continue without decussation, while the internal cross each other to the opposite side. A paralysis, temporary or continued, (like that of the *pes anserinus*, from exposure to cold) of separate portions of the optic nerves in their commissure, might perhaps explain the strange disease alluded to: *suffusio dimidians*.

Some of the deaths recorded of remarkable men have been supposed to prove that the higher faculties of the intellect have a greater power of triumphing over the effects of bodily disease than have those faculties and powers which we possess in common with the brutes. This is true only in a very limited sense; and the striking sentiments uttered by such men in their last moments are wrongly supposed to indicate the possession of greater mental powers, more independent of corporeal structure, whereas they indicate nothing but the simple fact, that one brain remains perfect to the last, although the disease in the other is imcompatible with life—the man dies from disease in one brain, but the other remains in full possession of all its faculties.

This was remarkably shewn in the case of the celebrated Dr. Wollaston, alluded to by Dr. Holland in a note, page 166, of *Medical Notes and Observations.* I have heard many minute particulars of the death of that very remarkable man, who seemed to possess the curious faculty of carrying out to perfection, and to a useful result, every idea that was suggested to him by another man, without being able to originate one himself. I believe that some account of his death was published, but after much search have been unable to discover it, and can therefore only give a few of the particulars which rest in my memory, and add to them the statement of Dr. Holland above cited. I hope, on a future occasion, to furnish the full details of a case which throws much light on the theory I am endeavouring to establish.

Dr. Wollaston died from disease of one brain, producing entire disorganization of it. He was aware, from a very early period, of the nature of his disease and of its inevitable result; he had first been made sensible of its existence on the occurrence of numbness at the end of his finger when out shooting. "He was accustomed," says Dr. Holland, "to take exact note of the changes progressively occurring in his sensations, memory, and voluntary power. He made daily experiments to ascertain their amount, and described the results in a manner which can never be forgotten by those who heard him. It was a mind *unimpaired in its higher parts*, watching over the physical phenomena of approaching death; and, what well deserves note, watching over the progressive change in those functions which seem nearest to the line separating material from intellectual existence."

It is much to be lamented that so accurate an observer, and so deep a thinker, as Dr. Holland, should have been suddenly incapacitated by dangerous illness from following up his attendance on Dr. Wollaston to the last moments of his existence. But for this interruption, I feel satisfied that he would have come to the same conviction from that single case, which has been impressed on my mind by a great number of similar instances of cerebral disorder, and that my theory would have thus taken its rise from higher authority and received a more able illustration. I cannot, however, agree with Dr. Holland, that the mind of Dr. Wollaston was unimpaired in its higher parts, more than the mind of any other man under similar circumstances. Disease so extensive must have produced complete prostration of all the animal instincts and propensities, which no longer required any effort to control them—they were not of sufficient force to disturb the judgment, because the vitality of the whole system was reduced to so low a state; but the spirit of selfishness, which is certainly not one of the higher qualities of the mind, survived almost every other sentiment, and it was only in his last moments that Dr. Wollaston could resolve to part with his profitable secret as to the management of Platinum, by which he had already realized an enormous fortune. I cannot but think it a duty to record all the selfish littleness of great men as a warning to others, and therefore do I put the fact on record. There is, however, another example of his full possession of some of the inferior mental faculties which is very remarkable. At a time when even his medical friends, Dr. Babington and others, supposed him to be so near death as to be perfectly unconscious, and when he was unable to speak, he marked down a few lines of figures on the slate and added them up correctly, as a signal to them that he was still quite conscious of his state, and therefore able to appreciate their services.

The view of the brain and its functions here presented may perhaps tend to a more compassionate and humane treatment of those minor degrees of imbecility, which are not usually considered to arise from disease or physical defect. Even an excessive degree of imbecility is compatible with great sensibility and the most exalted moral sentiments; yet I have seen such persons treated with injustice and cruelty instead of compassion, and a responsibility exacted for defective mental performances which it was as absolutely impossible for them to *perfect* as for their tormentors to invent logarithms. This kind of torture may be imposed thoughtlessly; but it is sometimes inflicted in the wanton triumph of superiority. Strange, that those who would hold it base and unmanly to ridicule a man for the minor calamity of a *club-foot*, should think it no shame to subject a fellow-creature to this mental misery who bears the vastly greater misfortune of a *club-brain*. Place one of these thoughtless or unfeeling men in the position of a schoolmaster, and see the horrible torture he will inflict on the most innocent and helpless of God's creatures.

It is a startling fact, that some of the greatest geniuses that have ever delighted or improved mankind have been remarkably dull and slow-minded in their childhood and youth, and that precocious and astonishing mental development that delights an unreflective parent, generally ends in a mature intellect of less than average excellence. That, in fact, great intellects are of slow growth, and long in coming to maturity. How many Addisons, Popes, Scotts, Byrons, Brunels, Davys, Cuviers, Faradays, and others, may have been spoiled by the absurd determination to force open every bud, that the whole of the roses may blossom at the same time.

Mr. Barlow mentions the case of an idiot boy, son of a blacksmith, who had been taught to strike perseveringly with the great hammer, and thus earned a subsistence, although he had not intellect enough to manage the most trifling affairs. In this, as in many other instances, there was a very high moral feeling. Having on one occasion accidentally killed a neighbour's goose, he was inconsolable, and could only be pacified by the fullest restoration to the owner. I know no argument so strong for the doctrine that different parts of the brain have different functions. An instance in exemplification of this combination of idiocy and pecuniary morality occurred to myself, many years ago. In passing into the Netherlands from France, I was stopped at the frontier at Quiévrain to examine my luggage. This being done, a handsome lad, apparently about seventeen, dressed in a blouse, came up to me, rubbed himself up against me, and in spite of my having repeatedly pushed him away, persisted in passing his hand over my person. I thought him drunk, and on his again putting his hand to the pocket of my pantaloons, raised my fist to knock him down, when the men of the custom-house called out, "Stop, stop, sir, it is a woman." I then supposed she had been inspired by an amatory feeling, but found on examination that she was in a state of imbecility, which I had not at first noticed, and that she was engaged by the custom-house people thus to search the persons of travellers to detect smuggling. She perfectly comprehended the object of this strange duty for a person with her limited intellect, and every evening carried the receipts of the day several miles to deliver them to the collector, she being more trustworthy than any sane person. She knew exactly the sum which they had received in the day, and the men said would have suffered herself to be cut to pieces rather than give up her trust.

Her history is rather curious, if the narrative they gave me could be depended on. She had been violated under circumstances of peculiar atrocity, by a party of Cossacks, and on recovering from the effects of their brutality, vowed that she would never again wear the dress of woman. She gradually sank into insanity, and thence into idiocy. It did not say much for the delicacy or humanity of the superior officers that such a person should be placed in such a position, but in those days honest people were rare.

How much of the moral aberrations of adults are attributable to the voluntary wickedness of the individual, and how much to the ungoverned and ungovernable impulses of diseased organs, can be known only to the Creator; but it cannot be unimportant to society at large, nor to our own self-respect and complacency of conscience, that we should be permanently aware of our ignorance, and that when we err in judgment it should be always on the side of mercy. We see a man, for example, of mature age, who has hitherto maintained an irreproachable character, and who possesses the respect of his fellow-creatures—who leads a life of order and sobriety, brings up his family with respectability, inculcates good principles, and sets a good example. We see such a man suddenly detected in some enormous wickedness—he has swindled or defrauded

—has openly set decency at defiance, or has been discovered in the lowest haunts of filthy and monstrous debauchery. It is said that "*Nemo repente fuit turpissimus;*" and if we exclude the effects of disordered brain, the assertion is true; but a small degree of *disease* shall change the whole character of the individual.

One of the most common effects of incipient insanity, arising either from disordered action of the brain or from the commencement of change in its structure, is a transition from the habitual affection for certain persons into positive hatred of them, often of the most intense description. If the cause of this change be temporary—that is, disordered *action*—the effect subsides in a few months, and the individual is restored to mental health; but if produced by an alteration taking place in the *structure* of the brain, it generally ends in permanent insanity or confirmed imbecility. The cases are very few where the commencement of disorganization has either subsided spontaneously,or the disease has been cured or materially controlled by medical means.

Is there any man of mature age, nay, of any age, who is not conscious of repeated changes of sentiment during his past life? Has he not at one time condemned and repudiated feelings and opinions which at another period he had held with complacency, or perhaps defended with obstinacy? Then, if he feel that his own mind has changed again and again, is he quite certain that his present conviction will last for the remainder of his life, and that he may not, from further experience, or from having looked at the same things from a different point of view, or from a physical change in himself, be induced to regard his present opinions as fallacious, like those which he has already abandoned? It is an unsatisfactory reflection but a wise one, to consider our existing convictions as liable to error, like those which have preceded them; we thus avoid the dogmatism which at once offends the self-love of others and makes them resist the consideration of our arguments, and we promote the reciprocal forbearance which forms the bond and blessing of society. When we reflect that a slight excess or deficiency of blood in a certain part of the brain—a slight excess or deficiency of vibration in a certain bundle of nervous fibres—a slight excess or deficiency in the quantity of phosphate of lime, uric acid, or ammonia, in the blood, shall make the same man at one time religious, moral, continent, and placable, and at another, irascible, unreasonable, licentious, and irreligious; that a blow on the head shall change a man of piety into a blasphemer, shall make an affectionate mother put to death her children, a tender husband destroy his wife; shall derange all the habits, feelings, sentiments, and convictions of one who is yet considered by his fellow-creatures to be entirely master of his own actions. When these things are taken into consideration, along with the fact, that there is every possible gradation between this state and complete responsibility, we shall be inclined to practise to its fullest extent the charity inculcated by Christ, and forgive the offender seventy times seven times, rather than risk the infliction of an unjust punishment.

It has been said that the only *perfect mind* is God himself. We know so little of the mighty maze of Creation, that there may exist beings as much superior to ourselves as we are to the lowest of the zoophytes. Between our degree of intellect and perfection, the space is infinitely greater than between man and the molusca; and the inhabitants of some of the myriads of worlds which surround us may possess a degree of intelligence which we are utterly unable to conceive. To them it may be given to know the mysterious connexion between the soul and the corporeal organs through which it is compelled to manifest its emotions; to comprehend why, for example, a spicula of bone should change love into hatred; but with such frail and imperfect beings as ourselves, it is only by the belief in a Revelation that these abstruse contemplations can be restrained within boundaries where alone they can produce a result. Happy the man who, either from early tuition or the natural structure of his mind, can rest on that for a solution of all difficulties. A full, unhesitating confidence in that which he has been taught—that is to say, *faith*—is the greatest of all blessings. The mightiest intellect that was ever conferred by the Creator, and that intellect cultivated to the highest perfection, can only lead its possessor astray when he attempts to penetrate by the aid of reason alone, through the moral wilderness which surrounds him. The man is happier who, in the faith of that which he has been taught, sits down at the threshold, and refuses to enter on the unprofitable investigation.

Even unbelievers cannot but envy the superior progress made in attainable knowledge by those who have resolutely shut up the path that leads to nothing; and have resolved not to waste their energies in a voyage of discovery which it is morally certain they can never complete, when, by appropriate employment in their proper sphere, they may make a substantial progress in things cognizable by unaided reason.

One of the most distressing forms of mental disturbance I ever knew, was in a beneficed clergyman of sincere piety, extensive knowledge, and unbounded benevolence. He came to me repeatedly to complain of trifling ailments; but although we were exceedingly intimate, and he bestowed his confidence upon me as to his worldly affairs to an inconvenient extent, I could always see that there was something in reserve which he could not make up his mind to communicate. The natural conclusion was that he had fallen into one of those entanglements to which clergymen are just as liable as the laity; and I endeavoured to pave the way for an explanation, by palliating the supposed infirmity. He always denied, however, that he had committed any indiscretion, and at last confessed to me the cause of his unhappiness and embarrassment. Never shall I forget the awful agitation and convulsive agony expressed in his countenance, as he with difficulty and with many interruptions at last completed his story. I will give it as nearly as my memory will serve in his own words, omitting, however, one remarkable and influential event of his early life, that the individual may not be recognised.

"I was brought up," said he, "with great severity; my father having been educated in the Presbyterian form of religion, and with all the bigotry of that harsh and intolerant sect. Every innocent joy was condemned as a crime, and the slightest expression of pleasure denounced as sinful. I became a morose and solitary being; and, when at college, made no acquaintances, but kept myself quite aloof from human sympathy. I took honours, and obtained ordination at the earliest period that it was possible. My father determined, as he phrased it, to *put me into harness as soon as possible, to keep me out of mischief by the feeling of responsibility*, and immediately procured me a curacy. My humble living was bestowed by my college as a reward of merit; and well it was so, for my father died penniless and insolvent, and for many years past it has been the sole support of my widowed mother and crippled sister. I became successful as a preacher, and have attained to a local eminence which promises to lead to a valuable appointment; but I am intensely miserable, and always ill from anxiety; at one moment tormented with the idea that I am preaching falsehood and encouraging delusion—Christianity appears to be a fable without a shadow of foundation, and it seems to me a wicked mockery of the living God to preach it as a truth; in these moments I determine to give up my living, and abhor myself for having so long accepted the wages of sin and deceit; then the thought of my helpless mother and sister comes over me, and I endeavour to endure the remorse for their sake; I think also of the injury of such an example, and how it would loosen the bonds which restrain the wicked, and I cannot resolve on the sacrifice. At another moment I have the most entire, unhesitating faith in the doctrines and in the authenticity of Christianity, and look with horror at my previous sceptical delusions as the instigation of the author of evil. I pour out my soul to God in prayer to be forgiven for having listened for a moment to the tempter; feel soothed and refreshed, and enter again on my duties with alacrity and zeal. This frightful alternation keeps me in constant alarm; and the terror I feel at the moment of full belief, lest Satan should again assail me with his suggestions, more than countervails the timid light that in my wandering moments tells me I shall again believe and be comforted. I feel the transition from one set of convictions to the other, and this state is the most frightful of all; seem as if I were two beings; and I am in momentary expectation of madness—God help me!"

Men will explain this state of mind in various ways, according to their own convictions. I can only conceive it to proceed from a discrepancy in the action of the two organs of thought—that, in fact, however incongruous the opinion may seem to those who have not studied the subject, *one brain be-*

lieved, and the other did not believe—a state which is a very common precursor of madness, if indeed it be not the first stage of it.

The further progress of this case, I purposely conceal. It was very remarkable; but were I to give the details, the individual would be recognised, and it would inflict unjustifiable pain on persons whose feelings I hold sacred. Analogous cases of slighter and varying intensity are by no means rare. On the subject of religion, as on politics, an alternation of partial convictions is frequently seen. Happy those who have no doubts, no hesitations, no difficulties; but repose in their quiet settled convictions—who have ceased to reason, and to weigh probabilities and evidence—and who once convinced, are convinced for ever.

Wait the Great Teacher Death, and God adore.

There is an interesting little story in the "Illuminated Magazine," shewing an entire change of character from a physical cause. It is narrated in too florid a style for a work of science, yet may convey some useful instruction. I knew the parties, and can vouch for the general accuracy of the narrative. The story may induce a parent to pause before he punishes a sudden change of conduct in a child previously virtuous and good.

"We are sent into the world (says a very learned and amiable friend of mine) to see what we are fit for." I believe that every man of superior intellect has his mission, and that to injure one of these minds is a high crime and misdemeanour against the majesty of human nature.

I consider that every species of cruelty to children of slow intellect arises from brutal arrogance. The very man who as schoolmaster, mechanic, or artist, will not tolerate anything but excellence in his pupil—will, when guided by the instinct of paternity, not merely be tolerant of imbecility but absolutely be unconscious of its existence in his own child. How often is a medical man subjected to the embarrassment of awakening the parents to the existence of positive idiocy in their offspring? Many years ago I was consulted about the bodily health of a young lady twelve years of age, and on asking how long they had observed the symptoms of imbecility, was answered that there was no imbecility whatever—that to be sure she was slow in learning, but remarkably acute—and they cited to me instances of cleverness which would have been quite in character, but not remarkable, in a child of four or five years of age. She was virtually an idiot.

It is true this is an extreme case, but in a lesser degree the same thing must have fallen under the observation of every medical practitioner and schoolmaster. The latter have often assigned the unreasonable blindness of parents to the imbecility of their children as an excuse for their own severity. The following is the story alluded to:

A gentleman, engaged in the higher departments of trade—a good man, an enlightened man, and an affectionate parent—had two sons, who at the time I begin their history, were respectively of the ages of five and ten. The attachment between them was so remarkable as to be the common topic of conversation among all their friends and acquaintance. The children were incessantly together; and to see them walk round the garden with the arm of the elder round the neck of the younger while the other, who could not reach to his neck, endeavoured to clasp his waist—with their long auburn hair, in the fashion of the day, hanging down in ringlets, and as the elder stooped to kiss his little brother covering his face, those who had seen them thus occupied, their lovely features beaming with affection, would have said that nothing on earth could give a more vivid idea of angels.

The children when separated for a few hours were miserable; and when the time arrived for sending the elder to school, it was a subject of serious reflection with the parents and friends, whether so intense an affection should be checked or encouraged: the former was decided on, and the elder was sent to a distance.

Both children were so exceedingly unhappy, that sleepless nights, loss of appetite, incessant weeping, and rapid wasting of body, made every one fearful of the consequences of prolonging the absence, and they were brought together again. Those who witnessed the tumultuous joy of their meeting, describe it as inexpressibly affecting. They soon recovered their health and spirits, and their mutual affection seemed if possible to be increased by their temporary separation.

The experiment, after a while, was again made, with similar results; and it was decided never to risk another.

An arrangement was now entered into with a schoolmaster to receive both boys, although contrary to the regulations of his establishment, which professed to admit none under ten years of age.

The two boys kept themselves almost entirely aloof from all the rest; the elder helped the younger in his education, watched him with a kind of parental solicitude, kept a vigilant eye upon the character of the boys who sought his society, and admitted none to intimacy with his brother of whom he did not entirely approve. The slightest hint of his wish sufficed with the younger, who would almost as soon have contemplated deliberately breaking the Commandments as opposing his wishes in the slightest degree.

Both made rapid progress in their education, and their parents' hearts were filled with thankfulness for the blessing.

In the midst of this happiness, news arrived from the schoolmaster that, from some unexplained cause, the elder boy had begun to exercise a very unreasonable and tyrannical authority over the younger; that he had been repeatedly punished for it; but although he always promised amendment, and could assign no cause—reasonable or unreasonable—for his conduct, he soon relapsed into his usual habits, and the schoolmaster requested to know what was to be done. The father immediately sent for both boys, and entered upon a lengthened investigation. The little one was almost heart-broken, and exclaimed, "He might beat me every day if he would but love me; but he hates me, and I shall never be happy again."

The elder could assign no reason for his animosity and ill-treatment; and the father, after many remonstrances, thought it right to inflict on him very severe corporal chastisement, and confined him to his room for some days with nothing but bread and water. The lad on his liberation gave solemn promises of altered conduct, but shewed little affection for his brother, although the latter used a thousand innocent stratagems to inspire him with tenderness. They returned to school. In a few days similar scenes and worse occurred; the boy was again and again punished by the master, again and again promised amendment, but in vain, and he was at last taken away from school by his father.

A repetition of severe punishment, long incarceration, and a rejection by all his relatives, had no effect in changing his disposition; his dislike to his brother became fixed animosity, and from animosity degenerated into the most deadly hatred: he made an attempt on the child's life; and, if he saw him pass an open door, would throw a carving-knife at him with all the fury of a maniac.

The family now resorted to medical advice, and years passed in hopeless endeavours to remove a disposition obviously depending on a diseased brain. Had they taken this step earlier, these floggings and imprisonments would have been spared, as well as the heart-sickening remorse of the father.

Still the boy was not insane: on every topic but one he was reasonable, but torpid; it was only by the sight of his brother, or the sound of his name, that he was roused to madness. The youth now advanced towards manhood. When about the age of fifteen he was taken with a violent but Platonic passion for a lady more than forty years of age, and the mother of five children, the eldest older than himself. His paroxysms of fury now became frightful; he made several attempts to destroy himself; but in the very torrent and whirlwind of his rage, if this lady would allow him to sit down at her feet and lay his head on her knee, he would burst into tears and go off into a sound sleep, wake up perfectly calm and composed, and looking up into her face with lack-lustre eye, would say, "Pity me; I can't help it."

Soon after this period he began to squint, and was rapidly passing into hopeless idiocy, when it was proposed by Mr. Cline to apply the trephine, and take away a piece of bone from the skull, in a place where there appeared to be a slight depression. "The indication is very vague," said he, "and we should not be justified in performing the operation but in a case in which we cannot do any harm; he must otherwise soon fall a sacrifice."

It was done, and from the under surface grew a long spicula of bone piercing the brain! He recovered, resumed his attachment to his brother, and became indifferent to the lady.

The disease which led to these terrible results had its origin in a blow on the head with the end of a round ruler—one of the gentle reprimands then so common with schoolmasters.

What must be the remorse of any father who, having exercised his right to inflict severe castigation for moral offences, finds, in the further progress of the case, that the depravity arose, *ab initio*, from disease within the skull! I cannot conceive a more intense anguish, except in the case of extravagant and ill-founded jealousy leading to the destruction of a faithful wife—when death has rendered compunction useless, and reparation impossible.

CHAPTER XVI: *Case of Mr. Percival; Reflections; Diseased Volitions*

In medical literature more or less directly treating of insanity, there is scarcely a book from which more instruction may be drawn by the physician, the moralist, and the philosopher, than the "*Narrative of the treatment experienced by a* GENTLEMAN *during a state of Mental Derangement.*" We rise from a perusal of the tale with additional convicion of the soundness of the common adage that "truth is stranger than fiction." The most vivid imagination never laid bare the human mind, and shewed its darkest recesses more perfectly, than this true narrative of mental suffering. I hope to make it conducive to important issues. Perhaps I feel still greater interest in the melancholy tale, from remembering the individual when a boy, and having formed an opinion of him at an early age. The work is published anonymously, but the author designates himself so clearly in the course of his narrative that there is no indelicacy in removing a veil obviously intended to be transparent. He is the son of the late Prime Minister, Percival, who was shot in the House of Commons by Bellingham, in the year 1812.

The work is suggestive of a multitude of reflections. It is, perhaps, the only instance on record where a madman was able to retain in his memory all the events of three years insanity and delusion; and had I no other example to produce of the duality of the mind, it would be conclusive of a fact, which, when thoroughly established in the public conviction, will lead to consequences of the highest interest and importance.

The author was, I know, educated with the greatest care, but being of a highly nervous temperament, that is, having a brain easily excited, and probably a sympathetic system with a natural tendency to disorder, required an education of a totally different character from that which he received. Had he been sent into the navy at an early age, I do not doubt that he would have escaped the awful visitation.

The work is written with talent, and is perfectly consecutive and consistent; but it is obvious that the writer, although restored to society, has not yet entirely recovered from his delusions. I shall quote his own words extensively, and make the application as I go on; suggesting in brackets what I conceive to be the nature and progress of the disease.

He was one of that not very small class at our public schools who grow up with an excess of religious feeling quite incompatible with *pari passu* cultivation of the intellect. This remark will not seem unmeaning to men of experience—strong religious enthusiasm is a very dangerous accompaniment to the pursuit of literature by a young mind—and either the intellect or the health gives way under the double cultivation. The religion of the young and uneducated ought to be a religion of mere acquiescence; the religion of the highly cultivated and mature, a religion of investigation: the young and fragile brain, as yet not physically developed, has not room for the rapid expansion which is produced by abstruse metaphysical and mysterious contemplation. The doctrines styled evangelical are so mystical and bewildering to the youthful inquirer, that a slight observation by parents and tutors would suffice to shew the very great danger of encouraging such incomprehensible abstractions. At twenty-five or thirty, when the brain is firmly formed, such speculations are comparatively harmless. I speak here alone of the effect on the physical organ in this examination of religion—the merits or demerits, truth or falsehood, of the doctrines, I do not attempt to decide. We see that men of the highest talent, education, and character, are about equally divided on the subject: one half strongly condemning, and the other half enthusiastically applauding these views of what is called Evangelical Christianity. We leave the decision to clergymen.

"At the age of seventeen," says Mr. Percival, "I left the public school, at which I had passed seven years, not without credit, and went to study with a private tutor." At eighteen he had a commission in a cavalry regiment, and afterwards in the Guards, where he passed his time quietly and unobserved. He had been brought up, like most of the sons of men of rank and fortune till near manhood, with scrupulous morality: the license of a mess-room shocked him. "I had at school three or four friends, and no very extensive general acquaintance. If I was remarkable in society for anything, it was for occasional absence of mind, and for my gravity and silence when the levity of my companions transgressed the bounds of decorum, and made light of religion, or offended against morality. In private I had severe conflict of mind upon the truth and nature of the Christian religion, accompanied with acute agony at my own inconsistency of conduct and sentiment with the principles of duty and feeling taught by Jesus and the Apostles. . . . After several years inward suffering and perplexity, I found at last, for a time, peace, and joy, and triumph, as I imagined, in the doctrines usually styled evangelical." He next begins to preach to the men, procures seats for them in a separate chapel, and harangues them. Remonstrances arrive from Colonel and Chaplains; he becomes more and more confirmed in his enthusiasm; is led by a passage in the New Testament, "*choose liberty rather than slavery*," and withdraws from the army. Goes to the University—forms acquaintance with young men of similarly heated imagination—attends Baptist and Independent meeting-houses—becomes a believer in miracles—sees visions—has spirits come to him—desires to go to Glasgow, to examine into the miracles of the unknown tongues which were performing there—wakes in the night to pray—expects the Holy Ghost to visit him—goes to the seat of miracles at Row—becomes acquainted with that strange aggregation of dupes and impostors—and along with that extraordinarily gifted man, Erskine, becomes decidedly deranged in mind.

"Ovid's description of the inspiration of Pythagoras," says he, "tallied with my experience; the voice was given me, but I was not master of it—I was but the instrument." He uttered ideas which seemed not his own, and even sang involuntarily. [One brain is now disordered and approaching to positive disease. Consciousness remains in the sound brain, which naturally judges that the involuntary suggestions of the other are *external*—an explanation of a thousand passages in the lives of the saints, etc.]

"I was *made* to open the Old Testament, and in the 28th chapter of Deuteronomy read, that I should be cursed in my family; in my going out and coming in, etc.; and the Lord shall smite thee with *madness*, and blindness, and astonishment of heart." He begins to know, by a sensation on his palate, throat, and hearing, whether he is speaking against the will of God, or in accordance with it. [That is, as I explain it, his sound brain is conscious when that which he utters is involuntary—and it was perhaps a fact, that the volitions of the diseased brain were really accompanied by those derangements of the organs of taste and hearing.] He says, "I was compelled either to hold my tongue, to speak as I was *guided*, or to speak my own thoughts." [He had still the power to be silent—even to exercise some control over the morbid volitions of the disordered organ; but, believing them to be of divine origin, he uttered them.] He is accosted by a woman of the town—exhorts her in the language of Scripture, and she leaves him. Five minutes afterwards another comes up, "and led me away to my destruction."

He becomes very ill; his sense of shame, of ingratitude, of remorse, of his guilt in bringing disrepute on doctrines which he was persuaded came from the Holy Spirit, completed the disorder of the brain; he becomes positively mad, and is put into confinement.

"A spirit came upon me, and prepared to guide my actions. I was lying on my back, and the spirit seemed to light on my pillow by my *right* ear, and to command my body . . . the guidance of the spirit left me, and I knew not what to do."

It is clear that the slightest breach of the consentaneity of the two brains must be destructive of the one sentiment of consciousness which has hitherto been the result of the perfect unison of action in both of them; just as one object of vision, one sound. This must be the inevitable result if the mind depend for its exercise on the perfect concord of the two. We see however that consciousness is not lost when one brain is injured or defective, consequently it must now reside in one of the two brains; the more perfect will no doubt possess it, and if that be the case the diseased suggestions of the disordered brain must appear to arise from some source external to the individual, consequently from other beings. If consciousness, which now cannot, by any possibility, occupy both brains, for they are not in unison, could be supposed to reside for the moment in the diseased organ, the conclusions of the *sound* brain would be held to be erroneous, as in the case of the madman who disbelieves the evidence of his senses; but the healthy brain is obviously more likely to judge of the disordered one, as is generally the case. The defective cannot exercise judgment, *because it is defective*. As I have already remarked, the sound brain, possessing the faculty of unclouded reason, can call in external aid, and, like a regular army, overpower the tumultuous mob of thoughts from the other.

"I looked down on my limbs, when one-half of my frame appeared in a state of scarlet inflammation. When I went to dress, this had again subsided."

He is now "commanded" to stand on his head and twist his body round; he tries it, but is afraid of breaking his neck. [His sane organ is becoming disordered, and has but imperfect command, though still sensible of the danger.] He is manacled, and fastened to his bed. [It is probable, from the propensities he now displays, that the disease is extending to the cerebellum, when uncontrolled muscular movements form the only relief.]

"My confined position and idleness of mind and body left me at the mercy of my delusions; my need of wholesome exercise and occupation was denied. . . . I had a species of doubts; but no one who has not been deranged can understand how dreadfully true a lunatic's insane imagination appears to him, how slight his sane doubts." [One brain still remains almost perfect, but the disorder of the other has increased till it is entirely uncontrollable, and it is only in the moments of its *collapse* that the sane organ can influence the will.]

"The act of mind I describe was accompanied with the sound of a slight crack, and the sensation of a fibre breaking over the right temple; it reminded me of the *mainstay of a mast giving way;* it was succeeded by a loss of control over certain muscles of the body, and was immediately followed by two other cracks of the same kind, one after the other, each more towards the right ear, followed by an additional relaxation of the muscles, and accompanied by an apparently additional surrender of the judgment!". . . . *Until now I had retained a kind of restraining power over my thoughts and belief; I now had none.*" [The disease now occupies both brains.] "I could not resist the spiritual guilt and contamination of any thought, of any suggestion; *my will to choose*, to think orderly, was gone."

He now has an impression, almost a conviction, of the possibility of being in two places at the same time!

"My brother was with me; I was seated in an arm-chair; a doctor entered. . . . I was condemned again to bed. I would have given my hand to remain up; my bed was a scene of horrors to me."

He is now fastened in a sitting posture all day to an iron-bar in a niche in the wall; he hears divine voices.

"My sense of feeling was not the same; my smell, my taste, gone or confounded." [The disease is now very extensive, and it is a matter of wonder that his memory should remain; it shews that one brain was still comparatively sound, and probably chiefly disordered by sympathy.]

"It was always a great delight to me to get my hand at liberty, and the first use I made of it was to strike the keeper who untied me. I was directed by my spirits to do so. I always attempted to wrestle with him, or asked one of the patients to wrestle with me.

"Another delusion I laboured under was, that I should *keep my head and heart together*, by throwing myself head over heels over every stile or gate I came to." [Additional proof of disorder or disease of the cerebellum.]

"It is no small duty of the curer of nervous patients to have regard to the regularity of the evacuations, and there is no point for which they more require all the liberty that can be granted them. There is a moment beyond which the retention of urine becomes very deleterious to the circulating fluids, and affects the nervous system with acute pains." [How often have we seen delirium produced by this cause in persons in health, who have been detained at a public ceremony for example. I saw several who were injured for life at Lord Nelson's funeral.]

"The system (of mad doctors) is a cruel mockery of the patient. He is professedly a pitiable object of scrupulous care—the innocent dupe of unintelligible delusion; but he is treated as if responsible, as if his dupery were his fault; and if he resists the treatment he is then a madman! And if, as in my case, he is agonized and downcast with continual and unmeasured self-accusation of his great guilt in being insane, he receives no correcting intimation that he has something to say for himself—that he is an appalling witness of the power of disease—no encouragement, etc.—the belief is, that lunacy cannot be subdued but by harsh treatment."

Happily this is no longer the opinion: the success of Pinel, Dr. Conolly, and others, has produced a host of imitators, and cruelty to the insane will soon be universally considered infamous and unmanly.

Some who are old enough to remember the Parliamentary investigation into mad-houses in the year 1814, may perhaps recollect the case of William Norris. The man had attacked his keeper; but as he himself stated the affair, he had only defended himself from what he considered improper treatment. He was, however, a dangerous lunatic, and confined in the following manner: A stout iron ring was rivetted round his neck, to which was attached a chain, with another ring sliding up and down on an upright massive iron bar fastened to the wall. Round his waist was a ring composed of an iron-bar two inches in diameter, and on each side of it an iron loop through which his arms were passed, and thus pinioned close to his sides. Two similar bars riveted to the waist-bar, at both ends, went over his shoulders. The iron ring round his neck was connected to the bars over his shoulders by a double link. From each of the bars going over his shoulders passed a chain to the ring on the upright iron post. He could not advance from the wall, for the chain was only twelve inches in length, and his right leg was chained to a trough which formed his bed. He was thus compelled to lie only on his back for more than twelve years! Gracious heaven! No doubt those who ordered and enforced this dreadful treatment, expressed due horror at the atrocious cruelties of the Inquisition! Yet this man was able to read books of all kinds and the newspapers, conversed with perfect coherence, and was much interested in the topics of the day and the events of the war.

It is not for the purpose of dwelling on abominations long since discarded that I bring forward this case, but to state that this man was perfectly conscious of his ungovernable volitions—that is, one of his brains remained healthy, but disturbed by sympathy, and unable to control the other. He said, "I know that I am a dangerous person, and should be sorry to be allowed to walk unmanacled in the gallery; but if I could be prevented from doing mischief to others, which I should not attempt unless provoked, I should consider the permission to take exercise a great indulgence." But to return to Mr. Percival—

"The lunatic, of whom it appears all possible moral perfections are expected, instead of allowance being made for all possible moral weakness, whilst he is cut off from all human aid."

In a more advanced period of his confinement, he says, "I was often prompted to throw Herbert backward; but although I was told (by the spirits) that it was what he desired, I could not conquer the fear of its causing his death," and he abstained. [He is beginning to recover, and the better brain is capable of ratiocination, and is resuming its power of controlling the other.]

"I used to throw myself forward flat on the face on the ground, and besides this the voices told me to throw myself to the right or the left, which I did repeatedly." [Cerebellum]

He hears the patients speak of a suicide. "I was considering also how a man could summon boldness to endure the bodily pain, as well as to obliterate moral feeling, when my right arm was suddenly raised and my hand drawn rapidly across my throat, as if by galvanism. I then (says he) justified our law, which acquits an insane man from the verdict of *felo de se.*"

He now speaks of his opposing convictions on the subject of religion, in a mode which shews clearly that one brain entirely believed in the truth of Christianity, and the other as entirely disbelieved it.

"An insane person (he remarks) is not always aware of anything but his delusions, and his delusions contending with his feelings for the mastery over him make him a madman.

"Some of my spirits, when I met the surgeon who had performed the operation in a brutal way, and without my permission, told me to resent it, but others desired me to forgive him. These on the whole prevailed, and I shook hands with him."

Can there be a more distinct expression of two volitions? At this time he is recovering, and obtaining clear ideas of his position. His anger with his family for not believing his statements, his indignation at the treatment to which he was subjected, seem to have superseded every other feeling; his pathetic appeals on behalf of his fellow-prisoners are very touching, though obviously the result of still-existing cerebral disturbance.

An attentive consideration of the case induces me to believe that judicious treatment at an early stage of the disorder would have so far strengthened the sound brain as to enable him, in a great degree, to overcome his malady; that gentleness, or even the *affectation* of sympathy, would have much modified the course of it; and that unlimited freedom of muscular motion would have carried off a great part of the superfluous excitement, and rendered him calm: he would thus have escaped that rankling feeling of indignation at intolerable constraint which retarded his cure.

Among other observations which give rise to serious reflection, he states that an old gentleman, a Roman Catholic, a patient in the house, used to take the Bible away from him, saying, "You have read enough of it—it is that which brought you here." Is it not strange that a patient in the most decided religious insanity should have been allowed to study the Bible?

Many who have looked down on the human race from the respective eminences of philosophy, religion, or social position, and have seen them foreshortened till they were hardly recognised as fellow-creatures, find, on descending to the same level, not only that they themselves are below the average, but observe important irregularities among mankind, not cognizable till thus placed where they could form a well-founded opinion. It is thus, when we look down from the heights of reason upon the unhappy lunatic. Let us for the moment place ourselves in imagination on the low level of the insane, and think how we would be "done by." Let a man reflect on the just anger he has felt at being wantonly interrupted, even in a yawn, which he had vainly attempted to suppress, and he will be partly aware of the serious aggravation of mind that must take place in a madman, from suppressing by manacles and strait waistcoat the intense desire for muscular action; caused, perhaps, by extension of disease or irritability to the cerebellum. Leave these poor wretches room for the exercise of their superfluous vitality, for till that be expended they cannot control the more disordered brain by the sounder one. Let the unhappy victims of the direst calamity that can befall humanity, indulge the impulse without restraint; and when they shall have brought on muscular fatigue, their minds will become comparatively tranquil. In the case of Mr. Percival, I firmly believe that, had this been permitted to the extent he desired, the diseased volition of the organ that dictated such a mode of relief would have been so far exhausted as to leave the better organ in a state to *listen to reason.* This may seem a strange assertion. What? Reason with a madman? Yes. Not in his paroxysm of ungovernable violence, but in the intervals of comparative rationality, when you have soothed him by suavity and respectful deference. Had these periods been taken advantage of *to suggest the reasons of his treatment,* I do most firmly believe that one brain always remained sufficiently healthy to comprehend them, and to aid in controlling the other. Had it been his happy fate to be placed under the action of the modern benevolent system, the confinement of three years in the intense misery of impotent indignation might perhaps have been reduced to six months of comparative tranquillity and happiness.

Could I hope to see such a man as Dr. Conolly invested with power at the head of a medical commission of similar men—and there are such to be found—to investigate, govern, and *absolutely dictate*, the treatment to be pursued in every madhouse in the kingdom, and know that I had efficiently aided the holy cause, I should feel that I had performed the task allotted to me, and that I had worked out the governing predominant idea which has possessed me through life—the desire to do some one decided act to benefit my fellow-creatures. I do not think that my life has been entirely useless in this respect: but there is so vast a field for the exercise of the highest human knowledge, wisdom, and goodness, in the management of the insane; in the due government of those who have a curable tendency to insanity, and in the early education of all, so as to eradicate that tendency, that were it duly cultivated, as I conceive it *ought* to be, and *might* be cultivated, and I could have the conviction that I had been instrumental to this blessed result. I should thank God for a mass of solid happiness in the few years that remain to me, more than sufficient to have gilded a long existence. We are in the right road, but we have only advanced a few steps. Should the benevolent men who are devoting themselves to this object not be permitted to do the good of which they are capable, God will, no doubt, in his own good time, raise up successors; but in the meanwhile the prospect is dark and cheerless, and thousands must endure a misery which it would be easy to annihilate.

To parody the Arabian prayer I have quoted in my preface: "Oh God! be kind to the insane, to other men thou hast been already abundantly kind, in giving them the blessed faculty of unclouded reason."

CHAPTER XVII: *Definition of Insanity; Comparison of the Watch; Dr. Conolly's Inquiry into the Indications of Insanity; Proofs of Double Mind in that Work; Examples of Rapid Transition of Thought; of Two Concurrent Trains of Thought; Forms of Mental Disturbance; Mr Barlow; Examples of Two Antagonist Volitions; Moral and Medical Objects of Dr. Conolly's Work*

In the moral as in the physical world, a small addition to the ordinary stature makes a great man. A man of six feet is not remarkable, but a man of seven feet is gigantic. It seldom happens, however, that either intellect or bodily frame is thoroughly well formed throughout. It is only in such cases as O'Brien and Sir Isaac Newton that nature puts forth respectively a physical and intellectual giant of eight feet, and uniformly proportioned, and it takes more than a century to temper the clay for such a man.

I have been led to this remark by observing, during my examination of works bearing on the subject of insanity, that authors whose dicta I have been accustomed to receive without examination, through deference for their reputed intellectual stature, are on a closer examination no taller than myself. The defective reasonings, the "inconsequences," as the French call them, are more glaring than I could have supposed, and it appears that the reputation of intellectual superiority is not unfrequently unfounded. I will not perform the ungracious task of exposing the absurd conclusions which some established writers on the subject of mental derangement put forth as truths, but will merely warn the reader to withhold his assent from their authoritative announcements; for, if he adopt their results as the foundation of his own reasoning, he will waste his time and powers. Like a man who should enter into calculations of the strength of the tortoise on which stands the elephant that supports the world, he had better first make himself quite sure that the earth really rests on the back of an elephant. A large proportion of the works on insanity are the most perfect trash that ever a man wasted his faculties in composing or his time in reading. I shall therefore confine my attention to a very few of better pretensions.

The word *insanity* means *unhealth*, and it means nothing more. Why the term should have been applied to the class of diseases which, by disordering the brain, disturb the intellect, I know not; but the consequences of such restriction of its meaning have been mischievous. We are set to seek the causes of insanity as if it were *a disease*, whereas it is the effect or result of many diseases. The physician is expected to cure a disorder of the *mind*, as if it were something quite distinct from a disorder of the body. This is exactly equivalent to the step of which I have elsewhere spoken, of addressing a watchmaker thus: "Here is my watch—the motion is wrong, and I have brought it to you to be put right; but you must not touch the works—all the wheels, pivots, springs, balances, verge, contract pinion, and so forth, are quite in order. I do not know the structure of a watch, for I have never taken one to pieces or put it together, but have read books on the subject, and from the knowledge thus acquired, am sure that there is nothing wrong in the machinery of that I am now putting into your hands; therefore I beg you will not touch the works, but merely set right *the motion*, for that is the only defect."

Every one perceives the absurdity in the case of the watch, but the belief of those who are *not* watchmakers has been allowed to influence the *watchmakers* in our own profession, and it is only of late years that medical writers have begun to shake off the prejudice thus confirmed by the ignorance of the public. We still find in some of them a hankering after the mysterious, and an attempt to explain *the cause* of insanity instead of the causes. To explain *the* cause of unhealth is absurd, but the attempt to ascertain which of the causes of unhealth exclusively or most frequently affect the brain, and interfere with the perfect exercise of its functions, is quite reasonable; and if a man choose to confine his investigations to one portion only of the causes of unhealth, there is no objection to it, if he will only bear in mind that the symptoms produced depend on the structure of the organ which is the subject of disease, rather than on the nature of the cause. Inflammation, for example, shall increase the functions of one part, but entirely suspend those of another. Although the brain be the direct instrument of mind, and specific disease of that part produce mental derangement, yet the same intellectual disturbance may take place from a distant disease or disorder, by the mere force of sympathy—a word we have invented to conceal our ignorance of the real nature of the mysterious connexion. I have seen madness as complete from distended bladder as from inflammation of the membranes of the brain; it ceased when the cause ceased, and so will that in the brain itself, unless during its existence it have produced an organic change in the structure of the part.

It is obvious then that the causes of unhealth or insanity must be infinitely numerous, and our main business in the investigation is to ascertain which of these numerous causes admit of alleviation, removal, or prevention. This is quite enough to occupy the greatest talents, the most untiring industry, and the longest life that ever was devoted to the welfare of mankind. I do not attempt anything so greatly beyond my powers; but I do firmly believe that I shall remove many obstacles to the progress of others, and point the way to further discoveries, though the short remainder of my life will not suffice to advance far on the road to them myself.

If I can succeed in shewing that many of the complicated forms of cerebral unhealth, or mental derangement, are only varieties produced by *the more or less perfect exemption of one of the brains from the disease affecting the other*, I shall have done much more than simplify the treatment and increase the number of remedies. I shall have done something towards removing the ignorance of the public in this most interesting department of medical research—an ignorance which, at every step, forms an almost insuperable obstacle to our success. If I only succeed in convincing well-meaning, active, energetic, philanthropic, and benevolent individuals, who interest themselves for the insane, that they are exerting their wrongly-directed and mischievous efforts so as entirely to thwart their own good intentions, I shall have rendered a very important service to my fellow-creatures; and if any such persons take the trouble to peruse these lucubrations, I have too good an opinion of my cause to doubt of success, however humble the qualifications I bring to the task.

The impression made on my mind, after an attentive perusal of Dr. Conolly's "*Inquiry concerning the Indications of Insanity*," is so entirely different from that made by the work of any other writer on the subject, that I hesitate in expressing my opinions, lest they should be considered exaggerated and insincere. Almost every other work on insanity (and I have read all, I believe, that deserve notice) left a conviction that the writers wore fetters; that, with every desire to investigate for themselves, they still held firmly in their astronomy to the one fixed idea that the sun moved round the earth; and that all, or almost all, looked on the mind as a *whole*, and were chiefly anxious to furnish the means of deciding whether it was disordered or not. Now if we consider the mind as the aggregate of the mental functions (which, unless we make the word synonymous with *soul*, we must do), to speak of it *as a whole* is almost a contradiction in terms, since minds not only differ in the nature of their ingredients or qualities, but in the quantity and number of them. The word *mind*, in the only sense in which it can come before the physician, is a congeries of phenomena, any one or many of which may be absent; there is, indeed, no one quality or function which may not be deficient, or absent, without the general observer attempting to deny that the individual still possesses *a mind*. The vast and unprecedented powers of a Newton form, in their aggregate, *a mind*; and the poor, imbecile, and arrogant animal who cannot even conceive or believe the existence of a Deity, has still *a mind*. The mighty genius which invented fluxions formed but a *mind*, and the poor savage who has not intellect enough to comprehend a number beyond five, or to make himself a hut to shelter him from the inclemency of the weather, has still *a mind*; if indeed you choose to give that name to a collection of mental faculties almost below that of the humblest quadruped.

The mysterious nature of some of the qualities with which that wonderful organ the brain is endowed, makes no difference in the simple fact, that all the faculties are the results of organization. That the organization may exist without those results flowing from it we know, for till God has "breathed into it the breath of life" it remains, however exquisitely constructed, but an inert mass of matter; and when it pleases the Divine power to withdraw the influence which gave it those faculties, it falls again into the mere clod of the earth, and is resolved into its elements.

But these considerations belong rather to theology; and in the examination of the physical structure of the brain, of its functions, and of the derangement of those functions, such inquiries are not necessary. We know the simple fact that all the manifestations of mind depend on physical structure; that every change therein is accompanied by a greater or less change in *the mind*; that its qualities, its sentiments, its opinions, its affections, its belief, its propensities, and its passions, are permitted to be influenced, strengthened, weakened, or perverted by disease in the physical structure of the system; that a blow on the head shall entirely alter the moral character of the individual; that slight inflammation of certain portions of its structure shall change modesty, reserve, and devotion, into blasphemy and obscenity; that a small spicula of bone, from the internal surface of the skull, shall transform love into hatred; that other diseases shall make the sober-minded man vain and silly, turn the hero into the coward, or the coward into the ferocious bully; shall make the tender mother destroy her own offspring, and the loving husband put to death the object of his long-tried affection. These are fearful subjects of contemplation, and there are few minds that would not be bewildered in the attempt to explain them, if they had not that absolute reliance on the ultimate mercy and justice of the Creator, which it is the purpose of religion to inspire. However mysterious and incomprehensible these apparent contradictions, the sincerely pious man has no fears and no doubts; he pursues the straight path of duty marked out for him, and leaves to the Deity alone the decision of the degree of guilt that stains the soul, from the performance of acts of wickedness uncontrollable by his own efforts. Theologians will surely allow that man will be held responsible only for the actions dictated by the healthy brain; and that when God has afflicted his creature with the disease which disqualifies him for correct judgment, He will not set down his bad actions to the great account. But I have treated this subject elsewhere in a mode that I hope will satisfy the most timid.

The existence of moral evil in the world has ever been a source of perplexity to the philosopher, but it seems no greater cause of embarrassment than the existence of physical pain. To see a poor innocent girl the subject of that terrific disease, *cancer*; to watch her tortures and her terrors month after month; to see the sunken face—the wasted frame—the haggard eye; to witness the patience, the reverent submission to the will of God, and resignation to unmerited suffering, and the humble hope that cheers the early death-bed; and then to pass, as I have so often done, to the contemplation of the bloated debauchee and drunkard, who, notwithstanding his detestable vices, retains the health which would seem to be incompatible with his excesses, sinking still deeper and deeper in the mire of sensual indulgences, and grudging the very necessaries of life to his dependents. It requires something stronger than philosophy to reconcile us to this unequal dispensation of worldly happiness.

My object in introducing these remarks is evident: it is my wish to make the subject interesting to the public; and although it is impossible to treat the matter otherwise than professionally, I still hope to make non-professional readers comprehend the object and the scope of my arguments, because it is my firm conviction that all our efforts to improve the treatment of the insane are vain, till the public mind is disabused of its erroneous prepossessions and prejudices on the subject of insanity, or disorder of the mind.

The following will be recognised by all those who have watched the delirious rapidity of thought which precedes some of the forms of insanity. The disorder may in many cases be prevented from advancing to that extent, and may be materially alleviated, or even entirely removed, by proper means; it is very often one of the forms of diffused gout.

"Bring the tea—tea comes from China—wall of China—wall, *mur*, *muraille*, difference between them in French—French habits—habit, a coat—long-tailed coats for soldiers—jackets—division of Spaniards into jacquitos and habitos—civil war—murder of Cabrera's mother—mother, a widow—

widows, suttee—incremation—Inquisition—Catholic faith—Pope of Rome—Capitol—Tarpeian rock—mode of punishing criminals—Central Criminal Court—Court of Victoria—visit to the King of France—Queen Bess—female sovereigns—lady who thought herself Mary Queen of Scots—Highland dress not ancient—introduced by an Englishman—Englishmen all over the globe—colonies best resource of the poor—new Poor Law—introduced by the Whigs—Whigs and Tories—origin of the names—surnames from trades—state of trade—Boards of Trade—Board of Green Cloth—green—composition of light—polarization—Poland—sympathetic nerve—nervous—strong and weak—nerves and muscles—poisoning from muscles—poisoning—Marchioness Brinvillier's wax-work figure—Burke and Hare—Italian boy—Savoy—Mount Cenis—climbing Mont Blanc—go higher in balloon—hydrogen gas—modern chemistry—alchemy—Scott's novels—new style of writing—printing has superseded writing—printing reports—cannon—attack on China—Afghanistan—progress of the British empire—emperor—Napoleon—snows of Russia—Russian leather—binding—Bodleian library."

Thus have I known more than once a recovered patient describe his thoughts, as with a rapidity in the succession ten times greater than can be represented by words; *screaming* with the agony of being unable *to stop them.*

This state resembles, in some respects, the common form of pervigilium, where an equal rapidity, not of *thought*, but *thinking*, takes place. The subjects are not just touched as in the above example, but each is for a few moments dwelt on and discussed; there is a regular transition in them, and they lead naturally one to the other. It is a frightful state, but rarely terminates in insanity. In one instance, a gentleman under my care (apparently in perfect health till worn down by the malady) was fifteen days without sleeping. He would get up in the night, and tire three horses with galloping, in the hope that excessive fatigue might compel sleep, but in vain. Ladurlad says:

> Lay on him the curse of the burning brain,
> And the curse of the sleepless eye.

Certainly one of the most awful afflictions which human nature can endure. I do not wonder that the sufferer sometimes takes refuge in suicide.

The course of ideas when (as I imagine) the two brains are in direct opposition, is sometimes like that represented in the following paragraph. Soliloquy does not strictly render the meaning, for it takes place with more rapidity in the presence of witnesses. I do not wish to be understood as affecting to give the exact words of a madman, for they are generally uttered with a rapidity that defies every attempt to write them down; but there was a time when I possessed an extraordinary power of remembering recent conversations, and after visiting patients the whole day, could have given not merely every word of every dialogue, but their succession. I believe, therefore, that a large part, if not the whole, of the following, is an exact transcript of what took place.

"1. You have heard of the insults to which I have been subjected—made to lie down at the word of command—I am a gentleman—2. The sun is my father—don't you see the rays of light from my head?—3. They bound me hand and foot to the bed—a gentleman, sir, through ten generations—Canaille—but I'll be revenged—4. I will rain down pestilence—dry up all their wells—give them *coup de soleil*—hats are nothing—burn them up—fry their brains—5. Wretches! to treat me in this manner—I was entrapped here—made to believe that I was going to an hotel in my own carriage—my own coachman that has lived with me twenty years—6. I'll rain down red-hot pokers on them—glorious vengeance—ha! ha! ha!—set fire to the woods—kill all the pheasants—7. Not trusted with my own gun—and you, sir, did you not give the certificate?—No, sir, I will not shake hands—it was treachery—basest treachery—8. I shall dine off a piece of lion—calves and lions—all the same—skins make carpets—all the books in my library began to dance—you've read the Battle of the Books—Queen Mab comes here—Shakspere is wrong—9. She is a great fat woman—they call her housekeeper—she is the only one who treats me with respect—my own little boy pretended to be frightened, and ran away from me—she never sits down in my presence—10. Shower-bath of oil of vitriol—send them to hell—the devil told me to kill myself—he's at my ear now—begone Satan—I defy thee."

It is useless to proceed with the incoherent rhapsody, which seems, at the first glance, to have no meaning whatever. Let the reader take the alternate passages which I have marked, and he will find that 1, 3, 5, 7, 9 form a tolerably continuous narrative of his injuries; while 2, 4, 6, 8, 10 are mere delusions. I confess myself utterly unable to explain these phenomena but on the theory of two brains. When the thoughts are distressingly discursive, it arises from both brains being occupied, and *not* on the same subject. When they are both employed consentaneously on one subject, the course is quite different, and *thinking* is an act of slow and laborious progression. It is not when we are studying, pondering, investigating, that we have the excessive rapidity of thought—such is, indeed, incompatible with the deep consideration in which we are occupying both brains with the same subject; the rapid shifting from one train of thought to another, is, in fact, the vivid and confused synchronism of the action of the two brains. It is not till we have reduced one of them to subjection and "acquiescence," that we are capable of commencing the process of deep reflection.

I feel quite satisfied that this "miraculous rapidity of thought" in the discursive exercise of the mind, is really the action of two brains; sometimes the ideas in one brain may be suggestive of ideas in the other, as well as in itself, and this may produce concurrent as well as alternate trains of thinking. Every man who has not been "fed on honey, and drank only rose water," but has tasted the bitters of life, must have felt this distressing balance of the mind, and how impossible it is to pursue any investigation, or arrive at any satisfactory conclusion, during the existence of such a state of cerebral excitement. Some persons find this form of pervigilium to be always produced by strong green tea; others experience the same effect from strong coffee; while others again find that these things increase their power of study. In general, the early stage may be subdued by a slight approach to intoxication with fermented liquors, which, by acting on both cerebra, supersedes, perhaps by substitution, the disordered discordant concurrence, and produces the requisite harmony of action essential to the prosecution of *study*.

"A medical gentleman for whom I have much respect, used often, when a student, to exercise his mental faculties to extreme fatigue; and in such states of exhaustion lost the power of perfectly commanding his attention, which was not only perceived by himself, in the want of power to continue his studies, but sometimes amusingly exhibited to his companions. On one occasion, when about to describe the situation of some town which he had visited, he spoke of it as being situated near the deltoid muscle." Thus far Dr. Conolly; now let us translate this into the language of duality.

The gentleman had been exercising what Dr. Conolly calls the *faculty* of attention for a long time; that is, he had been using the two brains concurrently and conjointly for the purpose of *study*. Subjected to equal labour, they were not equally exhausted—an obvious result from the usual difference of power in the two—like the difference which gives the superior skill of the right hand from the greater power of the left cerebrum. One of his brains carried on the conversation with his friends, imperfectly aided by the other, which from time to time reverted to the previous object of study; at momentary intervals the tongue was compelled to obey its influence, and in the case cited, gave the words "deltoid muscle," instead of the words "county of Warwick," which were dictated by the brain which was more especially occupied in conversation. The tongue could not obey the volitions of both brains at the same moment, but it gave them alternately. A similar imperfect concentration of cerebral functions, I think must have been experienced by every one; the few who have not felt it, at any rate have observed it in others: it is not till a physical or moral shock has completely dissipated the former train of thought that any emphatic attention, that is, any continuously concurrent action of the two brains, becomes practicable.

There is a form of mental disturbance, which every man accustomed to the society of the highly educated and the wealthy will easily recognise, and which exhibits the double mind in a very striking manner. Nothing can exceed the fidelity of the very graphic description of it given by Dr. Conolly. It is aggravated and confirmed, if not produced, by stimulating food and fluids—food highly concentrated and mixed with pungent condiments, such as is usually found at the tables of the rich. I think the disease is more common among the upper classes in Scotland than in England, from their habits of greater excess in drinking. The derangement of the mental functions comes on very slowly, unless there be, as in many of our aristocracy, an hereditary disposition to insanity produced probably originally by the same habitual indulgence, and the irritability of brain transmitted to the offspring. "These well known effects are curiously illustrative of the interruptions and modifications which a disordered body may cause in the manifestation of the mind, and of the external or corporeal indications of those effects. They are shewn most strongly in those who are constitutionally susceptible in a high degree of every kind of stimulus. Exempt perhaps for a time from all the vulgar consequences of excess, its stupor, its imbecility, its absurdity—they become the subjects of a series of mental and moral changes singularly amusing and curious. New intenseness is at first imparted to every sense, to every feeling, and to every faculty of the mind. A vivacity of attention, an incredible activity of memory, and an unwonted splendour of imagination, contribute to the delight of the individual and of those by whom he is surrounded. Nothing escapes him—every subject receives illustration from his lips—his observations on common things display unusual acuteness, his wit is irresistible and his sentiments are exalted. He marvels within himself that he is master of such vast and varied stores as are now revealed to him. From this state, which grave philosophers have condescended to speak of with praise, the step to that from which 'all consideration slips' is very short, and very soon made. *There seems to be an interval during which the man is composed of two beings contending for the ascendency*, and not being yet lost to reason, he is even somewhat amused to *trace the encroachments making by his imagination* over the natural strength of sensation and emotion."

All this is evidently drawn from nature, and is faithful to the minutest shade. I recognise the fidelity of the representation, but do not confine its origin to the cause stated. I have seen exactly the same train of symptoms, in a lesser degree, from a sudden accession of fortune, the accomplishment of some object of ambition, or from anticipation of happiness in an approaching union with the object of intense affection. I should, however, put the description of the *transition state* into other words, and am not without hope that, if Dr. Conolly honour these pages with a perusal, he may acknowledge the correctness of my hypothesis in the case.

No two parallel organs can be suddenly and equally affected by the same general cause—this is so true that it may be almost laid down as an axiom. The introductory stage in this, as in many other disorders, is one of increased activity of function gradually but rapidly progressing into disease. Now in the case just quoted, I should state the matter thus: The brain which is least disturbed is perhaps merely in a state of moderate excitement, and capable of observing correctly, though not of exercising control over the other, which is rapidly passing into what Dr. Holland happily terms "insubordination." The man is aware of his new mental powers, and feels himself in a manner two beings, consciousness being sometimes in one brain and sometimes in the other; he perceives so great a difference in his sensations and his judgments at different moments, that if he be in the slightest degree superstitious he considers the sensations and emotions of one of the brains as external to himself, and therefore the suggestions of a spirit, evil or good, as the case may be. I have heard a man in this state say, "My guardian angel I believe is taking upon himself the trouble to think for me. Such was the condition of the gentleman who destroyed himself, and whose case is already narrated. Gradually both brains partake of the disturbance, and then the insanity is almost established. The further series of events depends on the most capricious chance: "Accident now determines," says Dr. Conolly, "whether he quarrels with his best friend, or shakes hands a thousand times with a new one; slight provocations lead to high defiance, or soothing words produce tears and protestations of endless regard. Whatever temptation may assail him, whatever pleasure vice may offer him, or, in some cases, whatever crime may be proposed to him, he has little or no power of resistance left. . . . Throughout the progress to this dismal end, we see illustrations of the different degrees of mental impairment ending in complete but temporary insanity [exactly as in drunkenness], and it is perfectly plain that insanity begins at that stage in which comparison ceases to be exerted." The man is, in fact, now drunk, and conducts himself accordingly, and it matters not from what cause arises the state of brain which we recognise as intoxication—indeed this form of insanity is in every respect identical with that arising from spirituous liquors, except only in its origin and its duration.

Whatever may be the mode of action of fermented fluids on the nerves of the body, it is the effect produced on the brain which temporarily changes the mind and character of the individual; the impoverishment of the blood from the long continued suckling of a child, manifests itself in the brain, and consequently on the mind, in a manner almost identical with the indulgence in drinking, yet the origins are exactly opposite, and in this case a liberal allowance of wine removes it; and this effect on the brain and mind may doubtless be produced by many other causes. The result is insanity, varying no more in its modes than intoxication from excess in fermented liquids and stimulating food. One man becomes morbidly irritable and quarrelsome, another ludicrously affectionate, a third stupid, a fourth witty, a fifth obscene, a sixth sordidly avaricious, a seventh profusely generous, an eighth vain, a ninth silly, a tenth superstitious, and so on through every phase of real insanity; and we may almost pronounce that drunkenness is insanity and insanity intoxication.

Dr. Conolly goes on to say, that "in the common cases of defective judgment or erroneous opinion, of which few people in the world do not now and then exhibit instances, there is ordinarily no real impairment in the mental faculties, *but rather some carelessness or indolence in exerting them, or the comparing power alone is defective.*" Now I call this comparing power, or, as the phrenologists term it, exercise of the organ of comparison, the synchronous and concurrent action of both brains directed to one object, and cannot but think that this is more logically proved than the existence of a separate faculty of the mind called *attention*, contended for by many writers.

The "carelessness or indolence" depends generally on the want of that discipline which ought to have made attention easy and habitual, of which I have spoken in my propositions.

Dr. Conolly arrives at the conclusion that "insanity never exists without such an impairment of one or more of the faculties of the understanding, as induces or is accompanied by some loss of the power of comparison. The justness of this conclusion (says he) may now be tried by selecting different examples of insanity, in some of which one faculty, in some many are affected, and by observing whether or not the affection of one or more faculties would alone account for the insanity, or whether such affection is only followed by insanity when the comparing power begins to be injured; and whether the nature and extent of insanity depend on the nature and extent of that injury or impairment of comparison."

If comparison be the action of two brains concurrently exercised, it would seem to follow as a corollary that when one of them is destroyed there can no longer be comparison—that is, there can be no consciousness of consentaneity in the evidence afforded by the two brains, either in sensation or perception, or in pure exercise of the reasoning power; and that consequently, strictly speaking, one brain can *not*, as I have asserted, carry on *all* the functions of the intellect. I think this objection unfounded, for the following reasons:

No one imagines that when one brain is diseased to such an extent as to annihilate its functions, or is absolutely destroyed and absorbed, the individual can exercise the more intense functions of the mind—that he can guide the intricacies of a complicated suit at law, or follow out a new demonstration in mathematics with the same ease and precision that he would have done when in perfect health: the thing is a contradiction—his bodily health and mental powers are necessarily enfeebled by disease so formidable and extensive, and the man is "not himself." Nevertheless, in the same manner as we see that the eye, when its fellow is destroyed by cataract, and it has thus lost the power of measuring distances by the angle, becomes more and more perfect in measuring aerial perspective, and except in climates of extraordinary transparency, gradually makes to itself a mode of judging by a degree of distinctness of objects too minute to be cognizable by others; so in like manner I believe, or at least in a mode somewhat analogous, the single brain practises an attention to minutiae which was unnecessary when there were two healthy organs to enable the individual to judge with a facility resembling instinct. After the destruction of one brain, a man will give the most lucid instructions for his will, and make not merely a rational, but a sagacious disposition of his property. This may fairly be called an entire possession of his intellect, although the whole powers of the one brain would not have existed but for this gradual cultivation during the long and slow progress of the disease.

The alternations of sense and folly in some madmen seem to be no more than the alternations of delirium in patients subjected to intermittent disease. I knew the wife of a clergyman in Lincolnshire, a woman of very excitable and nervous temperament, who, during the hot paroxysm of ague, was always preposterously and ludicrously insane. I do not mean mere simple delirium; an hour afterwards, when the sweating stage came on, she recovered the entire possession of her faculties. There seems no reason why one brain should not, from some temporary cause, be for the time incapable of unison with its fellow, and so far incapable of comparison and judgment, and the patient therefore, in one sense, *mad*; but this is widely different from the disease that permanently, or for many months, produces the state of conscious or unconscious delusion, or from the state where the disturbance spreads to the other brain, and all power of correct judgment is lost.

I quote again from Dr. Conolly: "It is only on the supposition of the comparing power being lost that we are at all enabled to explain a phenomenon which can in no other way be accounted for, namely, that presented by a man labouring under an insane delusion and yet entertaining a belief entirely opposed to it, and of what is incompatible with the delusion, cherishing *two opposite sentiments in fact, or two opposite convictions at the same time*. . . . They will address those about them in harsh and cruel terms, and weep because they feel that they do so. A lunatic will say that he is very ill, but that it is strange he cannot persuade himself to believe it.

Truth and delusion seem in such circumstances contending for the mastery; but the strongest ally of truth, the power of making just comparisons, has deserted her standard, and unless her forces can be rallied, delusion finally gains the victory. . . . In this intellectual disorder, lunatics have committed atrocious crimes, feeling remorse even whilst committing them."

This figurative language is scarcely adapted to the discussion, and the author rarely gives way to it, although himself possessed of a vivid imagination. I would desire however no better proof that the two brains can carry on two *synchronous, opposing, concurrent* trains of thought, than is afforded by cases like these, of which I have seen several. On any other hypothesis they are utterly inexplicable; but once admit the fact, which it seems to me that I have demonstrated, that each brain is a perfect instrument of thought, feeling, and volition, and that when in a discordant state from disease the two give discordant impressions, and all the mystery vanishes. There is double mind—two minds, in fact—two identities; and consequently correct judgment or correct comparison, if the expression be preferred, is no longer possible. The victory of delusion over truth which Dr. Conolly speaks of is simply extension of disease to the other brain.

"If the practitioner," says Dr. Conolly, "is unacquainted with the varieties of the mind and their tendencies, and imagines that *insanity and sanity cannot be mixed up together in the mind as they are in the body*, he feels a degree of conscientious horror concerning any interference with an old gentleman who may be a little weak, but who he is quite convinced is no more mad than any of those about him." He then proceeds to describe the mischief that may arise from a neglect of coercion.

This is not the place to entertain and discuss the question of the exact point at which interference with the freedom of a man's actions shall become justifiable, but I beg to draw attention to the few words which I have put in italics. I do not hesitate to assert, in spite of the authority of Dr. Conolly, that sanity and insanity never co-existed in the same mind, that is, in the same brain. They may alternate almost as regularly as the successional symptoms of an ague. The duration of the fit of sanity or insanity may be prolonged, shortened, or anticipated and prevented by medical means, but the two states cannot co-exist in the same brain. The two brains, however, may not only *not* be in the same state, but they may be in opposing antagonist states; and this I conceive to be the true solution of the mystery which so often attracts our notice, of two opposing convictions, or that a man shall conduct himself with perfect correctness while conscious of being watched; but "if left to his own thoughts for a little while, and his attention not excited by those about him, his state will be evident enough; he will be seen to be wandering and lost in his recollections, will perhaps rise up and endeavour to make his way out of the room, without remembering the situation of the door, etc." That is, as I should explain the matter, he may by a vigorous effort of the sound, or comparatively sound, brain exercise temporary control over the other, and check its manifestations of imbecility; but when he thinks his object gained, he relaxes the painful effort, and shews the real state of his mind. Even in a state which no one calls insanity, or dreams of subjecting the patient to restraint, this different state of the two brains is observed—two minds, two convictions. "A mere catarrh will sometimes cause one ear to convey a different sound from that conveyed by the other; the same note, but in a different key; the same words, but as if from two voices, one an octave higher than the other. In paralytic patients all sensation is lost in one hand, one arm, or one half of the body. A patient told me that for a time after an attack of paralysis every thing appeared to him to be green; another said that he always seemed to have on one side of him a hill and on the other a deep pit. By others, I have known complaints made that all the objects on one side seemed to be quite close to them, in consequence of which they walked with a continual direction towards the side opposite." I give the above examples in the words of Dr. Conolly, as higher authority, although during the last forty years I have witnessed several similar examples. It is quite clear then, that in these cases one brain feels and reasons differently from the other; in the instance of paralysis we can ascertain which of them it is that acts wrongly, or does not act at all. There may be, as we know, also a difference in the news brought to the brain by the "up-train," as Mr. Barlow happily expresses it (*the nerves of sensation*), when the "down-train" (*nerves of volition*) performs its duty correctly; it is conceivable, and even highly probable *à priori*, that with both "trains" in due order other functions more stricty intellectual may be perverted in a similar manner in one brain, while the other remains perfect, and capable of fulfilling every exercise of a rational being. I proceed then to shew that such probable course of things is an established fact, and that from various causes one of the brains may entertain a conviction diametrically opposed to the convictions of the other; that such opposition may be shaded off through delusions, eccentricity, conscious delusion, and controllable delusion, into mere casual and temporary discrepancy, perfectly commanded by the will. Numerous examples of consciously imperfect self-control from double volition are cited by writers on insanity. To mention only a few:

A German girl, servant of Humboldt, who had charge of a child, entreated to be sent away, from fear that she should destroy it, as whenever she undressed it and noticed the whiteness of its skin, she was seized with an almost irresistible desire to tear it to pieces.

A young lady in a Paris asylum experienced, from time to time, a violent inclination to murder some one. On these occasions she always asked to have the straight waistcoat put on, and to be carefully guarded until the paroxysm was over, which lasted several days.

A celebrated chemist, of a mild and social disposition, committed himself a prisoner to an asylum to save himself from an intense desire to commit murder. Often prostrated himself before the altar to implore the Divine assistance to deliver himself from the atrocious propensity, of the origin of which he could give no account. He used on these occasions, when he felt the desire coming on, to ask to have his thumbs tied together—this was sufficient to restore his composure.

A countrywoman was seized with an intense desire to strangle her child, and she went out to get rid of the horrid thought, and went into a church to pray to be delivered from the frightful temptation; but every time she placed it in the cradle the same impulse came on, and was only prevented from passing into an act by the same means. Her time was passed in a constant struggle between the propensity to destroy and a dread of yielding to the impulse.

The wife of a butcher requested her husband to keep out of her sight, the knives used in the trade, and all the children, as she had an overpowering desire to destroy them.

Similar cases are innumerable. The phrenologist assumes the existence of an organ giving a propensity to destroy, and other organs restraining it; but how much more easily and rationally do the facts harmonize with my theory of two wills in two brains—a fact demonstrable and indisputable.

Dr. Burrows mentions the following case: "A lady of good family and most amiable character, aged forty-eight, with an hereditary predisposition, and who had been insane about twenty-five years before, became a good deal affected from a younger sister having suddenly manifested insanity. Shortly it was necessary to confine the elder to her room for the same cause. In a few days the younger sister, for want of due precautions, destroyed herself. The fact was concealed from the elder sister; but she likewise betrayed a suicidal propensity. She confessed the feeling and *reasoned upon it as an aberration of her mind*, and as sinful, and *entreated not to be trusted*. In fact, she made many attempts on her own life. She had many other delusions—one of which was, that *another woman was within her, and prompted her insane ideas and actions*. At times she was highly excited and would dance on the tables and chairs, tear her linen, and bite those about her, if permitted. . . . It was quite distressing to hear the occasional expression of her deep sorrow, that she was *unable to control her impious and immoral feelings and extravagant actions*."

If such cases as these, and others which I shall have occasion to cite, do not prove the existence of two minds—one in opposition to the other—of two volitions, concurrent and antagonist, quite independent of that kind of control exercised by the intellectual powers over the animal instincts—if all this fail to establish my propositions, then I must confess myself utterly unable to conceive the nature of moral proof, and connect the links of a chain of ratiocination.

Whatever may be the explanation offered by phrenologists, it seems to me that these cases are much more satisfactorily disposed of by attributing the conduct to disease of one brain, which on slight excitement gave ungovernable volitions, while the perfect brain was judging of and vainly endeavouring to restrain them—and that under such circumstances they are glad to be aided in their ineffectual efforts at self-command by positive coercion.

Similar instances of disturbed volition, attended by perfect consciousness that these irregular impulses are the effect of disease, are so common, that I should think there is hardly a practitioner who has not encountered examples of it.

I have met with more than one patient in private practice who would confess that his life had for many years been rendered completely miserable by the constant effort required to suppress these impulses, even when their manifestation tended only to acts of folly, and not of crime. A very active and meritorious clergyman, who expended a large portion of his small income in works of charity, told me in confidence that after hard study or want of rest, this double mind made him greatly apprehensive of insanity; and that often when preaching, there would seem to be placed before his eyes some profane book which the devil tempted him to read in lieu of his sermon. That the more he prayed for aid against the temptation, the more he found himself oppressed by it; and that at last he discovered that violent efforts for an hour with the dumb bells, or fencing, immediately before service, would entirely remove it. His great difficulty was to use the necessary exercise without attracting notice. A good gallop would have been the proper course, but the money which should have kept his horse he gave to the poor. A similar modification of diseased action in one brain controlled by the other is found in the propensity which some persons with a tendency to insanity possess, to blaspheme at church, and interrupt the most solemn part of the service by violent or obscene language. Such impulses are not known to others till they become ungovernable, but they exist in a slighter degree in some who are called sane. It has often, very often, fallen to my lot to listen to such communications. Perhaps other practitioners have been equally the depositaries of these unhappy confidencies, and they, like myself, suppose themselves peculiarly situated in this respect. I firmly believe that I have anticipated and prevented more than one case of double action of brain in the milder forms of hypochondriasis from terminating in positive insanity. I regret that our clergy no longer practise the duty enjoined by the Rubric, of listening to and encouraging the spontaneous confessions of their communicants, which they seem to abstain from, like Jack in the Tale of a Tub, lest they should have any resemblance to Peter. If endowed with a moderate share of knowledge of cerebral physiology and pathology, they might do incalculable good by turning over to the physician *in its curable stage* a malady which, from lost time, is almost entirely unmanageable when entrusted to medical care. I am not without hopes that even the present work may tend to produce a greater accord between the two professions on the practice to be pursued in such cases, which are found most frequently among the most virtuous, most amiable, and most interesting of human beings.

I could give numerous cases illustrative of this propensity, but foresee that my book will be much larger than I had planned it, and therefore abstain. I will only mention one, of which the circumstances are rather remarkable. A young gentleman of ancient family and historical name, of good general disposition and fair though neglected education had an ungovernable propensity to run up into an organ-loft in the middle of divine service and play some well-known jocular tune, attached perhaps to profane or indecent words. This he would do so suddenly, that it was impossible to prevent it before he had thrown the congregation into confusion. He was always sorry for it, and declared that he tried with all his might to prevent it; and he always abstained from going near a church in service time, though he would read the prayers at home with apparently sincere and tranquil devotion. If he accidentally passed an open church door, the temptation was irresistible, and he often got himself into serious embarrassment by indulging these freaks. He conversed with coherence and rationality, and in all other respects was perfectly sane; but he was subject to periodical epileptic fits, and the propensity was at last traced to connexion with this malady. Many years elapsed in this very mild and equivocal form of mental disturbance; he went abroad, and I lost sight of him, but was informed that he entered into great sexual excesses and sensual indulgence, his fits became more and more aggravated, and he at last died of what his friends called brain fever. The persons who attended him at the last moments knew nothing of his previous history, and the brain was not examined.

The moral object which Dr. Conolly seems to have had in view in his "*Inquiry concerning the Indications of Insanity*," was to exempt from the tender mercies of the law persons who, although eccentric in their habits and incapable of exercising all the mental faculties in due order and subordination, were yet possessed of sufficient self-control to avoid injuring others or themselves, which he very justly considers to be the boundary of the right of interference on the part of society.

I extract the following passage from his work, describing one of the forms of imperfect mind much more common than is generally supposed; but the alarm and consternation which it excites when it is only a temporary ailment, and the fear of being treated as insane, induce the patient to confine his confessions to a confidential medical friend; the public rarely hear of the malady. I have known a similar temporary form of disorder in rather a slighter degree to be apparently caused by a collection of wind in the stomach, and instantly relieved by the expulsion of it. Whether the influence of the pneumogastric nerve was, on this occasion, direct or recurrent; whether the brain disordered the stomach, or the stomach the brain, I do not pretend to decide. I have a strong opinion in favour of the latter explanation.

"A gentleman of considerable attainments, after long-continued attention to various subjects, found himself incapable of writing what he sat down to write; and wishing to write a cheque, could get no further than the first two words; he found that he wrote what he did not mean to write, but by no effort could write what he intended. This impairment of his memory and attention (1) lasted about half an hour, during which time his external senses were not impaired, but the only ideas he had *were such as imagination dictated* (2) without order and without object. He knew also, during this time, that when he spoke, the words he uttered were not the words he wished to utter (3). When he recovered, he found that in his attempt to write the cheque, he had, instead of the words, 'fifty dollars, being one half-year's rate,' put down 'fifty dollars through the salvation of Bra——,' but could not recollect what train of ideas had suggested the latter words, or what their meaning had been."

Now if I am correct in supposing that attention and memory (1), that is to say, memory in the sense of *voluntary recollection*, which is the faculty here spoken of, and which is quite distinct from the tranquil and spontaneous recurrence of bygone ideas—if I am correct in asserting that these two faculties are the voluntary concentration of both brains to the same subject, then it is easy to conceive that they should be impracticable while one of the brains was in a state of insanity—for true insanity it was, however temporary. The ideas suggested by this disordered organ were "such as imagination dictated" (2), that is, the sound brain was incapable of overpowering the diseased suggestions; "the words he uttered (3) were not the words he wished to utter." There was only one organ of speech, and it was compelled to obey the most tyrannic of the two discordant influences. Is not this an exact representation of the commencement of insanity, where the patient gives utterance to two trains of thought in the form of a colloquy? *The suggestions of the devil, the possession by an evil spirit,* are also merely different forms of this species of mental disturbance. In the case of Mr. Percival, which I have considered elsewhere, and in that of the gentleman who struck his head against the sofa, related by Dr. Holland, and indeed in a great number of other cases, the imaginary voices were supposed to be of several individuals. A slight difference from time to time in the imaginary pitch or tone of the diseased sensation, or rather of the imaginary voice the effect of such diseased sensation, will explain this.

The great *medical* object of Dr. Conolly seems to have been to shew the gradual loss or perversion of parts of the mind while the remainder was capable of all its ordinary exercises—in fact, to remove that line of demarcation, that imaginary boundary, between the sane and the insane, which has hitherto been the great stumblingblock in the way of medical jurisprudence. Had the public the same conviction as to bodily health, that every man is necessarily *well* or *ill*, and that there is no intermediate state, it would produce a similar confusion. We should be legislating about the right of a man to walk out of doors, or the necessity of compelling him to stay in bed. Men admit that the division into *well* and *ill* cannot be always made; yet, in general there is little difficulty in applying the terms. It is the same with illness of the brain, or insanity.

Dr. Conolly appears to resolve real insanity into the inability to exercise the faculty of comparison—that when he can no longer *compare*, the man is mad. I think, however, that it is hardly just to limit the faculty thus exercised by a word of so narrow a meaning; and that the word "comparison," in the sense he uses it, is really and truly synonymous with judgment. When a man can no longer exercise judgment, there is no question that he is of unsound mind; but the degree of judgment which shall constitute mental health must still be a matter of opinion, in which different persons will entertain different opinions, and the boundary is thus again transparent and invisible. It seems to me that comparison is the very essence of all *judgment*, and that it composes, either with physical evidence or with memory, the whole of the mental operation. Thus the distinction seems of impossible definition; although the cases which admit of doubt must be exceedingly rare with a man of mature experience and knowledge. Unless, indeed, the word "comparison" include judgment, it amounts to nothing. The indication of imperfect mind in persons who are always seeing a likeness when there is no resemblance, is still comparison—defective or erroneous comparison; but as the judgment is incorrect, we certainly do not consider that kind of comparison a proof of sanity. Comparison, then, in the sense in which Dr. Conolly uses the word, must be held, I think, to mean *correct judgment*, which, if a man possess, he is certainly not insane.

This comparison or judgment cannot well be made truly,

unless both brains are healthy and act consentaneously; but one of them alone may exercise the faculty to a limited extent, and be even conscious that the other brain is not in harmony with it, and that its conclusions cannot be depended upon; that is, there are erroneous impressions on the senses or erroneous ratiocination in one brain which the other is capable of correcting—conscious delusion of the senses, as in the case of Nicolai and Dr. Bostock; consciously defective ratiocination, as in the clergyman with two convictions. The sound brain is, however, not capable of any but the simplest mental operations, for want of the aid of its fellow-labourer.

CHAPTER XVIII: *Apology for Quoting Largely from Established Writers; Long Case of Moral Insanity from Dr. Pritchard; Remarks Thereon; Danger of Allowing Large Latitude to Equivocal Responsibility; Progress of Depravity; Other Cases from Dr. Pritchard; Dr. Hawkins; Early Inference Drawn by Myself from Similar Cases*

The references I am now about to make are essential to the train of reasoning. Were I to refer to the passages without citing them textually, the reader could not be expected to take the trouble of turning to the originals, even if he had them in his possession. There are few medical men, still fewer of the public, whose library has an ample supply of works on insanity. Men look on these works, and with some reason, as uncertain guides through the wilderness of mind—each professing that his own road is the straightest and the shortest, but none of them leading completely out of the marshes and quagmires of doubt and embarrassment, and placing us on solid ground, in a clear and well-defined open country.

I make this apology for inserting the following case from Dr. Pritchard's little work "*On the different Forms of Insanity.*" The reader is requested to bear in mind the letters of reference.

"Mr. W., aged about forty, was a corn-dealer and baker, a man of mild and retiring disposition; steady in business, regular and domestic in his habits—highly conscientious—religious, without ostentation—correct and cautious in his conversation, and kind and benevolent to all persons. His health was considered to be delicate, but he was never ill; and he avoided great exertion, feeling himself not equal to it. He was a married man, and had several children, of whom he was very fond. He experienced some severe losses in business, which weighed heavily on his mind, and he became exceedingly depressed. He made great efforts to recover himself from his despondency, and exerted himself with the view of recovering for his family what he had unavoidably lost. He was to a great extent very soon rewarded for his efforts.

"It was shortly afterwards observed by his friends that his increased exertions had improved his spirits, which it was remarked had become much more elevated than they were previous to his depression. He now began to extend his business, in which he was become more keen; he displayed more acuteness in buying and selling, and seldom trusted to others anything he could accomplish himself, and he was ever watchful of an opportunity to make purchases, or to effect sales to his advantage. These changes in his habits went on until the character of industry appeared to his friends to be over-performed, and they feared that he indulged something like unnecessary exertion and anxiety, and that his excessive activity of body and mind would destroy his health. (A) His journeys became longer and more frequent, and his nights were greatly shortened; and he was often absent from his accustomed place of worship on Sundays. After some months had passed, and while these changes were going on, his family ventured to remark to him that such extended journeys to transact uncertain business withdrew his attention from that at home, which was regular and profitable.

"For the first time he was then observed to speak in a tone of voice, and with an expression of feeling which had never belonged to him. (B) Still his family and friends had no fear of madness, but entertained a dread lest he should overstep the line of security in business, or undermine his bodily health by excessive exertion. His temper, which was naturally so mild, from this time grew hasty and irritable; he became incapable of bearing an opinion opposite to his own, and was irritated if a check was offered to his present proceedings. (C) Still he prosecuted the same scheme of business, without as yet deviating from his course; he extended, but did not alter his plans; and thus were more than ten months disposed of. A change now became manifest in his feelings towards his family; he frequently spent his evenings in the society of others rather than in that of his wife and children. (D) He spoke in approbation of all that he saw elsewhere, and found innumerable objections to what was done at home. His children were less engaging and intellectual than those of his neighbours, and his wife's domestic arrangements were less complete, and he was evidently less attached to her. He was at the same time in the habit of indulging freely in stimulating drinks, to which he had never been accustomed, and excused himself under the plea that his great exertions required support. (E) He became addicted to strange women, and the fact being brought home to him by his wife, brought on the crisis which had been long approaching. Having given vent to the most passionate expressions, and threatened violence of a serious character, he quitted his home, forsook his family and his business, wandered about the country, sleeping in the open air, and subsisting by the meanest artifices. (F) His friends at length found him, and consigned him to my care. Twelve months had fully elapsed from the time when they perceived a change in his natural habits.

"When I received him, the expression of his countenance was animated and lively. Great activity was indicated by the quickness of his eye, but the unsteadiness of his looks, together with a quivering smile playing about his lips, marked it as an activity without object or motive. His face was pallid, the conjunctiva finely injected, the pupil contracted; the head was hotter than the rest of the body, and the hair, which was thin, was crisp; the tongue was foul, and the bowels constipated; the hands and feet were colder than the rest of the body, and the former had that soft feel peculiar to the highly nervous; the pulse was slower than natural, feeling full and bounding, but it could be compressed, and the current of blood checked by the slightest pressure. The respiration was tranquil and regular, slow, and scarcely perceptible by looking at the chest. (G) In conduct and manner he was anxious; eager to be doing something; moving from place to place without apparent object; transferring every article of furniture that was moveable; abounding in speculations and new projects; proposing long journeys to be executed in haste; talking incessantly, but coherently, and for the most part rationally, upon a great variety of subjects. He used no expression of antipathy against his family, nor indeed against any person, but it was evident that the mention of his wife and children greatly increased his agitation. He had no fixed notion which influenced his conduct, and *no delusive ideas.* When addressed on the subject of his situation, he was fully aware of the place he was in, and knew the reason of his confinement. He attached no blame to any one for placing him under my care, and admitted that he had felt unlike himself for some months, but had flattered himself that his health was improved, and that his increased spirits were the legitimate consequences of this and of his improved finances. He was conscious of his conduct to his family, but neither blamed nor extenuated it. (H) On business he would converse most rationally, but if the opportunity had presented itself, would have expended his money in useless purchases (?). He was capable of making the nicest calculations connected with his own affairs, and was correct in all his dates when speaking to a second person; but when left to himself, his conduct and language were absurd in the extreme. (I) This person perfectly recovered in three months.

"I give this case," says Dr. Pritchard, "as one in which the deviation from healthful and natural habits was complete, and brought about in the most gradual manner. It is worthy of remark, from the momentary conviction which the individual obtained of his state when he ceased to direct his own movements and to be his own master. He often told us—after his recovery—that the idea that *he had been mad for some time* flashed across his mind at the moment he entered the establishment.

"Simple as this case is, and it is one of the most simple that we meet with, we yet find associated in it all the forms of moral debasement. Simple over-excitement was the commencement of the disorder; but a change in the habits of life and temper, a prostration of the natural feelings and affections, a loss of the sense of moral rectitude (J), and a complete deprivation of self-control, gradually followed. Of this description of cases I have met with very many instances, not among those who have fortunately been treated as insane, but among such as, remaining at large, have gone from one misfortune to another, till they have become beggared in estate and reputation, and sunk at length into a loathsome gaol or wretched workhouse."

Now I wish to speak of a man like Dr. Pritchard with all the respect that his great experience and various attainments so justly deserve; but I venture to say that to call this a case of insanity is a perversion of terms. If this man were mad, then there are a hundred thousand men in this nation who walk the earth unshamed, if not unblamed, and fulfill some of the highest offices, who are still madder than he, and yet pass on, unsuspected of mental derangement. Do I dispute the propriety and the justice of restraint in such cases? Assuredly not. I have already spoken of this form of disorder—if it can be so called—and shall here make it the subject of more detailed consideration.

It is, in fact, an exceedingly instructive example of mental disturbance, which is the very strongest term it deserves, and from the mode in which that expression is generally used, it is indeed almost too strong for the occasion. Let us examine it from the commencement, and see how it applies to the theory of the duality of the mental functions.

This man cannot be said to have lost the command over his volitions—he was to the last a responsible being; and, had his misconduct broken a positive law would have been justly liable to punishment.

He begins by excessive exertion to repair his losses, and, finding himself successful in his efforts, becomes more than usually cheerful, and probably enjoys better health in consequence of the change in his habits from a domestic occupation in an unhealthy atmosphere—as is necessarily the residence of a baker—to an out-of-doors life and *frequent* change of air—one of the most important of medical means. He feels the pleasure of the change, loses his domestic habits, and finds more gratification in varied society than in the monotony of home; forms probably some improper attachment, and in the early remorse of incipient guilt, becomes anxious and uncomfortable, and gives the impression to his friends that his unaccustomed exertions are more than his health will bear. (A) He absents himself more and more from his family, and feeling ill at ease, becomes irritable and peevish. (B) Loses his relish for home, and tries to persuade himself that he has valid excuses for his conduct; absents himself from his domestic circle, where all tends to remind him that he has lost his own respect. (C) Tries to drown his self-reproach in intoxication. (D) Becomes more and more indifferent to character; engages in gross sexual debauchery; and when reproached with his misconduct (E) is violent and abusive, and abandons his home. (F) Becomes reckless and a vagabond.

This is the common regular progress of depravity, and shews no other sign of insanity than is inherent in all vicious conduct. His brain becomes irritated and ungovernable through drinking, and one cerebrum necessarily gives way before the other, as in the case with all cachexial disorders—indeed it is scarcely possible to adduce an example of a general disease affecting equally and simultaneously the two halves of the body. The disorder gradually spreads to the other cerebrum, though only in a very slight degree; and the pressure of any powerful motive added to its resolves, enfeebled by drinking, would have sufficed to re-establish its command. This is prevented by his confinement in a lunatic asylum, where the absence of intoxicating fluids allows his brain to recover its health. (G) He uses no expression of antipathy against his wife and children, but the mention of them naturally agitates him with remorse for his conduct; his conscience is not yet seared, and having now the comfortable excuse for his past actions—the plea of insanity—he takes courage, has the grace not to palliate or justify his conduct, but quietly let the thing take its course. (H) When he is alone he *lets himself down*, and talks absurdly—not incoherently, be it remembered; but the trouble of controlling the still irritable brain by its fellow, scarcely yet recovered from the effects of habitual drinking, is more than he will put himself to the pain of exercising *when there is nobody by.* However, being debarred from drink, and compelled to lead a steady, sober, and quiet life, he is re-established in three months.

I cannot think, with Dr. Pritchard, that there was any other prostration of the natural feelings and affections than is common to all bad husbands, nor any loss of the sense of moral rectitude, although he had ceased to practise it, for he never attempted to justify his conduct.

Thousands and thousands of husbands go through all these phases without any one suspecting them of insanity; but I agree with Dr. Pritchard, that could a law be enforced to put such persons in restraint, many a family would be saved from degradation and ruin. It is a case of what the common people call "madness spelt with a *b*"—badness.

I have elsewhere spoken of the ancient "*Lettres de Cachet;*" originally as reasonable, as just, and as fairly exercised, as the "injunction" of the Lord Chancellor of England. Under a despotic government such a power became abused, like every other irresponsible exercise of authority, but in this country, with a jealous and vigilant press, there is no more danger of its being unfairly exerted than any other arbitrary act of the Lord Chancellor. We allow him to violate the most sacred feelings of human nature, and take away innocent children from a vicious father, and yet we will not allow him to take a vicious father from a virtuous wife and innocent children. Unless there exist the only sacred thing in the eye of "Equity," *property*, he is not allowed to interfere at all. *Poor* souls may go to the devil at their own good pleasure—*de minimis non curat lex*. Property, indeed! Property is a sacred thing souls may be damned without the intervention of the law.

The case I have just related is by no means unique. Many a medical man must have been placed once or more in his life in the painful position of being compelled to decide on the moral responsibility of an individual convicted of some gross offence, who had hitherto maintained an irreproachable conduct. Unless the physician's mind have been previously well exercised in the consideration of such possible contingencies, he will not only be unable to satisfy his own conscience, but he will not satisfy others and preserve his own character. The cases are sometimes exceedingly equivocal and embarrassing.

"Persons (says Dr. Pritchard) who had reached a considerable age with unimpeached reputation, and were highly esteemed by all their friends and neighbours as men of probity and high respectability, have displayed a total subversion of character; they have become loose in their morals, depraved, reckless, and devoid of all moral principle. An elderly gentleman, whose history was lately described to me by a near relative, had an attack of paralysis which affected his intellects; this he survived—his intellectual faculties were restored, but his character appeared afterwards to have become thoroughly altered. He was absurd and capricious in the highest degree; and in order to carry into effect the schemes which he laid down for himself, he declined no means, however nefarious—would break through the most solemn engagements and tell the most palpable lies, making at the same time high professions of devotion and strict attention to religious duties. Another gentleman, who had been for many years a magistrate, and was highly respected in his neighbourhood, became at a later period of his life an altered man, and addicted himself to all sorts of evil practices; the change in his character was a matter of common notoriety and common wonder. He continued during the remainder of his life, or to a late period of it, to be considered a worthless, depraved person, lost to all sense of shame and propriety. Some traits of eccentricity were observed in his conduct, but these never gave rise to the notion that he was insane till after his death, when so many singular particulars were discovered, that the suspicion of mental derangement gained ground among his acquaintance." And, is that all?

The writer is rather too ready to allow this excuse of insanity in cases of perverted moral conduct. It is a dangerous doctrine to promulgate; and it behoves every man to be cautious of countenancing such a feeling, for if it were generally prevalent it would dislocate the whole frame of society. With deference for the opinion of Dr. Pritchard, I cannot think that any one of the three cases of depravity can be justly allowed the shelter of irresponsibility. In the first of the two cases just cited, I would so far admit the influence of disease as to acquiesce in the belief that the paralysis had injured that brain which had been accustomed to exercise control over the other, and thus made him in some degree incapable of resisting temptation. In a court of justice, if he were on trial for positive crime, I would certainly have laid full stress on the effect of the disease, but am by no means sure that the man deserved the same consideration on the part of his friends and relatives; and I should have given a very doubtful testimony before a commission of lunacy, believing that in the former case it is the duty of a medical man to lean to the side of mercy and risk the escape of the guilty, and in the latter to promote personal restraint—it being virtually of no importance whether the defective self-command depend on want of will or want of power—the subjection to confinement being a slight evil, and, strictly speaking, no injustice, although the insanity were doubtful; but in the other it behoves us to be almost *more* than certain before we condemn a man to infamy.

In the second case, as in the instance of the corn-dealer, I cannot see any ground for exoneration. Among the very wealthy and the very indolent, similar examples of depravity are common; and I have often felt disgust and indignation at the toleration by the public, of the grossest criminality in such persons;—indeed, of the most impudent defiance of decency and decorum, which, in one of humbler station or scantier fortune, would have been visited by the severest censure, or perhaps would have justly incurred condign punishment. In the great majority of cases the parties have been habitually vicious, till impunity has brought about its natural consequence—carelessness in precautions; and it is the exposure alone which is sudden, not the depravity. Unless the symptoms of cerebral disease can be clearly ascertained, it is highly probable that the previous good conduct was only masterly hypocrisy.

The qualifying circumstances which attenuate the guilt of those who have been habitually correct in their moral conduct, with occasional, but not excessive, variations, are spoken of hereafter. I would sum up with the advice to a young medical man: always to lean towards impunity, when the person is accused of crime in a court of justice, but to lean towards restraint in a commission of lunacy. It is God alone who knows the absolute truth. No doubt many a sane man has been led into the commission of serious crime suddenly, on the accidental combination of numerous improbable contingencies presenting to him an overpowering accumulation of motives, who, in his deliberate moments, would have contemplated the crime with abhorrence, and would not have believed it possible that he could ever be guilty of it.

The infallible Court of Appeal is not in this world!

The following cases are cited by Dr. Pritchard. Several similar instances of double volition in things less criminal, as well as things atrocious, have come within my own knowledge; but I prefer to give these striking examples from authority already recognised, and can only express my surprise that a writer so well informed could have missed the inference which seems to arise so naturally from the premises.

"A countrywoman, twenty-four years of age, of a bilious, sanguine temperament, of simple and regular habits, but reserved and sullen manners, had been ten days confined with her first child, when suddenly, having her eyes fixed on it, she was seized with the desire of strangling it. This idea made her shudder; she carried the infant to its cradle and went out in order to get rid of so horrid a thought. The cries of the little being who required nourishment recalled her to the house. She experienced still more strongly the impulse to destroy it. She hastened away again, haunted by the dread of committing a crime of which she had such horror. She raised her eyes to heaven, and went into a church to pray. This unhappy mother passed the whole day in a constant struggle between the desire of taking away the life of her infant and the dread of yielding to the impulse," etc.

Dr. Hawkins relates the following:

"E. B., a young and hitherto healthy woman, the mother of two children—in humble life, but not in indigence—applied at the Hitchin Dispensary, in consequence of the most miserable feelings, accompanied by the strong and almost irresistible propensity (or temptation, as she termed it) to destroy her infant. This feeling first came upon her about a week before, when the child was a month old; and she was now sunk into an extreme state of dejection, and she beggd to be continually watched, lest she should yield to this strange propensity."

Now, to destroy one's own child is not a natural propensity which can be assigned to a separate phrenological organ, even if there be one; it is not an instinct; it is not an animal impulse; it is no part of the natural mind, requiring, like the sexual and other propensities, to be constantly watched and controlled, and prevented from passing into excess, by the exercise of the higher intellectual powers. It is a diseased action of a whole brain, which cannot at the same moment have this propensity and a wish to prevent it; cannot be in two opposite and antagonist states at the same moment; the thing is a manifest contradiction in terms, and as impossible as that yesterday should come after tomorrow; but it is very possible that as one brain alone is a perfect organ of thought, feeling, sentiment, and volition, one brain may have the morbid propensity from disease or disorder, and the other be perfectly healthy and occupied in watching and controlling the insane desire. All this seems to me so clear, so perfectly conclusive and satisfactory, that I really cannot conceive the state of mind which could refuse assent. One brain *can* act alone—one brain *does* act alone in the ordinary business of life, in *my* opinion. It is proved that it does so when the other is destroyed: there is no other mode of explaining the matter without arbitrary assumptions which shock the reason; and this mode explains it entirely.

For more than forty years I have been familiar with the manifestations of disordered intellect, having at a very early period of my life had an opportunity of watching the phenomena. This form of unhealth always presented great attractions to my curiosity, even before I became acquainted with the structure of the brain, and while I was chiefly impelled to observe such cases by a superstitious interest. I cannot remember the period when I did not notice two volitions and two minds, nor could I even in my earliest years accept the solution which at that time explained every phenomenon so satisfactorily; namely, that the devil was speaking as well as the sufferer, and that the dialogue which the maniac carried on was between that personage and his own soul. I have a vivid recollection of many of these monologue dialogues when I was only sixteen years of age, and can perfectly remember the *gush* of convictions which took possession of my mind about five-and-thirty years ago, when, having learnt the anatomy of the brain in the imperfect mode in which it was then taught, I was all at once convinced of the truth of my present propositions; not perhaps to the full extent I now enounce them, but quite satisfied of the existence of two minds, though unable and indeed unwilling to work out the theory, because of the unsatisfactory moral corollaries which seemed to be attached to it, of which I have already spoken in the introduction. Whether I may convince others depends on many other things besides the truth of my doctrines. I have myself no more doubts on the subject than of the circulation of the blood.

It would be easy for me to cite examples which have come under my own observation, and which all tend to confirm my doctrine; but, knowing how little I have myself been inclined to place confidence in the assertions of unknown writers, I do not bring them forward. The unsupported narratives of men not attached to a public institution, and who, therefore, can give no guarantee for their veracity, still less for their exemption from prejudice and partiality, weigh very little with the profession, at least with such of them as choose to reason only on premises thoroughly established by educated and competent observers, and who look on all argumentation as pure waste of time, till the data are past dispute. Such is my own feeling, and I take for granted that a similar feeling pervades others. It is for this reason that I have made so large a use of the testimony of men already known to the profession. Should my present work excite attention, I cannot but think that there is, throughout, a vein of honesty which will induce the public to give me credit for sincerity and truth. Should my speculations be accepted as well founded, I have many corollaries to draw, and applications of the theory to work out, in medicine, morals, jurisprudence, education, and the management of criminals; on which it would be useless to enter till I know whether my doctrine be admitted or rejected.

CHAPTER XIX: *Progress of Insanity; Unimportance of the Mode in which it is Manifested; Varieties in the Condition of the Blood; Miracles; False Perceptions; Nature of Insanity; Catalepsy; Ganglionic System; Rarity of Insanity; Moral Reflections*

I must not be supposed to assert that, because disease of one brain is a cause of conscious delusion, and the extension of it to the other a cause of unconscious delusion or insanity, that this is the general and uniform origin of mental aberration. On the contrary, we sometimes see extensive disorganization of one brain without any delusion whatever. Disease of what are called the convolutions of the brain even is by no means necessarily accompanied by important error, either in the special senses or in the reasoning powers. The organs being dual, the functions are taken up by the healthy brain; and, as in the ordinary exercise of them only one brain is energetically used, the transposition does not attract notice. It is only when we want to use both of them, in the act of study or serious consideration, that we perceive the defect; and as such defect sometimes takes place from temporary causes, as gout, etc., we are conscious only that there is "something wrong in the head," as it is usually expressed, which produces the confusion of mind. A great number, and indeed a large proportion, of cases of insanity manifest, on dissection, inflammation and thickening of membranes, effusion of water, tubercles, abscess, cancer, softening, atrophy, paralysis, ulceration, tumours, and various other diseases; but these latter are rather to be considered as concomitants or sequents, than causes; since we know that an alteration of structure so minute as to be sometimes incognizable by the eye shall be sufficient to destroy the mind, or pervert one or more of its faculties; although the destruction of the mind, or of the power of reasoning correctly, is by no means incompatible with life—for we have examples of men remaining insane for more than half a century, and enjoying good health during the whole period. Decidedly, however, the tendency of the disease which destroys the intellect is generally towards those disorganizations which destroy life; and there is no disease, local or remote, which may not have the effect of producing insanity. I have elsewhere pointed out the circumstances under which alone we can hope to obtain positive information on the seat and extent of the disease which is incompatible with sound mind.

The want of the due influence of a healthy brain on the vital organs to which its nerves are distributed, or from which they arise, renders some insane persons liable to a great number of diseases, and completely removes the old conviction, that the mad and the gouty live longer than the average. Offices for the insurance of lives never partook of the delusion, and continue to reject steadily all who cannot prove themselves exempt from such maladies.

From the reciprocal influence of the brain and the internal organs, it is not extraordinary that diseases of each should affect the other, as we shall have an opportunity of noticing when we come to explain why one brain only should be first affected by causes which are common to both halves of the body.

I speak now only of the first stage of insanity; for it is pure waste of time and thought to discuss incurable diseases, of the nature of which we can really know nothing till after death. We only know that the brain is *spoilt*, and that is all that is of importance; for in this stage we might as well attempt to reduce the boiled white of an egg to its original transparency as to restore the reason.

In the first stage then, the *form* it shall assume is of very trifling importance. When the friends of a patient wish us to listen to a long detail of the fancies that occupy the mind of a person in the delirium of fever, or the commencement of insanity, we may reply, "Of what importance is it to know the detail? all that is required is to ascertain the fact of the discourse being rational and coherent, or not." If supposed to be the erroneous judgment of a sane mind, one might attempt to reason with the invalid; but if it be cerebral disturbance, such a proceeding would be absurd. Much stress is generally laid on the estranged affections of the patient; but if the natural and healthy action of the brain be that of affection towards the wife or child, what more obvious than that the altered *action* should be altered *affection?* and why should this be of more importance than the dislike of a sick man to some article of diet for which he had previously a great relish?

There is one observation to be carefully made whenever the case comes under treatment sufficiently early, but this rarely happens—namely, to notice whether, in moments of peculiar but temporary tranquillity, there is a clear conception of things as they are and a reasonably sound judgment formed of them, and especially if the patient suspect that he is possibly under delusion. If this be the case, then I consider that one brain only is diseased; and that, independent of all the medical means in our power to remedy an impoverished blood as after excessive lactation—or unhealthy blood as in cachectic diseases—or an excess of acid in the blood as in rheumatism—or an excess of alkali as we sometimes see spontaneously, and exactly similar to that produced by long continued use of the liquor potassae for the cure of gravel—or that peculiar state of the blood caused by the continued use of pork (well known to experienced practitioners)—or the dissolved state of blood from confinement to salt-meat and inability to obtain vegetable food, as in scurvy (which very much resembles the alkaline state spoken of above)—or in purpura—or gouty matter in the blood in a state of solution, of which we have abundant proof—or imperfectly elaborated blood, from dyspepsia—or blood defective in fibrine and red particles, as after excessive hemorrhage. All these states, and many others well known to every observer, besides such alterations and changes as are the subject of legitimate inference, though not universally acknowledged, are to be noted and acted on; and every reasonable attempt made to remove the disordered states which we know to be frequent causes of insanity, and always aggravations of it. Besides the use of all known methods of curing the physical disorder, there should be a careful selection of all the motives that can be assembled—even sometimes, though very cautiously, *fear*—to induce the sounder brain to exercise and strengthen its power over the other.

That mysterious and incomprehensible thing, the *will*, has, we know, an important influence on the whole animal economy, and many instances have come before us where it has staved off insanity; others where it has aided in restoring health. I will cite a case which is well known to me and which exemplifies this action, although unconnected with insanity. A celebrated man of literature, dependent for his income on the labours of his pen—feeding his family,as he jocularly calls it, out of an inkstand—was in the advanced stage of a severe illness. After many hesitations, he ventured to ask his medical attendant if there remained any hope. The doctor evaded the embarrassing question as long as possible, but at last was compelled sorrowfully to acknowledge that there was none. "What!" said the patient, "Die! and leave my wife and five helpless children! By——I won't die."

If there be oaths which the Recording Angel is ashamed to write down, this was one of them! The patient got better from that hour.

The numerous miracles performed by Prince Hohenlohe (himself not even a believer in Christianity), are evidence of this extraordinary power. I remember more than one example which came under my own knowledge, but it would shock the feelings of some pious friends to cite them as arising from natural causes. Such persons are entirely convinced that the miraculous recoveries were the results of the immediate interposition of the Divine will, and graciously permitted to take place in a Protestant country, in order to hasten the blessed Advent of univeral religious concord.

Whatever be the nature of nervous influence—whatever be its real essence, the words fluid and circulation seem to be just as good explanations as any other, as they are in electricity and magnetism, whose essence no one supposes to be *fluid* in the popular sense of the term. I wish then, to be understood in this sense, when I suggest that the violent effort of the will restores the circulation in the nervous tubes or fibres. We have many instances of torpid bedridden persons suddenly able to rise at the cry of fire; and of others who have been as suddenly re-established by the influence of strong faith, of which I have known two very remarkable instances. The case of the power of speech suddenly bestowed by strong volition, already narrated, is only one of the many examples of the influence of the brain, even to the restoring or creating functions, an influence which, in the ordinary state of those functions, escapes observation. It is an established fact, that men, inspired by intense desire to perform the mother's office to a child, have been able to create milk in the breasts, and furnish it with abundant nutriment. Those medical men who practise among the wealthy, the idle, and the voluptuous, must have observed how much the constant determination of the thoughts to the seat of a trifling ailment will aggravate or modify its progress; and that the disease which would have passed away spontaneously in the clerk, becomes formidable in the retired tradesman.

The false perceptions of the insane are not so difficult to account for, as they would seem at the first glance. Whatever impression be made on the mind by external objects through the medium of the special senses, whatever sensation be thus conveyed, *the act of perception* must be some kind of movement in the organ of the mind; whether it be undulation, vibration, oscillation, circulation, or any other of the million changes which we may imagine but to which we cannot give a name. The sensation of pain, for example, communicated from a diseased toe to the brain, must be some kind of movement in the nerve leading from the part to that organ; and the perception which follows thereupon must be also a movement in the organ perceiving it. We know that the sensations conveyed to the brain from the diseased toe will be continued after the removal of the limb; that the nerve will still send information, which is now *false*—the patient feels the toe as distinctly as before the operation; that is, the habitual vibration of the nerve continues, and his perceptive faculties are not yet sufficiently educated on this subject to distinguish between a sensation at the extremity of the nerve, when the nerve terminated in the toe, and a sensation in the extremity of the nerve now that it terminates a little below the knee; thus the sensation continues when the cause has ceased to exist.

A similar process probably takes place in the exercise of the mental faculties. I will take the simplest example of it—the impressions conveyed by the eye. I have seen, for instance, the Emperor Alexander at the head of his troops in the Place Louis XV at Paris; the impression made on my brain, which gave rise to the reflections of my intellect, was produced by some kind of movement in the retina and optic nerve which conveyed the idea to the mind. Now, in like manner, as the nerve from the diseased toe conveyed the sensation of pain to the sensorium when the limb was amputated, the retina and optic nerve may take on the same movement when the Emperor Alexander is no longer present, and I may fancy myself still looking at the pageant. If this take place with both brains, I have no means of knowing that it is a false impression, unless the higher intellectual organs are sufficiently healthy and perfect to induce me to acknowledge the testimony of other persons, as more worthy of belief than that of my own senses. If the morbid or *false* sensation exist in only one brain, *I know with the other* that it is a delusion; nothing being accepted as proved by a sound intellect on self-judgment which does not receive the concurrent assent of the two. The assent which is accorded to the testimony of others is through a totally different process—called Faith.

Every idea, every thought, every sensation, every perception, every act of judgment, may be renewed by that most wonderful and mysterious faculty—the memory; the slightest and faintest renewal of the slightest portion of any previous perception or judgment in one of the brains may, by the equally mysterious and incomprehensible power of volition, be set up fully in *both* brains, till the whole is brought back to the mind. This is called recollection when voluntary, simple memory, if involuntary.

Whatever be the process thus voluntarily performed, it must, I repeat, be a movement of some kind and in like manner as the false report from the sentient retina and optic nerve, or from the stump of the amputated limb, is conveyed to the brain, and excites a corresponding movement of cognition therein—so may the movements of simple memory or of recollection excite the mental conviction that things are then existing which are only remembered.

If these movements depend on the circulation of a fluid in the minute nervous tubes in the brain (of which hundreds are required to make up the size of a hair), or if these tubes be merely hollow fibres producing their effect by vibration or movement of any kind, it is not difficult to conceive that, instead of acting together in the regular *fasciculi* which constitute the established and true functions of the healthy mind, they may act irregularly or singly, or in erroneous combination, and thus create false ideas. If this take place in a small portion only of the brain, it may produce morbid perversions of the faculties of that part alone whether affective or intellectual—perceptive or reflective—propensities or sentiments. If it take place in one brain only, it may be so slight as to be perfectly controllable by the other, or it may be in a corresponding part of both brains from sympathy of action. If this take place among the organs of the lower propensities, it may require all the power of the higher organs to keep them in check, and this power may be insufficiently exercised, or may not be exercised at all. It may be exercised at irregular or regular intervals, and may be alternately exercised and abandoned with all the periodicity of an ague, or of the peculiar functions of the female. I have given an example of this.

We know that by a blow on the head, as in the case of the butcher's son, by a violent shock from terror, or by nervous apoplexy, the functions of some portions of this complicated structure, or the whole of it, may suddenly cease, without the organ being irreparably injured. A moral influence, such as that, for example, of sudden detection in a crime, extravagant grief, or other causes, may produce a state of cataleptic apoplexy, which, after continuing some time may suddenly terminate in complete restoration.

There does not seem to me any difficulty in conceiving that, as it is clear that portions of the brain may *act* singly, portions of the brain may *cease* to act singly, and having continued torpid a considerable time, some counter shock may effect an instant restoration to mental health, of which we have many examples in the insane. I cannot think it an extravagant supposition that the transition, alternation, or interchange of activity and torpidity of different portions of the whole cerebral mass ministering to the intellect and the affective faculties may by sufficient to explain all the varieties of mental derangement which excite our wonder by their extravagance and absurdity. In the cases where there is no organic lesion portions may be in the torpor of deep sleep, as the whole of them are placed for a part of every twenty-four hours, and the changes of mental manifestation produced by such causes in parts so various, added to those which arise from the existence of two perfect thinking apparatus, may have effects so various and extensive as to account for all that we witness among the insane.

No physician who has attentively watched a case of genuine catalepsy (it has been my fate to see three such, which is I believe a large proportion), but must be conscious that large portions of the brain, or, as a phrenologist would say, a great number of the organs of the mind are in a state of perfect torpor while others are in unnatural activity.

A lady, about forty years of age, whom I knew, was actually placed in her coffin in the belief that she was dead, yet her sense of hearing was preternaturally acute. She declared that, in her chamber on the second floor, she heard her character discussed by the servants in the kitchen. When her brother, a solicitor in the City, came to see her at Camberwell in this state, and declared that she should not be buried till putrefaction took place, she felt intense gratitude and a gush of tenderness, but was unable to manifest it even by the motion of an eyelid. Suddenly all her faculties were restored to her

I visited the Countess Escalante, one of the Spanish Refugees, who remained in a similar state for a shorter period, during which she saw her husband and children, was quite conscious of all they did and said, but did not recognise them for her own—was absolutely without the power of moving a finger or opening or shutting her mouth. She was instantly restored to full consciousness; and this attack recurred suddenly at intervals of ten days or a fortnight, and was succeeded by an equally sudden restoration.

The late lamented Malibran afforded another example of this temporary suspension of some of the faculties; but in her case it generally lasted but a few hours, till, on the last fatal occasion, the mistake of the unfortunate bleeding, not being allowed to be remedied with cordials and restoratives by her homeopathic attendant, the torpor passed by an easy transition into death.

Whether the explanation I have attempted throws any real light on the subject is for others to determine; any mode of accounting for the phenomena of insanity without the aid of metaphysics or theology, must, if established in the convictions of the public, lead to important and useful consequences. While looked on as a disorder of *the mind* alone—whatever that may mean, I confess myself utterly incapable of comprehending the expression—all attempts to establish a sound theory are vain; but if we consider the deranged manifestations to depend on physical causes, gross or subtile, we have some hopes of a real result. Some of these physical causes are so obvious that they require no demonstration to convince the most ignorant; it is when they depend on nervous influence in its mysterious variety that we require to bear in mind the absolute fact that we have to do with a physical disorder, however obscure; and that, like many visible disorders of the body, it is sometimes to be let alone till it gets well; sometimes its spontaneous removal is to be facilitated by abstracting every thing which could tend to prolong or aggravate it; sometimes the distant disease, which by sympathy excited the disturbance, is to be gently led to a favourable termination; and sometimes we are to use the most active, energetic, and persevering efforts, and all the resources that art, science, and experience can afford, to overcome a positive, visible, and tangible disease.

There are some corollaries which only need to be named, and their truth is so easily comprehended as to produce instant assent. If, for example, as I have so often stated, and now again repeat, one brain be a perfect instrument of thought—if it be capable of all the emotions, sentiments, and faculties, which we call in the aggregate, mind—then it necessarily follows that man must have two minds with two brains; and however intimate and perfect their unison in their natural state, they must occasionally be discrepant, when influenced by disease, either direct, sympathetic, or reflex.

Direct, from disorder or disorganization in the brain itself, or from the supply of blood to it being defective, unhealthy, or in excess.

Sympathetic, from disease or disorder in some other part, as a collection of hardened substances in the folds of the intestines, inablility to empty the bladder, etc.

Reflex, from disorder or change of structure in portions of the ganglionic apparatus—that wonderful system of what may be strictly called *little brains* in the interior of the body, connected together by a complicated web of nerves, which produce a complete intercommunication—connected also with the brain through the medium of the true cerebral nerves of the neck. The object of this curious apparatus is to supply nervous energy to those organs which are obviously intended to be out of the control of the will—the heart, for example, whose functions could not be interrupted for a minute without causing death. We may conceive that disorder of stomach, or other organs, may be accompanied by change of action or of structure in some of these ganglionic nerves. We have several examples of such alteration of structure in them and the nerves leading from one to the other, and we know that there have been instances also where their powers have been so changed as to make them instruments of the will, as in the well-authenticated examples of men who have been able to control the action of the heart, and thus produce temporary or permanent death by a mere effort of volition.

If such changes can take place, if nerves of mere vitality can become nerves of volition; there is every reason to believe that they may also become nerves of sensation, and make the brain morbidly conscious of the processes going on in the body. This would be an easy explanation of the extravagant fancies of hypochondriacs, who suppose that they have a live animal in the stomach, and so forth. I cannot but think that many of the extreme examples of such delusion, which virtually amount to insanity, have their origin in this change of function or of structure; which it is clear may be either temporary or permanent. While the cause lasts, such persons are objects of compassion; but as these peculiarities are sometimes assumed, and some of them are of so slight a nature as to pass away if the mind be properly occupied, it is not right, on all occasions, to indulge such persons with the expression of great sympathy. A thousand examples are on record where the mere habit of self-contemplation indulged in by the idle and the wealthy has created such delusions, which at the touch of poverty vanish. I know no more fitting object of contemptuous compassion than a wealthy voluptuary of either sex, who has "intensified" self-attention, till the practice has entirely destroyed all sympathy for others, and reduced the voluntary invalid to a very incarnation of selfishness.

A principal object of the ganglionic system would seem to be to carry on the functions of life during sleep, like the additional spring to a watch to enable it to go while winding up. It is the imperfect repose of the cerebral system, with the intermixture of the influence of the ganglionic, and the difference in the degree of somnolency of the two brains, which I conceive to be the cause of the phenomena of dreams and somnambulism. The shock, the confusion of mind, and the headach, of which all must be conscious, on being suddenly startled from profound sleep, are thus explained, and it requires some time before the transposition of the two nervous systems can be placed in due balance and repose.

A man who has been studying hard for some time; that is, who has been occupying both brains equally and *intentionally* in study, till he has induced fatigue of both, *never dreams.* It is only where the previous train of thought has been discursive, or where a reverie has been indulged, either painful or agreeable, that this strange phenomenon takes place; except, indeed, when it is produced by indigestion, or some internal disease, and then it always takes on the same character.

I have some curious speculation and a multitude of interesting facts and inferences with respect to somnambulism and dreaming, but this is not the place to produce them. I have just touched on the subject elsewhere, and hope at a future day to throw some light on this very dark and intricate subject on which no modern writer has been able to add to our scanty stock of information—but I wait for statistics.

In summing up what has been said, I think it may be assumed without risk of contradiction, that the fact of each brain being a perfect and complete instrument of thought is abundantly proved. That each, while in health, corresponds entirely in action with its fellow, is obvious from the fact that this unison and correspondence give only one result, as in the case of the two eyes producing single vision. That when from any cause one brain is disordered, a discrepancy in the two processes of thinking takes place. That the healthy brain (aided by the action of such of the organs of its fellow as are not affected by the disorder which disturbs the others) can, in nearly nine hundred and ninety-nine cases in a thousand, according to the usual proportion in this country, control all manifestation of morbid emotion or judgment, but that the thousandth case is the madman.

Is it not then a matter of wonder and admiration that with all the disturbing causes, moral and physical, which the ignorance of man causes or omits to obviate, the proportion of the insane should be so exceedingly small? and is it any objection to the belief of a superintending Providence, that, in a world obviously intended for progressive education, one single case in a thousand is permitted to be beyond the control of our faculties. The advance of science has already shewn us the means of obviating many of the causes of mental derangement, and there is strong reason to believe that we shall yet make extensive progress in the same direction. I please myself with the hope of being instrumental to this blessed result.

While diseases are permitted to afflict every other part of our bodies, it is not surprising that so complicated an organ as the brain should be liable to the same influences; and there seems no reason to doubt that, in the wonderful system of which we form so insignificant a portion, physical evil and imperfection, as well as physical pain and moral obliquity, are permitted portions. The inequality in the functions and powers of the two thinking organs is the very essence of that variety of character and conduct which makes the world what it is.

Without the existence of much evil, a large portion of the good that ennobles humanity could not be called into action—were no offence ever given, there could be no forgiveness—did no one fall into misery, benevolence and compassion would lack their object, and charity would be unknown—were all wise and prudent, there would be no need of guidance and control—were the child's brain perfect at first, all the duties of the parent, the proper exercise of which is his occupation and his happiness, could not be required. Patriotism, honesty, veracity, self-restraint, humility, perseverance, fortitude, self-denial, courage, and a hundred other virtues, must be unknown, if their corresponding defects did not exist. No! "All worketh together for good." *The world neither may, might, can, could, would, should, or ought to be anything but what it is.* It was intended to be exactly that which our limited faculties observe, but can neither entirely comprehend nor fully appreciate. Let us be careful to fill our own part in it, and leave the rest to Providence.

CHAPTER XX: *Difficulty of Deciding the Point at Which Insanity Begins; Mathematicians and Artists; Increase of Mental Powers; Madness of Volition; Negligent Volition; Power of Controlling Hereditary Tendency to Insanity; Self-Control of Lunatics; Medical Jury*

The embarrassment of a young practitioner on being called to decide on the fact of insanity in a patient is one of the most anxious and distressing things he will ever have to encounter in the course of his professional life; and it requires a greater degree of moral courage than falls to the lot of most men to make such a decision as he can reflect on afterwards with satisfaction. I was very early placed in this painful position, and could not even then, reconcile it to my sense of justice that a man's liberty should be entirely dependent on the intelligence, or even the honesty, of a youth of three-and-twenty. I believe myself to have always acted impartially on these occasions; but can perfectly remember the shame and annihilating self-abasement with which I listened to the reproaches of a venerable gentleman thrice my own age, whom I had entrapped into a madhouse under the pretext of taking him to visit a friend. I have never been able to persuade myself that such stratagems are ultimately beneficial, for the just indignation felt at the deception neutralizes the benefit of restraint, and is a great aggravation of the patient's unhappy lot. On other occasions, before I was five-and-twenty, I had to give written answers to interrogatories from Doctors' Commons on twenty abstract propositions respecting the nature and essence of insanity, when not only was I entirely ignorant of the modes of deviation from reason, but of almost every one of the causes of aberration; yet, on these answers of a flippant young man depended the liberty, and more than the liberty, of a fellow-creature.

I speak now of a period five-and-thirty years ago, when the treatment of insane persons was so brutal and senseless, that condemnation by a medical certificate amounted to the infliction of a punishment greater than that which the law imposes for serious crimes. Dr. Conolly has well described the effect on the patient's mind, on the first dawn of reason, when thus confined; and justly dwells on the distressing importance of a decision which was to be attended by consequences so formidable. The abstract question of sanity or insanity was a trifle compared with the question, "Shall this man be subjected to loss of liberty and to brutal cruelty?" It is a slight thing in the present day for a medical man to be called to pronounce a case to be or not to be hydrophobia, but at the period when the affirmative was followed by the infliction of suffocation (as I have heard an old gentleman say he twice witnessed), it might well give a man pause ere he pronounced an opinion which virtually amounted to the awful sentence of death.

These strange and inconceivable anomalies in our law have been ameliorated, but not entirely removed. I do not doubt that some thirty or forty years hence men will look back with incredulous wonder at the history even of the present day, in respect to the whole management of the law of lunacy, just as we refer with horror to periods within my own time, when twelve, fifteen, and on one occasion, two-and-twenty persons were hanged in one morning at the Old Bailey, many of them for crimes which would now perhaps be expiated by six months' imprisonment and the treadmill; yet in those days these sacrifices to the *violated majesty of the law* (as they were called) excited horror in very few minds, and the abolition of the practice would never have been effected, but by that small and powerful instrument—the *goose-quill.*

The line of demarcation between insanity and reason is like that between soberness and drunkenness. It requires no sagacity to distinguish the extremes, but the gradations are infinite, and the boundary evanescent or imperceptible. Yet it is not so difficult to decide the point at which it is right to interfere. A jury "*de lunatico inquirendo*" declares the time arrived when the patient shall not be entrusted with the care of his own property—the policeman pronounces the same verdict when he takes charge of the purse and watch of the man he finds drunk in the street. In the latter case the period of recovery is known, and it is known that the recovery will be complete; but in the former case the assumption of the right to control the actions of the man with disordered brain is, I believe, for life, and does not admit of being superseded by his recovery; if so, it is a great defect in the law. We require an inquest with temporary powers long before the case arrives at the point which justifies perpetual restraint. The "*Lettres de Cachet*," in their origin (before they were abused for political purposes), were only granted on a petition of the man's family, setting forth that he was a wantonly extravagant spendthrift and was dissipating the property of his wife or children in foolish and blameable self-indulgence—that is, that he did not *exercise* self-control; and this, for all social purposes, justified personal restraint just as much as if he had absolutely *lost* it. If such a law could be executed in this country, how many families might be saved from disgrace and ruin, and how many men prevented from disgusting the world with the exhibition of their shameless vices and filthy depravity? When both brains are disordered from self-indulgence and excess, or when the control of one brain over the other for moral purposes is lost, or so weakened as to be useless, or when from neglected education it has never been acquired, or the whole moral sentiments have been contaminated by a putrid moral atmosphere, society has an indefeasible right to interfere and exercise the control which the individual no longer possesses.

Thus much, however, may be confidently asserted, that the portion of brain, or distinct organs (if they exist), which give the moral sentiments, may be thoroughly diseased or at least extensively disordered, while the intellect remains clear and unclouded, and the reasoning powers even unusually acute. The intellect, that is, the organ devoted to the exercise of intellect, may be as actively employed in defending evil acts as good ones, like an advocate in a court of justice—the *fee* is the *self-indulgence*, regardless of the consequences to others, as in the unhappily too notorious case which shocked the moral sentiments of the nation a few years ago, where the barrister (after the culprit had confessed to him the horrid murder he had committed) actually endeavoured, not only to screen the miscreant from just punishment, but to throw the guilt upon others whom he knew to be innocent.

This form of mental derangement was first named by Dr. Pritchard *moral insanity*, and the term is now generally adopted. It expresses very clearly a state of mind, more frequently seen in its early stage in our courts of criminal justice than before a lunacy commission, where it is seldom brought till a very advanced period of the disease, and after it has been allowed to inflict poverty, misery, and disgrace on those connected with the patient by ties of blood.

The gradations of disease up to the point of moral insanity are infinite, and lead to a variety of crime, ranging from the forgery which merely anticipates the arrival of property necessarily coming to the offender in due course of law (and which is in one sense his own), to the deliberate murder of a benefactor to hasten the enjoyment of the fortune he has bequeathed. The intellect can find reasons to excuse, to palliate, or even to justify the act.

A writer in the "*Quarterly Review*" (vol. ii, p. 158) remarks, that the "reasoning faculties have probably little or no influence on insanity, except as adding vigour to the mind by their moderate exercise and enabling it to resist the diseases of the body, or as weakening the nervous system by excess of fatigue." It is obvious that the writer is here thinking of erroneous perceptions, not the madness of volition nor moral insanity.

Many writers remark that mathematicians are less liable to insanity than any other class of men. Making allowance for the fact that mathematicians are one of the very smallest classes of society, and that therefore the number of insane of that class must be exceedingly limited, I yet believe the fact to be correctly stated, and that it is scarcely possible for a good mathematician with an originally healthy brain to become the subject of mental derangement. I explain this from two causes, both of them in perfect harmony with my theory. The originally fragile or imperfect structure of one of the brains which leads to this disease and which is so frequently hereditary, prevents that complete command of the volitions and concentration of thought I have before spoken of, as the characteristic of a well-disciplined scholar, and thus incapacitates for the study of a science requiring the absolute dismissal of all other thoughts during its acquisition. Thus a person with a brain liable to insanity cannot well become a mathematician.

On the other hand, the study of mathematics increases in a remarkable degree the command over the volitions, and strengthens the intellectual power of concentration, by establishing an absolute tyranny of one brain over the other, when they are originally of unequal power—the want of which tyranny is probably the reason why hypochondriacal and fanciful delusions terminate in insanity.

Artists, on the contrary, and men who cultivate the fancy for professional purposes, are for this reason more liable to insanity; they lay down the reins in order to witness and profit by the gambols of the unrestrained imagination, and then find it difficult to resume them. For the most part, such men are incapable of profound study; they use only a portion of their faculties at a time, and never acquire the intense power of concentration required by the others. Thus when disappointments and misfortunes occur, one or both of the thinking organs falls into disorder, which, if slight, forms only a whimsical delusion, or passes gradually on into hypochondriasis, monomania, or madness; because the governing brain has lost its power, or has itself become diseased, and thus self-control is destroyed, which is insanity.

The increase of the mental powers is noticed only, I believe, in those cases where the inflammation, undulation, vibration, or irritation of the nervous structure (whatever be its nature) extends to the two brains simultaneously, or perhaps commences in some of the bodies at the base of the skull which are common to both cerebra, as the pineal or pituitary glands, for example. Whenever disease commences in one cerebrum, and gradually extends to the other, there is a period of moody, equivocal sanity, during which great efforts are made, at least by educated persons, to overcome the morbid delusions; but in the other cases, hypothetically assumed by me to arise from disorder or disease in a part common to both sides, there is an extraordinary activity of intellect and increase of rapidity in the conceptions—"a fertility of imagination which changes the character of the mind without remarkably distorting it;" according to the expression of Dr. Abercrombie. "The memory (says he) is entire, and even appears more ready than in health, and old associations are called up with a rapidity quite unknown to the individual in his sound state of mind." Dr. Willis speaks of a gentleman, subject to periodical attacks of insanity, who always expected the paroxysms with impatience, because he enjoyed during them a high degree of pleasure. "Every thing appeared easy to me; no obstacles presented themselves either in theory or practice. My memory acquired all of a sudden a singular degree of perfection. Long passages of Latin authors occurred to my mind. In general I have a great difficulty in finding rhythmical terminations, but on these occasions I wrote verses with as great facility as prose."

Pinel says, "I have often stopped at the door of a literary

gentleman (who during his paroxysms appears to soar above his usual mediocrity of intellect) solely to admire his newly acquired powers of eloquence. He declaimed on the subject of the Revolution with all the force, the dignity, and the purity of language, that this very interesting subject would admit of. At other times he was a man of very ordinary abilities."

Dr. Conolly has given a description of this state—this very brief state of luxuriance of the mental powers before their extinction; he has described it so completely and so graphically, that nothing is left to be added by any subsequent writer. I have quoted his description elsewhere. It is one of the most painful objects that can be contemplated by a physician conversant with insanity. Where others feel nothing but admiration, he experiences great alarm, and foresees terrible consequences; and when in this state of preparation for oblivion, the mind suddenly takes an erotic turn, the individual is perhaps plunged in a moment into everlasting disgrace—the subsequent mania is considered to arise from the shame of detection, and it requires a good deal of moral courage on the part of the medical attendant to endeavour to place the defence on its proper ground; it is an ungracious and painful subject.

Unless my theory be adopted to explain the class of cases mentioned above, we are utterly at a loss to account for this great variation in the states preceding insanity. In the one case, morose and gloomy thoughts and stern self-control; and in the other, gaiety, with wit, memory, and increased general powers of the intellect—the former lasting for several weeks, the latter only a few days, or even hours.

In the diminution or destruction of the power of one ear, or of one eye, from a disease unattended by pain, the patient is scarcely ever aware of the loss till some accidental circumstance interrupts the full power of the other —a slight inflammation in the eye that is not affected with cataract, or a cold caught in the sound ear, first makes him conscious of his misfortune. In like manner, when one brain is injured, it is not till something occurs requiring *study* that he is aware, or that others are aware, of the defect. The difficulty of *recalling* a train of thought is, I believe, one of the invariable accompaniments of insanity, for it is an act in which both brains are concerned. Shakspeare, who seems to have known by a kind of intuition what it takes other men enormous mental labour to acquire, makes Hamlet say—

> . . . . bring me to the test,
> And I the matter will re-word, which madness
> Would gambol from.

I cannot remember to have seen a single instance of insanity, however slight, and however incognizable by any but an experienced medical man, where the patient, after relating a short history of his complaints, physical, moral, or social, could, on being requested to repeat the narrative, follow the same series; to repeat the same words, even with the limited correctness of a sane person, is, I believe, always impossible in the very mildest case of insanity. The point where this inability begins, however difficult to ascertain exactly, has always seemed to me the point at which strict responsibility for our actions ceases and the exercise of restraint by others becomes a right and a duty. In a large proportion of cases of madness of volition—that is, where one brain is disordered or diseased, and the other exercising over it an imperfect control—the patient is conscious of the approach of the period when this limited degree of self-command will be overpowered, and is anxious to place himself in a position where his own efforts will be aided, if necessary, by positive coercion. "Many of the articles in Aikin's Biography were penned in a lunatic asylum. The writer of them being subject to occasional attacks of insanity, and having warning of their approach, he was in the practice of giving himself up to the custody of an experienced keeper of a madhouse, prior to the full development of the disordered state."—*Quarterly Review*, vol. xxiv, p. 191.

This state of mind is so common that no person at all conversant with the management of the insane but must have met with many instances. I could enumerate eight or ten examples of it—the most remarkable of which is the following:

I was once visiting at a very respectable establishment for

persons of deranged intellects of the upper class, when the house was suddenly disturbed in the middle of the night by the violent noises and language of a young gentleman who had been long an inmate, and whose disease assumed a character of periodicity. There was a kind of cycle, beginning with intense despondency, passing on to composure, to cheerfulness, hilarity, boisterous gaiety, violent and convulsive mirth, extravagant volubility and wit, gross and monstrous obscenity, incoherence, and thence into the most furious mania, requiring coercion. This gradually subsided into melancholy, left him two or three weeks in a state of tranquillity, and then went again its miserable round. On the present occasion the patient insisted on seeing the head of the establishment, but as he was manacled by both wrists to the bed, it was not thought necessary to comply with his demand. The violence of the efforts he made and his furious screams, at last alarmed the attendants lest he should break a blood-vessel, and the gentleman was called out of bed. On approaching the patient, who had become instantly calm when told that the doctor was called and would come to him, he said, "What is the reason of this disturbance, sir; and why am I called out of bed at this unseasonable hour?"

"Don't be angry, doctor," was the reply; "I wish to tell you that I can get my hands at liberty. You see how small they are. You must send to the ladies' establishment for a smaller pair of manacles."

"There is no danger whatever of that, sir; you are perfectly secured: lie quiet and go to sleep."

In vain did the patient urge with increasing violence the necessity of securing himself more firmly. The doctor refused; when the young man succeeded in extricating one hand, and gave him a violent blow—"Do you believe me now?"said he.

This was an irresistible argument; a pair of ladies' manacles were sent for, and securely fastened. The patient pulled in all directions for some time, and finding himself quite unable to get his hands out, said "All right, now I am quiet. While I knew that there was a possibility of extrication I could not restrain my propensity to kill somebody. I am sure I should have done it, though I tried so hard to prevent it. Now that I know myself secure, I am quiet. Now do, my dear doctor, sit down and have a little chat with me. I have thoroughly waked you up, and it will be charity to bestow half-an-hour on me."

The gentleman told me that his conversation was then exceedingly witty and agreeable, and that only on a few occasions did he utter any incoherent expressions, and those only when the conversation flagged and he seemed to be off his guard.

The next day he had his usual paroxysms of violence, passing on into furious mania.

I cannot conceive any other mode of explaining this but on the supposition that one of the brains was in vain endeavouring to control the other, felt its authority slipping away, and was desirous to have the aid of positive restraint in an effort hourly becoming weaker and weaker. On this theory all the phenomena are simple and consistent.

The instances of men who have been kindly and judiciously treated in a lunatic establishment, voluntarily returning there when apprehensive of a renewal of the attack, are extremely common. The feeling which dictates the conduct is exactly the same as that which suggested to the young man the necessity of smaller manacles. The fact of the conviction of the absolute *impossibility* of committing a certain act of wickedness, or indulging in a certain depraved gratification, taking away all desire for it, is not confined to the insane. Revenge, for example, will sleep till it is extinguished; but unexpected possession of the means of its gratification will suddenly revive the dormant passion and render it uncontrollable.

I *know* that the continuous conviction of a man vowed to celibacy, that the indulgence of the passions is not only criminal, but morally and almost physically impossible, will in the end annihilate the desire for its gratification. This is a much more common state than is believed by Protestants. I have had much professional conversation with monks, and repeat that I *know* the fact medically, in a way which cannot deceive me.

Foville mentions the case of a young girl confined in an asylum for the insane, to whom it was considered necessary to employ the actual cautery (red-hot iron) to the nape of the neck. The girl was so intensely alarmed at the first touch of it, that although she had not previously had an instant of reason, she made violent efforts, and succeeded in escaping from the hands of several persons who vainly endeavoured to restrain her; she addressed them in perfectly rational language and entreated to be spared the horrible remedy. Mr. Esquisol consented to delay it, if she would conduct herself rationally and set herself to work. She promised to do this, and kept her word. She was immediately transferred to the convalescent side of the establishment, and soon became perfectly restored.

I consider this to be one of the cases of *negligent* volition. When a disordered brain has been allowed to escape from the control of the sound one, the process of government has been found to be increasingly difficult and troublesome, and a feeble sound brain has gradually relinquished its task and neglected its duty—desuetude has completed the insanity. Roused to action by the pain of the remedy, the brain has been suddenly placed in the state in which we sometimes find bedridden persons on the alarm of fire, and firm and influential effective volition is re-established. I do not recollect if the previous state of the patient is described, but perhaps it might have been general torpor alone of both brains, as we sometimes see in a more limited degree in a wealthy voluptuary.

It is probable that it was the occasional occurrence of a case like that just related, which seemed to justify the cruelties practised on the insane in former days, for we can hardly imagine human beings to have inflicted the horrible tortures then so common, out of pure delight in cruelty.

Of the power of strong moral feeling and volition (created, or increased and confirmed, by a sound religious and moral education) to control an hereditary tendency to insanity, we have numerous examples in the more elevated ranks of life, and in the class immediately below them, that which may be called the upper-middle class. We see the sons entering into the most enormous sensual excesses, exciting the disgust and abhorrence of their fellow-creatures, degrading themselves below the level of beasts, and ending their days in madness or idiocy—while the sisters, with the same, or even still greater fragility of brain, shall lead lives of exemplary virtue and self-restraint, and at most only shew the hereditary taint by slight peculiarities of manner, unless indeed an injudicious clergyman have had the management of their religious education, when the enthusiasm he has excited produces the same lamentable effects as are caused by their brothers' excesses in sensual indulgence. How *good* many of these women are, when judiciously educated, cannot even be *conceived* by the mass of mankind; but if I were seeking examples of the most exalted virtue and meritorious self-restraint that can dignify our "chetive" nature, here would I look for them; and not among the apathetic inanimate beings, whose negative merits are merely owing to the entire absence of motives to evil. It is no merit in a man who does not possess the sense of taste to abstain from gluttonous and epicurean indulgence in his food.

The examples of temporary self-control in the insane are extremely common. There is scarcely a writer on insanity who does not cite many instances. Dr. Abercrombie mentions a clergyman in Scotland who was brought before a jury to be declared incapable of managing his own affairs, and placed under the care of trustees. Among the acts of extravagance alleged against him was, that he had burnt his library; when asked by the jury what account he could give of this part of his conduct, he replied, "I had imbibed early in life a liking for that most unprofitable study, controversial divinity. On reviewing my library, I found a great part of it to consist of books of this description, and I was so anxious that my family should not be led to follow the same pursuit, that I determined to burn the whole." He gave answers equally plausible to all other questions, and the result was, that the jury found no sufficient ground for declaring him incapable of self-management, and he was dismissed. In the course of a fortnight from that time, he was in a state of decided mania. He had been able to exercise continuous control while he had an object to gain—the preservation of his liberty; but when this was accomplished, he laid down the reins; after a very short cessation of the self-restraint, he could not resume it, and became positively mad.

It would be tedious to narrate a greater number of cases. I wish only to shew that the self-control here spoken of, is a very different process from the control of the propensities and passions by the understanding and moral sentiments. It is strictly the coercion of one brain by the other; the influence which the sound mind exercises over the unsound mind; in which it is aided by such portions of the disordered organ as are not implicated in the specific mental disturbance which constitutes the delusion. This is more especially the case when it is a delusion of the perceptive faculties, as in the instances of optical deceptions and spectral illusions.

It is said that, if we were to admit so great a latitude in judging of immoral actions, if we were to allow impunity on the ground of insanity in cases of atrocious crime, there would be thousands of impostors ready to take advantage of the doctrine; and that when a man contemplated the commission of some act of violent wrong, he would previously take care to manifest extravagance of manner and language, which might induce a jury to excuse him from punishment should he be detected. This is a valid objection and deserves consideration.

It is certainly true that the point at which one brain is no longer capable of exercising control over the other can never be exactly ascertained; neither can we draw an absolute line between the degree of intoxication which makes the destruction of a fellow-creature an act of mere homicide, and that which leaves the criminal guilty of murder. Each case must be judged of alone, and by its own attendant circumstances. The equivocal cases must be exceedingly rare; and there is one consideration which seems to have been overlooked in estimating the probable effects of allowing impunity to crime, on the presumption that the brain was in a state of mental aberration. It is this: The great difficulty of ascertaining the existence of insanity in an early stage (when the patient has a strong motive for concealing it, and one of the brains stills remains a perfect instrument of volition) has been supposed to imply an equal difficulty in ascertaining the truth of assumed insanity; a difficulty, however, which does not exist. The best actor that ever lived would be detected in an hour's examination by a medical man of moderate experience and ordinary sagacity. Having been several times placed in this situation, I know the facility of detecting such assumption; it is much greater than that of detecting the real illness of a soldier who dislikes the compound nitre powder and leaden pills of the battle-field, or of the man drawn for the militia and claiming the benefit of some defect or disease as a ground of exemption. In both these cases there is sometimes serious difficulty, which, when decided against the applicant, leaves on the mind a very painful dread of having committed an injustice: but in fictitious insanity there is no such doubt; every one attempting the deception *overdoes* the character; he only knows the grosser outlines of such cases, and in his attempt to fill them up he often *reverses the shadows*. It is, besides, impossible to keep up the character when the muscles of the face become fatigued, and if closely watched, and his attention suddenly called to another subject, he has not the madman's rapidity of transition; before there is time for consideration and decision he has let fall the mask and is detected. Even the sullen look of melancholia requires a painful effort of the muscles of the face, which cannot be long kept up voluntarily. There is, I think, no danger whatever of success in any such attempt at deception, if the case be referred, as it ought to be, not to insulated individuals but to a medical jury—conducting the examination in their own way in private and not in the present absurd mode of cross-examination in public before men necessarily ignorant—not merely ignorant of the best mode of ascertaining the fact, but wanting even the rudiments of that preliminary knowledge, which is a small, but essential part of the investigation; and besides, ignorant of the habits, modes, and peculiarities of mental aberration. The judge and counsel are generally almost as incompetent on these subjects as the jury, and quite as incapable of an enlightened decision.

CHAPTER XXI: *Distinction Between Folly and Imbecility; Possibility of Cultivating an Imperfect Brain into Average Intellect; Education Not to be Hurried; Frauds of Tutors; Precocious Intellect; Examples of Cruelty in Forcing Premature Development; A Peculiar Form of Cerebral Irregularity*

There is no more common error than to suppose a person whose conduct is uncontrollably foolish and language silly, to be unable to judge correctly of the conduct and language of others. We see numerous examples of men who are frequently committing acts and uttering sentiments of excessive folly, from vanity and conceit, yet in their sober moments, and after deliberate consideration, can put forth words of wisdom and make shrewd observations, which must have been preceded by a long train of ratiocination. Nay, there are short periods when such persons will converse with an acuteness and a power equal to men of acknowledged sense and discretion. The phrase, first applied I believe, to Goldsmith—"inspired idiot"—refers to this peculiar structure of mind. Professionally, I have more than once heard a conversation between two such persons, who have separated with profound reciprocal contempt, and have made afterwards the most acute remarks on each other's folly. Men of sense and acquirements often *let themselves down* in the society of these foolish persons, whose intellect they despise too much to be on their guard before them. I have known one instance where a well-concocted scheme was rendered abortive by the *paulo-post-futuro sagacity* of one of these habitually silly persons.

This discrepancy may be thus explained—but this is of course hypothesis. My note-book contains several examples and observations on the subject; and I have no doubt of producing conviction, should there be a future opportunity of detailing them. In these cases I suppose the most active brain to be that which is the least perfect in its structure, and that the volition of the other is not sufficiently powerful to control it, either from want of cultivation or natural deficiency.

Imbecility and folly are by no means convertible terms, nor are they, indeed, merely degrees of defective power. Folly seems to reside generally in one brain only, and to be perfectly compatible with the possession of another brain of ordinary vigour and perfection. When the weaker brain becomes exhausted by its incessant exercise, perhaps through the day, and by the excitement of events, it will at night, in silence and solitude, remain passive, while the sounder organ takes a calm review of the follies it has been unable to prevent; a feeling akin to remorse will arise with strong resolutions of better conduct in future; and if the *then* thoughts be committed to paper, we are surprised how so silly a person can write so sensibly. This I imagine must have come to the knowledge of every one. I know that it formerly gave me the conviction that the person thus acting foolishly and writing wisely had been aided by others in the latter process; and it was not till after many conclusive proofs of the fact, that I allowed it to remain in my mind as a settled conviction, that *the same person may be exquisitely silly in conversation and in actions, and yet sober and wise in his closet*.

Imbecility is a different affair; it is an imperfection in both brains, and graduates down to idiocy. It may obviously be increased or aggravated by mal-practices and want of cultivation; but the mal-practices are more frequently a consequence than a cause: neither do I believe them so common as they are represented, especially among the poor and ill-fed. It is the idle, luxurious, high-fed, motiveless animal, that most frequently gives way to excesses reflexly injurious to the brain. Among the lower class of criminals the evils of solitary confinement are not so great as those of free volition in the reckless habits of the class to which they belong by birth, or to which they have associated themselves on the old principle of *similes similibus gaudent*.

Innumerable examples are on record, however, where a judicious cultivation—or even the careful exclusion of bad cultivation—shall entirely change the character of the young by changing the state of brain which gives rise to that character—at least, if the care thus bestowed be not delayed till after the period when the brain has acquired its full growth, and either adapted itself to the shape of the skull which contains it, or compelled the skull to make a similar concession. I know families where the characteristic of the children up to the age of sixteen or eighteen, may be designated imbecility—not *folly*, but a real defect in the powers of ratiocination; yet at five-and-twenty they possess the common average degree of intellect. One family especially there is, of which every member was, at the age of seventeen or eighteen, positively silly, yet they have all made their way in the world to positions of eminence, necessarily implying the possession of fair intellectual powers.

A single instance comes to my recollection, so remarkable and so conclusive as to the possibility of cultivating an apparently hopeless brain to the full exercise of the powers of a rational being, that I much regret the necessity of concealing the minute details, out of delicacy to the individual and to his family. All I can venture to say is, that at the age of sixteen he could not count ten, except by rote, for if interrupted in the series he was compelled to recommence; and if five shillings were put into his hand and he were made to return two of them, he could not have told how many remained had his life depended on the issue. He was carefully and tenderly watched by judicious parents, and a discreet medical adviser. No attempts were made to force open the bud and thus risk the destruction of the rose; the intellect slowly and gradually improved—motives were gradually and carefully presented to him, such as would have stimulated the exertions of a child of four years of age—the indulgence of the pleasures of the palate, for example, was made contingent on the acquisition of certain lessons—as he advanced, other lessons and higher motives were substituted, and thus were employed four or five years of quiet and gentle study. Every month shewed an improvement; and at the age of two-and-twenty he was on a fair level, not certainly with men of his own class of that age, but with other persons of inferior station and neglected education. About five-and-twenty the process was aided by a virtuous attachment, the highest of all merely human motives, and at seven-and-twenty he was a clever man. At thirty he became eminent in the department he had selected—has since made a splendid fortune, and now enjoys his *otium cum dignitate*, and the respect of a large circle of elevated companions. Here was "a brand snatched from the burning."

I know no example so strong, of the truth of the axiom and advice of Confucius, which I have so often quoted elsewhere, "Cultivate every soil; if good corn produce nothing but straw, it will at least prevent the growth of weeds."

How many youths are there among the higher classes whose brains being thus late in their development, the development still further retarded by ignorant or injudicious cultivation, pass on from a state of imbecility through all the roads of vicious indulgence of the grossest animal propensities, till they terminate their short and disgusting career in idiocy or madness. How many of these might have been saved and made to occupy a respectable station with honour, had they been entrusted to the exclusive care of an enlightened medical philosopher. How often has my heart ached at witnessing this wanton destruction of a mind—arising most frequently from the criminal indolence of parents—who seem utterly unconscious of the deep responsibility they thus incur to the Creator for the degradation and destruction of one of his creatures committed to their care. Yet such parents are often enthusiastically religious.

I conceive it very possible, to a man fully possessed with the idea of the two brains (as I have endeavoured to explain the doctrine), and in other respects fitted for the office of instructor, to exercise such a control over the development of the mind of his pupil as to change an intellect of very humble power (and which, if managed in the ordinary way, would terminate in imbecility), into one of fair average capacity. He would attempt this by the slowest process, as is done in the teaching of mathematics, where each step is so exceedingly small as to be ascended almost without a mental effort. It is the keeping back the mind rather than urging it forward, that leads to success in such cases. Had the gentleman just spoken of been subjected to ordinary discipline, he would most certainly have turned out an idiot. I have seen instances in high life where, from the impatience and unreasonable exactions of parents, a youth, whose brain might have been so cultivated as to produce a fair crop of intellect, has been utterly ruined by being taken from one tutor to another till a man has been found who would promise *to make a scholar in a short time.* In two instances I have seen *themes* sent to the parents as the production of the pupil (a lad of seventeen or eighteen), which it was absolutely impossible that any man of average talent could produce before the age of thirty—which the supposed author could barely read, and was quite incapable of comprehending. The tone of the composition implied a person of mature age; but the stratagem was successful, and in one of the instances the praises bestowed on the son excited so strong a feeling of gratitude in the parents as to lead to the high advancement of the tutor. A more impudently fraudulent scheme I never knew. The pupil was, to every eye but that of the parent, manifestly imbecile, and, cultivated as he has been, will remain so for ever—his brothers had the good fortune to fall into better hands. The clergyman who perpetrated the fraud cannot, however, be dispossessed of the preferment thus erroneously bestowed; and would perhaps, in his convivial moments, shelter himself under the advice of Solomon, "Answer a fool according to his folly;" and I dare say entertains an ample share of contempt for his profitable dupe, whom he regards no doubt as a spider regards the race of flies—his appropriate food.

It is to me an incomprehensible feeling on the part of parents, this unwillingness to believe in the existence of any positive defect, either mental or corporeal, in their children. You may prove to a man that his son is one of the vilest scoundrels that ever disgraced the earth, and though he is offended, he is not so hurt as by the suggestion that the youth is deficient in intellect. He may have the most loathsome acquired disease, and it is more tolerable to the parent than the accusation of a tendency to scrofula. A man will put forth to observation, without any feeling of humiliation, a leg mutilated by an accident, and rendered absolutely an object of disgust; but a trifling natural deformity he will take enormous pains and incur unbounded expense to conceal. I cannot account for this. I have known a gentleman with club-foot, a man of high accomplishments and strong mind, allude in an under tone to his "accident," and then blush with shame at the silly lie, uttered to persons who he well knew were aware that it was a connate deformity. It is a curious chapter in psychological history, which I leave to others to explain.

We have numerous examples of hereditary fragility of brain leading, on any sudden shock, to temporary or permanent imbecility. In one instance two brothers were drawn for the conscription, and one of them being killed in battle, the other, who was by his side, was instantly struck with perfect idiocy. On being sent home another brother was so affected by the sight of him that he was as suddenly seized in the same manner, and both were received at the Bicêtre and never recovered. I have cited another case, of the Indian minister, and have myself known two examples of death preceded by imbecility from sudden terror; but there is a still stranger form of cerebral malady, where almost without a metaphor the fibres of the brain may be said to be thrown into cramp, and at the end of many years, either spontaneously or from fever, or some sudden impression, the spasm ceases, and the individual instantly recovers full possession of his reason. Five persons were received into the Bicêtre in this state, all of whom recovered. Rush mentions a case where a gentleman, on some sudden pecuniary losses, was struck instantly with idiocy, remained in that state five years, and as suddenly recovered; and Dr. Holland speaks of others. Of this also I have seen an example, on it being announced to a gentleman that a docket of bankruptcy had been struck against him by a man on whom he had conferred great obligations. After the expiration of rather more than two years he recovered suddenly, apparently from striking his head against a low doorway. We know that nerves *may* be seized with cramp, as in toothach, and I can see no reason why the nervous fibres of the brain may not be subjected to a similar morbid action from physical or moral causes. If in the sudden spasm, or whatever it may be called, which takes place, they are mechanically injured, the idiocy may be permanent; if not, it may cease on any sudden movement in a different direction, as in the spasms of muscles. This is, no doubt, pure hypothesis, but it is so probable as to be almost certain.

The shock sometimes leads to effusion and destroys life in a different manner. A gentleman took his two children into the belfry of a church to shew them the prospect; they were in perfect health, and highly enjoyed the extended view; came down again in the highest spirits, and while examining a gigantic bell, it tolled the hour one. Both children were rendered speechless by the shock, were seized with illness, and in a short time died from water in the brain.

In a manner perhaps analogous to the cramp of a muscle, the nerves of volition (especially) *may* be put into a state of inaction, temporary or permanent, and through the cervical nerves a similar influence *may* be conveyed to the ganglionic nerves, and destroy life.

Now it is easy to conceive that a modification of this influence may excite into active obedience nerves over which there was previously no command, as in the case I have cited, where the power of utterance was instantly bestowed on a youth previously dumb.

I consider the state of torpor above described to be very similar, if not identical, with that produced by physical concussion, differing only in degree, and I give it the name of *moral concussion*.

The effect of sudden terror on the healthy brain may instantly reduce it to a state of cataleptic spasm. I knew a person who, standing in her kitchen with her child, saw its clothes take fire, and was instantly seized in this manner, and remained motionless till it was burnt to death, although there was within reach a tub full of clothes soaking in water, what would generally be called a providential means of safety. She made the most strenuous efforts to reach them, but in vain. Her arms were as absolutely uncontrollable by volition, as if they had been paralysed.

I have also seen two instances of sudden death from terror, where a similar cataleptic paralysis took place, and was succeeded by the voidance of immense quantities of the serum of the blood from the bowels, with congestion of the heart and great vessels; the blood being rendered too thick for circulation, life was soon extinct, under circumstances precisely similar to the progress of cholera. Indeed, I would defy any one to distinguish (by the symptoms alone) three modes of death: poisoning by tartarized antimony, Indian cholera, and the effect of overpowering terror, such as I have just described.

In cultivating a brain of retarded development, I would strongly recommend to begin with arithmetic by very slow degrees, and learning by heart verses, or short sentences, and to leave the imagination unfettered by any restrictions. Give an abundant supply of travels, romances, stories, and pathetic tales, in which the patient may luxuriate without limit; but by no means attempt abstractions even of the humblest kind, and make no appeal whatever to the reasoning powers. It is scarcely metaphorical language to say that the fibres, whose action is to produce the argumentative functions, are not yet disentangled, and the attempt to force them into action is accompanied by great risk of injuring them for ever. The only coercion used, should be for the purpose of enforcing *obedience*, and *never* to enforce *study*. A habit of obedience, more especially in trifles, it is of the highest importance to establish; and if well considered, the reader will perceive that such a habit implies the cultivation of self-control in its safest form. But time must be given—to hurry the development of such a brain is to kill the goose for the golden eggs. I firmly believe that I have seen youths who might have been cultivated into average perfection, tormented into permanent imbecility by the natural, but fatal determinatin to place them on a level with other boys of their age (for this state of things is exceedingly rare with the other sex). Every man of experience must know more than one family where the children advance very slowly to intellectual maturity, yet give no reason to doubt of its certain, though late arrival.

The reverse of this state of things, the *precocious* intellect, is unfortunately too well known. It is not always possible to keep it in check by the most judicious proceedings, for its is generally caused by a preternaturally rapid growth of the convolutions on the surface of the brain, incompatible with great physical vigour; but unfortunately such premature intellectual powers are so flattering to the vanity of parents that it is scarcely possible to convince them of the danger of their early cultivation. The child learns with such ease, its acquisitions are made with so little effort, that the fond parent cannot believe in the predictions of the medical friend, and spurs the willing steed to leaps beyond his strength, till the brain fails under the effort. Knowing these things, having witnessed the miserable consequences, I could not read the correspondence between William Pitt and his father without a feeling allied to terror. Never did man go so near to destroy the intellect of his son by over-excitement as that arrogant, unreasonable and imperious, and much over-rated man, the great Earl of Chatham, as he is called. "Courage, my son," said he, in one of his letters, when the poor lad was complaining of the enormous variety of topics urged on his attention; "Courage, my boy; remember there is only the Cyclopaedia to learn." William Pitt was very near falling a sacrifice to his father's ambition. Great as were his talents, I do not doubt that they would have been much greater had they been more slowly cultivated, and he might then have attained the ordinary term of human life, instead of his brain wearing out his body at so early an age. To see him, as I have done, come into Bellamy's after the excitement of debate, in a state of collapse, that with his uncouth countenance gave the air of insanity, swallow a steak without mastication, and drink a bottle of port wine almost at a draught, and be then barely wound up to the level of ordinary impulse—repeat this process twice, or I believe, even three times in the course of the night—was a frightful example of over-cultivation of brain before it had attained its full development. So much had its excitability been exhausted by premature and excessive moral stimuli, that, when his ambition was sated, it was incapable of even keeping itself in action without the physical stimulants I have spoken of. Men called the sad exhibition the triumph of mind over matter; I call it the contest of brain and body, where victory is obtained at the sacrifice of life.

It is not *parva componere magnis* to speak of similar examples in humble life, for the soul of the lowest mechanic is as important in the scale of creation as the soul of the king. I have seen the same wretched results in the case of a little boy in the shop of a draper, perched on a desk as the accountant, and attending in rapid succession to forty or fifty young men who bring their notes of sales to him to be verified and registered —to give correct change to every one while his attention is solicited by half-a-dozen at a time, and rendered responsible for the slightest error on pain of dismissal, perhaps to a miserable and sordid home; he strains his faculties till they almost burst with the effort, and goes to his bed at night in a state of collapse and exhaustion much worse to endure or to witness than the most excessive bodily fatigue; by-and-by he finds himself unable to wind up his brain to the daily task without the aid of spirits—the habit is begun—it will never be discontinued—he becomes confused—cannot make his accounts agree—falsifies them to avoid rebuke—is detected, disgraced, dismissed—becomes an outcast—seeks refuge in the habit of drinking—drops down from vice to crime—and thence to infamy and a premature death. Such cases are common.

In the state of transition which now exists throughout the whole social structure of this nation, and which has so entirely unhinged society by changes against which no prudence can guard and which no sagacity can foretel, the most remarkable of all the accompaniments is the universally prevalent excess of labour of mind and body to which every one is compelled to submit; all are in a mad gallop, and he who does not keep up with the rest is trampled under foot. It is difficult to predict the consequences of so unnatural a state of things. If it end in good, it can only be after the hopes and happiness of millions of human beings have been sacrificed in the struggle. I must own that I look with envy upon the tranquil life and scanty industry of other nations, even though accompanied by the stolid indifference of ignorance, and cannot but wish with Lord John Manners that we could resume some of the holidays of the Romish Church—they are the only protection to him who has nothing but his physical strength to exchange with his fellow-creatures for all the needs of life. The enormous accumulations of wealth in this country may add to the dignity and power of the nation, but they do not contribute to the happiness of the labouring classes. A man who has to compete with the steam engine enters on a fearful contest; and whatever may be the ultimate benefit of the triumph of mechanical power, generations of human beings must be crushed under the wheels of the mighty Juggernaut of Science while the process goes on. I cannot but look with apprehension at the irregular developments of human intellect which necessarily accompany the mighty change; and now that the mind can, by means of the press, make its sentiments vibrate in the heart of millions, should any unscrupulous man, of gigantic intellectual power, happen to hit on one of the chords which, when struck, find an echo in every dissatisfied mind, it depends on the most trivial accident whether the movement he excites advance the interest or prostrate the hopes of mankind; whether the mighty progress recently made be guided to a happy result, or the whole scheme of civilization be pushed back for centuries.

A ridge tile of a cottage in Derbyshire, says Mr. Gisborne, decides whether the rain which falls from heaven be directed to the German ocean or the Atlantic!

There is another form of cerebral irregularity, of which I have seen examples. A child from two to three years of age will manifest all the ordinary faculties which are expected at that period of life; nay, will sometimes, in the opinion of the parents, exhibit signs of precocious intellect, and the father and mother will express their exultation at the premature display of talent. Gradually all the persons, except the parents, observe that the child makes no progress; it advances rapidly in physical development; enjoys perfect health; but the intellect remains stationary, and at the age of ten or twelve it becomes obvious even to the parents that the child is imbecile.

Now there is a real distinction between this case and that of genuine idiocy: the faculties, however inadequate to the purposes of that age, are still complete, if we could suppose the child no older than the period at which the progress was arrested; and if we compare its manifestations of intellect with those of that period of life, we shall find that they are nearly equal, and have not materially retrograded; it is the incongruity between the infantine ideas and the size and age, which gives the impression of perfect idiocy; the countenance has not the vacant stare of the idiot; the voluntary movements of the limbs are still under the perfect control of the will, there is no dangling of the wrists (a hopeless symptom); there is no contrivance, no comparison, no strong thinking process perceptible; but sensation and perception exist in a high degree, and if you listen to the babble without looking at the child, you would scarcely perceive any incongruity or deficiency of intellect. If this state of things be allowed to pass on to the age of fourteen or fifteen without any enlightened efforts being made to call into action the dormant faculties, the case is then almost entirely hopeless; but in the early stage I have seen two examples of entire success, one of which is already narrated. Those portions of the brain which minister to the higher faculties of the intellect have simply ceased to grow, as we see the body cease to grow in some dwarfs, without deformity.

I have never had an opportunity of examining the brain of one of these beings; indeed, I cannot remember an instance of death at a sufficiently early period to make it possible to draw useful inferences from the inspection, for they are generally endowed with remarkable health. If the examination be delayed till the bodily development be complete, the state of the brain does not differ in any cognizable degree from that of ordinary persons.

Men of the present day can hardly conceive the obstacles which impeded the researches of anatomists forty years ago, and how dangerous to the success of the practitioner was the reputation of a desire for these inspections. I consider the operation of the New Poor Law as likely to lead to the most important results in this respect—when a higher class of men shall be appointed to the medical care of Union Poor-houses, as will certainly be the case gradually, not by increase of salary perhaps, but by the honour and influence of the appointment, rendering it (like the office of surgeon or physician to a hospital) an object of ambition to men of superior attainments—when from an improvement in the regulations as to the election of medical officers to these institutions, such election shall become a positive test of ability and acquirements—and these men be so situated in point of fortune as to be able to bestow *scientific* attention; I believe we shall have a body of medical statistics, so vast and so various, that a great number of the *vexatae questiones* of our *ars incertissima* will be finally set at rest; and that the road to knowledge will be straightened and shortened, to the great relief and advantage of the students who are now beginning to con their Latin accidence, or perhaps undergoing matriculation in the mysteries of the alphabet.

Dr. Haslam, in his little book called "*Sound Mind*," has some observations on the faculty of *attention*, through the whole of which runs a transparent vein of fallacy, if my view of the physiology of the brain be correct. He, like many other writers, attaches an importance to etymology of which it is in general quite undeserving. It adds no force or distinctness to the meaning of the word, to know, for example, that *succinct* took its origin from the tucking up of the apron and making themselves ready for business, among the Roman slaves; nor that *calculate* arises from the Roman children using pebbles for learning arithmetic. As unscientific words are generally formed from some loose analogy between a mechanical process and a mental operation, and are chiefly invented in days of barbarism and ignorance, it rather confuses than aids our reasoning faculties to bring before us a crude derivation which has been long superseded and forgotten. The meaning of the word *attention* must be thoroughly understood in its own modern sense, before a man can even comprehend the explanation given of its etymology; and when we speak of "a stretching forth of the mind to the object," I cannot but think, with Corporal Trim, that "the interpreter is the harder to be understood of the two." In the present day, new expressions are more precise; and when we talk of *getting up the steam*, for example, as applied to courage, we use a very short and very significant and appropriate metaphor, which saves much circumlocution.

Dr. Haslam, in speaking of *attention*, says, "Indeed something of this nature actually takes place in the organ [the brain]. In minute examinations by the eye, we actually strain and stretch its muscles, and feel the fatigue which results from over-exertion. When we listen, the neck is stretched forward, and such position enables us to collect those vibrations of sound that would otherwise be inaudible; but to infer that the mind itself was capable of being extended, would be to invest it with the properties of substance, and at once plunge us into the grossest materialism.

"According to the nature and constitution of the human mind, the effective duration of the attention seems to be very limited. If the eye be steadily directed to any particular object, after a few seconds it will be found to wander; and if the mind be exerted on the subject of its recollection, there is very soon experienced an interruption, from the intrusion of irrelevant thoughts. The effective duration of the attention will much depend on the superior capacity, nature or constitution of the intellect itself, but still more on the manner in which these habits of attention are exercised; for *by proper cultivation its duration may be considerably protracted.*"

The habit acquired by practice, of concentrating the attention of both brains to the same subject, is the faculty here spoken of; the *irrelevant thoughts which intrude*, are obviously a separate process of thinking in one of the brains, which resists the will of the other.

I here venture the hypothesis that the most unmanageable brain is that which most nearly approaches its fellow in power; that two brains nearly equivalent are almost necessarily accompanied by vacillation; whereas when one of them is decidedly superior in power (as I believe to be generally the case with the left), in this case the right brain aids and corroborates its fellow, as an assistant aids a workman; and more is done by the two directed by one will than both could have executed separately.

This suggestion will, no doubt, seem to the reader a very extravagant supposition, but only for a short time. I have had many proofs that, if steadily considered, it will be not only plausible but even convincing, so far as a mere hypothesis can produce conviction. I have alluded to the superior efficacy of the right hand as an instrument of volition, being dependent on the superior power of the left brain; but at present my statistics on the morbid functions of the two brains are too limited to admit of elaboration into proof. I beg the reader to believe that the hints thus thrown out are not the inspiration of the moment, but have been reflected on for years, and are put forth in the hope that the attention of anatomists may be drawn to the subject, and the result of future dissections recorded. There is a mine of discovery here, if it were properly worked, by a man well placed and capable of communicating an impulse to others.

"Let two ordinary persons," says Dr. Haslam, "A. and B., take a map of a district with which they are unacquainted, and let each be allowed half-an-hour to study the map. Desire A. to fix his attention undeviatingly on the map for the time, and at its expiration request him to put on paper the relative situations and names of the different places, and for the performance of this allow him another half hour. As the experiment has been repeatedly made, it may be confidently predicted that A. would exhibit a very incorrect copy of the original map. Let B. take the same map to study for the same time; but instead of keeping his eyes undeviatingly fixed to the object, desire him to view it only for a few seconds, and then, shutting his eyes, let him endeavour to bring the picture of the map before his mind: his first efforts will convey a very confused notion of the actual and relative positions, but he will become sensible of his defects, and re-inspect the map for their correction. If this successive ocular examination and review by the mind by continued during the half-hour, or even for a less period, B. will be competent to make a drawing of the map with superior accuracy to A., who endeavoured to fix his attention for the whole of the time allotted. In conducting this experiment some very curious phenomena may be observed. If A. had directed his eyes to the object intensely and undeviatingly, and especially in a strong light, and had then covered or shut his eyes in order to recollect the situations on the map, the straining of the organ to the object would defeat his endeavours, and instead of being able to bring the picture before his mind he would be annoyed and interrupted by the intrusion of ocular spectra, undergoing the succession of changes described by Dr. Darwin. Thus there are limits to the duration of our effective attention: if the organ of vision be too long directed to the object of perception, ocular spectra arise, fatigue and confusion ensue in the other senses, and if the subjects of recollection be too long and intensely contemplated, delirium will supervene."

Now, for a man who attaches so much importance to the precise meaning and etymology of words, Dr. Haslam is one of the most careless in the use of them, and there is great difficulty in comprehending his meaning. His analogy between a process of reasoning and an endeavour to obtain a mental picture (*an idea*) through the medium of one of the senses, will not hold at all; the processes are essentially as different as the organs by which they are exercised. The organ of vision is accompanied by a muscular apparatus, and like all other muscular structures, becomes fatigued by continuous exercise. Were the map no larger than could be comprehended by a single view, and could the eye be kept perfectly steady, so far from continuous attention being incompatible with a correct *idea* of it, there is, under such circumstances, a real picture of the object preserved on the retina, and transferred to whatever smooth unoccupied surface we may afterwards look at; so that it is easy for a person even unacquainted with drawing to trace the outlines. This fact has been familiar to me, as the experience of my acquaintance and myself, for nearly half a century, and was the subject of a paper by Sir Charles Bell more than thirty years ago. It is produced by the activity, repose, or exhaustion of sensibility in that portion of the retina on which the outlines fall, according as they are formed by light or the reverse, and which thus makes a similar outline on the paper we look at. The process described by Dr. Haslam is a sort of *getting by heart of the idea*, and is one of the very humblest of the mental functions. The exercise of continuous attention on any subject strictly intellectual, is in fact the only way to investigate; and it is the difficulty of accomplishing this object which is remedied by practice, and which gives the great superiority to the man who has been regularly taught the art and has continued to exercise it.

It is told of Sir Isaac Newton, that when asked how he had ever been able to *conceive* his doctrine of fluxions, he replied, "By continuing to think at it,"—the mode, indeed, in which every great invention has been accomplished. To think *of* anything is an easy process, cursorily performed by both brains, probably in alternate succession; but to think *at* a thing is a severe voluntary effort, only leading to a successful issue when it is the result of considerable mental power duly cultivated; and this is what I mean by the superiority of the disciplined scholar over the self-educated man. There are very few human beings who are capable of teaching themselves the painful process. In the beginning it is accompanied by what may be metaphorically (I almost think literally) designated a *mental cramp*—enough to deter most men from following up the process to a result.

"However great the pains which an individual may take to fix his thoughts to the examination of a particular subject, he will find that the effective duration of his attention is very limited, and that other thoughts often wholly unconnected with the subject will intrude and occupy his mind. On some occasions they are so prevailing and importunate that he loses the original subject altogether."—*Haslam.*

This is natural enough with two brains; inconceivable with only one. I dare not say that such fixity of attention would be the consequence of one brain being destroyed, because under such extensive and formidable disorganization, the whole intellectual functions must be languid and feeble—that the remaining brain may find any one subject burthensome is natural, and that it may from time to time discontinue and resume the process of thinking, is to be expected. Neither is it strange that in the healthy state of both organs one subject should suggest another collateral to itself, or connected by some mere verbal resemblance in sound or shape; but this is a different process from that to which Dr. Haslam alludes, and of which every one must be conscious in his own person: the intrusion of another totally different train of thought, which the first did not suggest, and is unable entirely to overpower, although it can for a considerable time pursue the new one to the exclusion of the former.

"It is acknowledged (adds Dr. Haslam) that the soundest and most efficient mind is distinguished by the control it is capable of exerting on its immediate thoughts."

The soundest and most efficient mind is that in which the

intellectual faculties have the strongest power over the animal impulses and propensities; and this depends chiefly on cultivation, but is also influenced by the respective original powers of the two classes of organs. The soundest and most efficient mind is also dependent on the cultivation of the reciprocal influence of the two brains, and the establishment of a permanent resolve to let no volition pass into action that has not the full consent and approbation of both of them—a rare accomplishment.

In taking leave of Dr. Haslam's work, I venture to express an opinion which, were he living, I should withhold in deference to the feelings of an old man—there is now no longer any necessity for reserve.

I can only account for the favourable reception of his crude opinions and reasonings and for the respectful allusion to them by modern writers on the ground that the subject of insanity was, at the time he wrote, almost entirely new. His defective education, and the utterly illogical and unphilosophical structure of his mind, are shewn at every page, and his want of power to observe and to reason, renders his assertions and his inferences utterly worthless. To cite him as an authority on any point whatever tends to retard the advance of sound knowledge on the nature and treatment of insanity. It is like appealing to a church-clockmaker on the structure of a chronometer.

The perfect consentaneity of the two brains, so necessary to the deep consideration of a subject, and the exercise of sound judgment thereon, may be interrupted by very trifling causes. The process, though strictly under the control of volition, it is volition duly cultivated and habitually exercised which alone possesses the power of resisting the interruption.

One of the strange phenomena of the mind and which has produced great embarrassment in the discussions on the nature and extent of the intellectual powers, one which philosophers have lamented their inability to comprehend, is that wonderful faculty by which we can select a subject of contemplation to the exclusion of others—can say, "I will think no more on this subject," or "I will think of nothing else but this." All attempts to explain this, which have come to my knowledge, have been merely the re-statement of the fact in different words, or a mystification from which nothing could be gathered.

The theory I am endeavouring to establish seems to afford a perfectly satisfactory explanation of this valuable mental power.

"It requires *two* persons to make peace (says Franklin), but *one* can make war." Concede the existence of a train of thought in each brain, and the thing is perfectly plain. If either brain wills *not* to entertain the subject, it is quite sufficient to destroy for a time that unison or consentaneity of the two which alone constitutes study or deep consideration, the essence of which is the application of both brains to the same subject at the same time; but until one or the other of them has started a new subject of sufficient interest to engage in its turn the attention of both, and establish a new object of *study*, the consideration we have not concentrated, becomes diffused on a variety of subjects, which are entertained with that discursive and imperfect attention which we employ in common uninteresting conversation—as in the exercise of vision, we look without seeing—we take in and languidly comprehend, all the objects before us; but when we wish to *examine*, we direct the axes of both eyes to one specific object, or one minute spot on that object, and then we not only *look* but *see, we examine*. We have sensation, perception, cognition, reflection, comparison, and judgment—the regular series ending in a result.

So it is with the two brains—each in the ordinary exercise of its faculties *looks* at subjects, but barely *sees* them, much less *examines* them; but when some one object has attracted the attention of both, if the consideration of it be painful, one of the brains can *will* the interruption of the conjoint process, *can make war* and if the subject have not been long enough under contemplation to defeat the attempt to discard it, we can "call another cause." In like manner we can choose among the topics before us that which we *will* to consider, and the more energetic brain can control the course of thought in its fellow; we then ponder, investigate, or study.

It appears almost certain that sensation and perception are not performed by the same organs which exercise the purely reasoning faculties, from the consideration that while we are fully exerting the latter, the former are in a great measure suspended, and their impressions cease to influence the intellectual machinery. I have elsewhere alluded to the well-known fact, that when both brains are deeply engaged in study we are almost unconscious, not only of every thing which is passing around us but even of internal sensations, or rather of phenomena which under ordinary circumstances would excite sensation. A man speaks to us, we do not hear him; we look at him but do not see him; we are subjected to cold or hunger, or we have an uneasy seat which gives at other times positive pain, we do not feel them; an offensive odour pervades the room, we do not smell it—or rather, we do not perceive it—although an impression made on this last organ will sooner recall our scattered thoughts than any other. The organ of smell is, of all the senses, the seat of the most powerful associations; forgotten scenes are brought back to the mind more vividly and intensely by an odour to which we have been long unaccustomed than by all the other senses put together. I can well recollect, at the age of fifty-five, a long train of events, persons, and conversations, brought back to mind with a flash, by the odour of Mareschal powder (formerly used to imitate red hair, then in fashion), when these impressions had been utterly forgotten and extinct for five-and-forty years. Had any portion of the conversation I had heard so long ago been related to me previous to the perception of the odour, I should have denied its truth. I remember a very affecting incident of this kind betraying the long kept secret of a lady of rank by the ungovernable impulse it created; but the parties are living, and I forbear.

The enormous relative magnitude of the olfactory ganglia in the horse, compared with the same organ in the hare-hound, and other animals which track their prey by the scent, would seem an argument against the connexion of size and power so strongly contended for by phrenologists.

CHAPTER XXII: *Hysteria; Hypochondriasis; Hydrophobia*

The disease called Hysteria, a word which originally signified that it was confined to females, is well-known to be occasionally inflicted on the other sex. We sometimes see this affection in young men of sedentary and studious habits. It is probably a disturbance of the brain from reflex action, and in both sexes mainly under the control of the will. Men are taught to be ashamed of any manifestation of this malady or passion as *unmanly*, and the efforts they make to overcome it are generally successful; but many a man of acute feelings must remember instances in his own person where the effort has been one requiring extraordinary energy and perseverance—success often doubtful and sometimes impossible. Among females of a certain age, just advancing to womanhood, the disorder propagates itself by sympathy with great rapidity, and will spread in a short time throughout a large school, if the head of the establishment be a feeble-minded person, or the medical attendant of too suave and timid a disposition. On the other hand, I know more than one lady in that position, who makes it a point to declare to every new comer that she "does not allow hysterics," and by throwing a very large bason of cold water in the face at the first symptom, drenching the clothes, and making it necessary to change every article of dress, establishes such a wholesome terror that the disorder is entirely expelled from the school.

I believe this form of disease to be generally the consequence of reflex action of the great ganglionic centres on the brain, excited sometimes perhaps by a trifling disturbance in their functions, or even by irregularity of digestion; and that, except where such a temperament has been criminally encouraged, the affection is always controllable by the will. That, in fact, such control is one of the habitual offices of the brain; and that, were not the attention occupied by the necessity of earning a living or attending positive duties, Reason would be very often temporarily unseated from a perfectly avoidable cause. This also is one of the forms of what Mr. Barlow describes as "Man's power over himself to prevent or control insanity."

Whatever be the temporary state of the sensorium produced by this

> "Monster ill, that mimics all the rest,"

it may become the permanent state of the mind by neglect; and my own opinion is, I think, confirmed by that of Dr. Conolly, that the loss of reason, the loss of power to control morbid influences and volitions, is much more frequently attributable to desuetude than to disease.

The *moral* treatment of the insanity that is not idiopathic or sporadic—that is, not depending on actual disease of the organ of thought, nor on the peculiar brain of the individual—is therefore of more importance than the strictly medical treatment; and it is on this ground that the medical superintendent of an asylum ought to have the entire selection of his agents—a subject on which I have much to say, on a fitting occasion.

In the first Livraison (Plate III) of Cruveilhier's great work, is a representation of the entire disorganization and enormous enlargement of all the cervical ganglions of the sympathetic on the left side, down to the arch of the aorta. The ganglia are transformed into a fibrous mass of from ten to twenty times their original size, and so hard that, as M. Cruveilhier expresses it, "*ils crient sous le scalpel.*" These strangely decomposed bodies were connected with all the cervical nerves in their course, which nerves, however, exhibited no signs of disease.

I would dwell a little on this case, for I am much mistaken if we cannot draw from it valuable inferences, which have not presented themselves to the narrator. It is most unfortunate that no account whatever could be obtained of the previous state of the patient. We will suppose then that these ganglia, which were of the consistence of hard cartilage or of the prostate gland, had long ceased their peculiar functions, and could not convey any impression whatever to the brain; still, if they are intended by nature to convey any impression whatever, there was a time at the commencement of disease, when they must have conveyed disordered impressions and produced disordered sensations by reflex action, through the cervical nerves. May not analogous maladies in their early stage, cause many of those anomalous symptoms which hypochondriacs vainly attempt to describe? and may not at least one of the cerebra have been so far injured or disturbed by the further progress of disease or disorder as to give the state of *conscious* delusion? thence pass on till it defies the control of the sound cerebrum, and the malady takes on the form of monomania or of permanent delusion? for the brain reasoning from wrong premises necessarily draws false inferences. Making still further progress, may it not advance to confirmed and probably *incurable* mania? These things appear to me the natural sequence; and how seldom is any part of the body of an insane person examined with attention, except the brain and its membranes, or perhaps, at the most, the organs of respiration and digestion. I can conceive that a great number of the more fantastic forms of hypochondriacal insanity may be explained on this hypothesis; and that to an advanced period of disease, the morbid sensations, or more properly the morbid convictions thence arising may be controlled by a sound cerebrum duly cultivated. A friend of mine in the country, a lady of independent fortune, high mental cultivation, and great vigour of mind, apparently in perfect health, was the subject of strange and indescribable internal sensations intensely distressing, and often prophesied that she should die—a prophecy ridiculed by all her acquaintance as well as by the medical attendant. She bore their incredulity with great complacency, and in the apparent exemption from all bodily ailment, died. "Something wrong in the chest" was the dictum of the man who performed the "post mortem"—an explanation which perfectly satisfied the impatient heir, and saved the reputation of an ignorant practitioner. Quere—was it like the case of diseased ganglia just recited?

Cerebral disturbance, from disease or disorder in the great ganglionic centres, must then, I think, be taken into account among the numerous causes of partial, temporary, total, or permanent insanity. It would appear from the researches of physiologists that the ganglia of the grand sympathetic are really so many reservoirs or manufactories of nervous influence, of which the main project is to render organic life independent of animal life, and (as expressed by Erasmus Wilson) "to produce a separation necessary for the preservation of the animal without involving his integrity"—thus the animal system being injured, the organic system may be preserved, while the mutual dependence of the whole is maintained. The grand sympathetic is then a depôt for the supply of nervous influence, when from accident or disease (and especially in sleep) there is an interruption to the current from the cerebro-spinal axis. Like a town on the banks of a river receiving its habitual supply from its own side of the water and keeping always a large reserve, but in case of siege and interruption, obtaining succour by the bridges which connect it with another territory.

In an early period of my professional studies I had, with the natural conceit of youth and with a large stock of the presumption of ignorance, investigated the testimony in favour of the existence of hydrophobia. It happened at that time that an epidemic terror, a panic, spread over the land, to an extent of which we have had no subsequent example. Under the direction of surgeons of established character for skill, good sense, and humanity, I had assisted to mutilate many unhappy individuals who had been bitten by dogs (that they were mad was never doubted), and the word went forth throughout the land, "war to the dogs." Strange to say, the dogs disliked being killed! especially by persons with whom they were not acquainted; and had the audacity to stand on their defence. Here was proof, superfluous proof, that they were mad, and they were therefore massacred without mercy. In these conflicts the attacking party was often wounded, and it was the duty of the dresser (*élève interne*) to cut out the bitten part extensively, regardless of the injury inflicted by the operation—like the flogging of the insane, which, if it killed them, at least saved them from further evil. An exemption from the awfully mysterious disease, hydrophobia, was thought to be cheaply purchased by a mutilation that almost rendered the man a cripple for life. I have sometimes even fainted in the execution of the cruel orders given, to which by-the-by (such was the intensity of terror pervading the public mind) the patient generally submitted with alacrity. I at last refused to be any longer the instrument of such cruel delusions and, affecting illness, withdrew from my duties.

By a very natural process in the human mind, like that which takes place with those who having witnessed the mummeries and cruelties of superstition, reject religion altogether, I reasoned myself into a conviction that hydrophobia was a non-existent disease, and exactly on a par with witchcraft in its claims to belief.

So strong was this conviction, and so conclusive did my arguments seem to myself, that I wondered at the infatuation of the public which could resist them, as expressed in the many letters with which I wearied the editors of newspapers. Becoming more and more strenuous as my reasonings were more and more condemned, I at last proposed that a dog, decidedly mad in the opinion of others, should be allowed to bite me in any fleshy part of the body. To this trial I was perfectly ready to submit, and preparations were made for the experiment. I bound up my arm with bandages of such a thickness as to be a defence against the teeth of the dog, leaving only a small portion naked, but quite sufficient for the experiment. When the time approached I was "talked down," but not convinced; and the affair dropped for some years.

Seeing afterwards the genuine disease in its most aggravated form and advanced stage, my disbelief was so far shaken that, when a short time afterwards a case came under my own care, I was induced to watch it with an attention that could not have been exceeded had my own life depended on the issue. I have since that time closely observed the phenomena of two other examples of this frightful disease, and I now proceed to explain the object of this long digression.

In the early stage of the disease it appeared to me that one brain was decidedly attacked before the other, and that there was a period of indefinite length during which all the morbid volitions were under the control of reason, or as I should say, of the sound brain. In the case which came under my care, the patient, who was a man of great intelligence and of middle age, had entirely forgotten the bite of the dog, and it was his constantly recurring observation to me that he feared he was going out of his mind—that he had an uncontrollable rapidity of thoughts, and mental delusions constantly obtruding themselves on his attention, which he found it impossible to dismiss, and which he in a manner believed, although he knew them to be groundless.

It may be supposed that he was practising a very common deceit, and had all along a suspicion of the cause of the disease, but independently of the fact that we were too intimate to make concealment probable, I was present when the suspicion first suggested itself to his mind. *I saw the awful idea steal slowly over his countenance*, and it was a study for Garrick himself. When this conviction established itself, the self-control, which had hitherto enabled him to suppress his emotions, seemed to me to be laid down as deliberately and intentionally as a man might lay down the reins when driving; and he went immediately over the precipice.

Up to this stage there is a very strong analogy between madness and hydrophobia; but the further progress, although resembling the furious delirium of maniacal patients, and still more strongly that of delirium tremens, is accompanied by symptoms peculiar to itself, and affords no further instruction to a student of insanity.

The instances must be exceedingly rare where any physical malady whatever can attack both cerebra simultaneously, and the progress of cerebral diseases (such as atrophy, softening, etc.) is so slow, as to allow a considerable period of time during which the patient might be conscious of antagonist volitions, diseased propensities, and disordered ratiocination, yet perfectly able to control them till the mental functions in the disordered brain were quietly and insensibly abandoned to the other cerebrum.

"When inflammation," says Bouillaud, "only occupies a part more or less extensive of one of the cerebral hemispheres, and when the other hemisphere is in a healthy state, the intellectual and moral functions, at least ordinarily, present no notable lesion. It seems that in this case the healthy hemisphere suffices for the exercise of these functions. [Certainly, because it is a perfect organ.] But if the inflammation of one hemisphere [this unlucky word!] spreads itself over the other hemisphere, a delirium of variable form occurs; [when the organ is no longer complete, the function is necessarily imperfect] according to the extent and intensity of the inflammation, *and perhaps also according to the part affected either in one or the other hemisphere.* A general delirium always exists when the partial irritation generalizes itself, an accident unfortunately often seen."

Here is the difficulty of ascertaining the pathology of the early stage of insanity—delusion; and the still earlier stage—*conscious* delusion. It is not till the disease spreads itself to both brains, and perhaps produces extensive organic changes, that we have an opportunity of obtaining physical evidence. Were it possible to make experiments on human beings in the same manner and to the same extent we make them on the inferior animals, we might obtain a degree of knowledge which would furnish better means of controlling the curable stage of insanity. We know nothing of the state of the brain positively till the disease has long passed beyond it. All that we can previously know is from inference alone.

I am not without hope, however, should my speculations be received, that having laid down the coloured spectacles which shewed them only one thinking organ in the two hemispheres, men may observe more accurately the changes which are occasionally to be tested in the suicides and accidental deaths of the insane.

Except in the case of accidents causing death to persons in the very early stage of incipient insanity, no opportunity is afforded of examining the state of the cerebra and their membranes till long after the disease or disorder has spread to both of them (which seems to me the very essence of confirmed insanity); previously to that event, the sound brain could exercise control over its fellow to such a degree as to prevent the manifestation of mental disturbance to others, or if the state of the mind were occasionally detected by some impulse coming on too suddenly to permit a successful effort at concealment, the character of the disordered action would be that of delusion or whimsical opinion. So long as the vague and irrational, or at least unfounded, ideas arising in one brain are under the command of the other, no one would apply to such a state of mind the term insanity.

There is nothing contrary to analogy in disorder first taking place in one brain. We see gangrene from a general cause commence first in one limb, and small-pox manifest its pustules at first on one side, which I have noticed to precede those on the other side sometimes by twenty-four or forty-eight hours.

CHAPTER XXIII: *Difficulty of Obtaining Information of the Early Pathological State; Dr. Greding's Reports; Impropriety of Classing Idiots With the Insane; Attempts to Educate Idiots; Opinions of Georget on Disease of the Brain as the Cause of Insanity.*

It is a remarkable proof of the little dependence to be placed on the assignment of specific localities for specific functions, that the most extensive disease shall be sometimes produced without any lesion of the intellect, and the most extensive lesion of the intellect exist without disease of the brain, or a disease so slight as to be scarcely cognizable on dissection. It is true that in the immense majority of cases there is more or less of injury to that organ or its membranes; but this is the gradual progress of the disease which ultimately destroyed life, and the appearances on opening the brain are, at that stage of the malady, no test of the degree of disorganization or disturbance which sufficed to interfere with the due exercise of mind, and especially *conscious delusion*. This can only be ascertained in the rare cases of accidental death during insanity in its early stage, and the attention has been so little directed to the subject that such cases have been generally overlooked, and the opportunities lost. I hope to excite attention to the subject, and to point out the means of rectifying the omission, for, if we are ever to possess positive evidence of specific local faculties it can only be from this source.

Even in death from those diseases of the brain which are directly destructive, of which so many examples are given by Dr. Abercrombie, there is, in almost every instance, an entire omission by that writer, of even the slightest notice of the mental functions; yet the variety of diseases enumerated must surely have afforded cases of mental disturbance. He gives examples of abscess of the corpus striatum—of the medula oblongata—of the cerebellum—destruction of septum lucidum —fornix—ulceration of the convolutions—tubercles—encysted tumours—softening—and various other diseases, but scarcely ever does he allude to the state of the intellect. Future observers will, I hope, bear this in mind, and remedy the omission.

Dr. Greding (cited by Dr. Pritchard), physician to a public hospital for lunatics and idiots, states as follows: "Out of 220 examined, the forehead was contracted, the temples compressed, and the occiput large and expanded. In a few, the head was elongated, and compressed at the temples; some had a head almost round, or of a square shape—these were epileptic idiots. Two had small heads, quite circular—these were epileptic madmen. Of 216 cases, including madmen, idiots, and epileptics, the skull was unusually thick in 167; this fact was also observed in 78 out of 100 cases of raving madness, and in 22 in 30 of idiocy. In many cases the cranium was remarkably thin. Holes were observed in the inner table of the skull in 115 out of 216 cases (!), in other instances bony projections from the inner surface. Cerebral substance softer than usual in 118 out of 216 cases; soft and pulpy in 51 out of 100; also in 19 out of 24 of melancholia, 8 out of 20 epileptics, and 16 out of 30 idiots. Dura mater adherent in 107 out of 216, in a few instances was of a blueish black, thickened and partially ossified. Pia mater thickened and opaque, 86 out of 100, beset with small spongy bodies 92 in 100; these bodies often united to the surface of the brain, and in some instances the seats of ossific deposits," etc. etc.

Strange! that the collectors of these useless statistics should not have borne in mind that *the disease the patient died of* is not *the disease he lived with*; for it was the change either in character or extent which caused the death of the sufferer. As well might we shew a gangrened limb as a specimen of inflammation. Neither was the disease (the visible organic lesion) of which he died, the disease which caused the insanity; for extensive disease is compatible with correct intellect. It is *the kind*, not *the degree*, of *alteration*, which renders the organ unfit for the manifestation of mind. I have already spoken of the circumstances under which alone the state of the brain, as shewn by dissection, is any index of the cause and nature of insanity.

Much confusion has been created by the habit of classing idiocy among the forms of insanity or dementia. There is no more resemblance between them than between the state of a man who has lost his legs from mortification and of another who is born without legs. Idiocy seems hardly worthy of attention at all; the animal is born imperfect, and is to be provided for as a human being, and furnished with such moderate physical enjoyments as it can appreciate. The organs which should furnish *mind* do not exist. This condition would be utterly unworthy of scientific notice; but that the gradations between the slavering idiot and the best indued mind are so minute that it is impossible to draw the line between them, and that, in the next place, it is just possible that a few of those in the equivocal territory might possibly be cultivated into a slightly greater degree of intellect, as some of those on the other side of the arbitrary boundary might, by neglect and desuetude, lose the few faculties they possess.

Insanity supposes the possession of average intellect, that is, of organs of the average degree of completeness, and that, when disordered or diseased, their disturbance may be rectified by art or be restored by the spontaneous *vis medicatrix naturae*, that is, *by time*. It is, therefore, worth while to examine with attention, and ascertain if we can guide or aid the process of cure.

To mix up idiots with the insane in public establishments only mystifies and vitiates the statistics. It would be just as rational to send all those who are born without fingers to a hospital for the treatment of the frostbitten, and then to draw inferences from the proportion of the whole number cured.

The experiment now making in Switzerland, of which I have but an imperfect knowledge, shews that there are certain degrees and modes of defective brain which admit of cultivation, so as to bring the possessor into the category of rational beings. Those who are familiar with the Crétins of the Vallois, must have observed, as I have, that there are all gradations of intellect among them, from that which places them scarcely higher in the scale of creation than the moluscae, to that of mammalia, and that there are even some who approach to the dignity of manhood. If the great experiment now making by the philanthropic gentleman who has undertaken the arduous task of educating these miserable abortions, can succeed in increasing their happiness, it is well; but I much fear that his humane efforts may end in only making them sensible of their miserable position.

M. Georget, of whose opinions I was entirely ignorant till this work was nearly completed, is one of the few writers who have expressly noticed the want of uniformity in the two sides of the skull in the insane. I believe that should attention be directed to the subject, much confirmation of it will be brought forward. M. Georget says, "We remark some skulls of the insane to be unequally developed, one of the sides being larger and more arched than the other—it is the right side that I have generally found with this disposition. Some skulls are as if they were twisted in such a manner that one side of the head is too forward and the other too much behind; there are some which have not the antero-posterior diameter more extended than the lateral—the cavity of these is elevated very much, especially in the posterior part. The cavities of the base of the skull present likewise irregularities—those of one side are sometimes larger than those of the other."

There are important inferences to be drawn from the fact, if established, that it is generally the right side which is affected by malformation, but my ideas on this subject are not quite matured, and I wait for statistics. I cannot but think, however, that the almost universal preference of the right hand (from its greater strength and more perfect obedience to volition) arises from the superior power and energy of the left brain. I believe that the inferior capacity of the left hand is not the effect of education alone, and I suspect that in the case of left-handed persons there is a transposition of the relative power of two brains.

It is well known that, in the instance of cataract occurring in one eye, the patient is rarely conscious of the defect while it is gradually taking place, but the other eye as gradually takes upon itself the duties of both. When deafness occurs from age, or from any cause which slowly diminishes the power of the nerve in one ear, there is a similar unconsciousness of the existence of the defect—the other ear, *pari passu*, taking up its duties. I was not in the slightest degree aware of it in my own person, till reminded that I was in the habit of turning my left ear when spoken to. In like manner I conceive that the loss or diminution of the power of one brain is imperceptible to the individual, in consequence of its fellow exercising the normal faculties by itself alone; but the power of hard study is gone, and the memory materially impaired. I believe that in all cases we instinctively use most freely the organ which is most powerful, and that some make most frequent use of the right cerebrum, some of the left, as that feeling predominates. These, however, must be received as conjectures only, put forth as suggestive to other minds in the hope they may lead to a more accurate examination of mental phenomena in cases of diseased brain.

Should the preceding remarks be ridiculed as the gambols of my hobbyhorse, I will console myself with the recollection of Sir Humphrey Davy's condemnation of Mr. Winsor's delusion, that it was possible to light London with coal gas: he pronounced it absurdly impracticable, and in twelve months after the sentence it was accomplished. Dr. Lardner, too, proved not only to his own satisfaction (which is an easy task at all times), but to the satisfaction of the world, that to traverse the Atlantic in a steam-boat was physically impossible—this also was shortly afterwards accomplished.

There is but little analogy perhaps in my illustration, but I must venture on another hypothetical credo. We see a whimsical person, with a tendency to hypochondriasis, one day timid, apprehensive, and cowardly—the next day bold, decided, and courageous; and this in some degree dependent on the weather—like the man and woman in the Dutch barometer, one character coming out in fine weather, another in rain. Ridiculous! Don't be too certain, reader, on this point—it may happen to prove that the two brains are in the habit of relieving guard, and that it is not the same sentinel who is on duty to-day that kept the post yesterday. There are stranger things in the brain than are dreamt of in your philosophy.

Let us now take a glance at the pathological doctrines of M. Georget, which Dr. Pritchard thinks worthy of quoting at full length.

He says, "Insanity is a disease of the brain; it is idiopathic—the nature of the organic lesion is unknown.

"The first proposition results from the following considerations:

"1. The essential symptom, *intellectual disturbance*, depends on a lesion of the cerebral functions.

"2. It is always preceded, accompanied, or followed by other important cerebral or nervous disorders.

"3. The disturbances of the other functions are neither constant nor severe; they are besides precisely similar to those," etc. etc.

To shew the absurdity of this definition, and the utter waste of time and thought of which such a mode of interpretation is the cause, let us take another subject and treat it similarly—the analogy is perfect.

Lameness then, we will say, is an idiopathic disease of the lower part of the body—the nature of the organic lesion is unknown—which is about as true of a lameness as of insanity.

1. The essential symptom, inability to walk, depends upon a lesion of the locomotive functions.

2. It is always preceded, accompanied, or followed by other important muscular, glandular, nervous, or articular disorders.

3. The disturbances of the other functions are neither constant nor severe; they are besides, etc. etc.

We will enumerate a few of the causes of lameness: rheumatism, gout, dislocations, ischias, calculus, lumbago, sciatica, diseased kidney, fracture of tibia, fibula, femur, metatarsal bones, tendo achillis or plantaris, ulcers, debility, fever, apoplexy, drunkenness, small-pox, etc. etc.

Is this *information* or knowledge? The causes of insanity are *not* unknown; some hundreds of them are perfectly known—fever, drunkenness, anger, of temporary causes—inflammation of meninges—habitual intoxication—reflex action from the womb—the great ganglionic centres—scybalae—malformation—spicula of bone from the internal surface of the skull—softening of brain, deposits, abscess, ossification—grief, joy, starvation—inflammation of substance—diseased temporal bone—cancer—atrophy—gout—scurvy. The list is unlimited of *known* causes of insanity, besides the myriads that are unknown or irrecognisable during life.

When M. Georget ends with saying, "The natural terminations of insanity are permanent disease of the brain;" it is almost equivalent to saying, "the natural terminations of lameness are disease in the lower half of the body." The expression is either decidedly opposed to fact, or has no meaning. Lameness and insanity get well often spontaneously, or are cured by art; and when they do not, it is because of the nature, extent, and duration of the disease spoiling the organ which caused the lameness or the insanity.

An old nurse came into the room where a medical consultation was being held, and said, "Pray, gentlemen, will you please to tell me how long my master's fever will last?"—"Why, nurse," replied the doctor, "that depends on its duration." "Thank you, sir," said the nurse, grateful for the information, and went away perfectly satisfied. Now the pupils of M. Georget have about equal reason to be thankful, and satisfied with the information afforded in this description of insanity.

There is so strange a discrepancy of opinion among writers on insanity as to the employment of bleeding, that one is surprised the public places faith in medical management of mental derangement.

Pinel says bleeding is always injurious.

Cullen approves of bleeding.

Esquirol condemns it.

Haslam recommends it.

Rush bleeds to the extent of thirty or forty ounces at a time.
Foville doubts about it, but uses it in the intermittent form.
Joseph Franck has a high opinion of it.
Fodéré, I think, condemns it.
Hitch and Dr. Shute proscribe it.
Pritchard approves it.
—Delightful harmony!

Now, it appears to me that to recommend bleeding in *insanity*, is exactly equivalent to recommending bleeding in *illness*. Mental derangement is caused or accompanied by so many disorders, that bleeding must be sometimes highly necessary, and sometimes decidedly injurious. The practitioner must decide on the whole case. Among this multitude of discordant counsellors, I may venture to suggest that a few leeches to the inside of the nose, where the patient will submit to it, will often give great relief, when he would be absolutely prostrated by the loss of a pint of blood from the arm. This is more especially true in persons past the middle age and of a gouty diathesis.

To what can the strange discrepancy of opinion as to the effect of bleeding arise? Such absolute opposition of sentiment is little calculated to inspire confidence in the medical men who are devoted to the subject of insanity—when we find Rush stating the beneficial results of an abstraction of blood, amounting to from twenty to forty ounces at a time, taken from the patient while in an erect position; that he had taken away two hundred ounces of blood from a man sixty-eight years of age in less than two months, and from another man four hundred and seventy ounces in the course of seven months, one is struck with a wonder, which is certainly not admiration, at the audacity of the practice; and we should be extremely unwilling to subject a patient to his tender mercies. Such a mode of treatment would kill nineteen out of twenty of the ill-fed herbivorous Frenchmen of the Salpetrière, however it might be sustained without instant destruction by feeders on flesh.

All that we can conclude from such lamentable discordance of opinion is, that bleeding is proper or improper in insanity, just as it is in other cases, and that we are not justified in resorting to it for the mental disturbance, except in the cases in which we should bleed without reference to it—plethora, inflammation, congestion, suppression of habitual sanguinous evacuations, and such analogous affections as would require the abstraction of blood were the mind in its natural state.

CHAPTER XXIV: *Change in the Brain from Exercise of its Fibres; Instinct and Reason; Jacobi's Remarks on the Intellect of Insects; Ratiocination of an Elephant*

When we observe the wonderful dexterity of a juggler, acquired by long and laborious practice, we cannot but acknowledge that the skills we admire must be accompanied, if not caused, by some change in the muscles of the arm, which render it more rapidly obedient to volition. We can hardly suppose it to be a more rapid volition, for volition itself is so inconceivably swift that it seems to require absolutely no appreciable portion of time. The sensation of pain from heat, its transmission to the brain, its perception there, the transmission of the will to the organ endangered, and its withdrawal from the danger, are manifestly successive events; yet the whole take up (according to our senses) no portion of time; and this in muscles or brain not yet educated. It is probable, therefore, that the innumerable volitions exercised in the complicated movements of the conjurer are rather alteration of the muscles of the limbs in obedience to volition, than education of the exercise of the faculty of volition itself.

In like manner we may suppose that it is owing to the education of the cerebral fibres in the various acts of the understanding, which, as for example in arithmetical calculations, are at first accompanied by positive pain as well as difficulty, that they become so easy as to be accomplished without a perceptible effort. I imagine then that a real physical change does actually take place in the parts of the brain exercised, as indeed phrenologists assert, and shew alterations in the external form of the skull, which there is every reason to believe to be the result of such exercise of certain fasciculi of nervous fibres in the brain. The head of the man who has called into action, to their full extent, the faculties bestowed upon him by the Creator, assumes a very different shape from that of the man who has "wrapped his talent in a napkin."

The brain of the man of education and skill, who has stored up a large quantity of acquired knowledge, who has used the faculties required in the process of adapting means to an end, may be fairly presumed to be, in some sense, of a different physical structure from that of the unexercised brain; as the muscles of the arms that have been cultivated incessantly by the juggler are, in a similar sense different in physical structure from those which have been always left in torpid repose.

Now, in estimating the wonderful sagacity of insects and birds which exercise a constructive skill, that, to us who are intended only for progressive education, seems absolutely to require a long series of instruction and practice, are we not justified in supposing that it may arise from the bestowal on them all at once of exactly that structure of their organs of intellect which, in corresponding portions of the brain in the progressive animal, is the result of long practice and gradual accumulation? We cease then to be surprised that the first nest of the bird should be built as skilfully as the tenth, and that every animal should be thus placed.

> "Just in the niche it was ordained to fill."

At whatever period the world was formed — that is, at whatever period its present arrangement, as presented to our senses, began—the trees created must have possessed those concentric rings which we know to be *now* indications of annual growths, although the tree had not existed a single day. The plant must have had the cotyledons attached to its stalk, although the seed of which they are a part had never existed. The animal must have had at once the horns which we now see to be slowly formed from a little jelly.

In like manner the surface of the earth—the soil we cultivate—must have possessed all those metallic oxides and other substances which we know *now* to be the slow results of chemical changes. The mountains must have had the same stratification and the same alternations of different metals, earths, and other combinations and superpositions, which we know to be *now* the results of successive deposits from fresh or salt water, of volcanic fires, of long series of convulsions and displacements. Whatever be the state of the physical world which fits it for the present race of beings, it must have been bestowed at once, or the races just created must have perished.

In like manner, the intellectual organization of the bird, the insect, the quadruped, or the fish, not being intended for progressive development and indefinite advances towards perfection, as that of man, was probably created complete at once. If the animal were not intended to advance, it would be formed at first as perfect as it was intended to be; and as all those sagacious instincts which excite our wonder are absolutely necessary to the welfare, and indeed, the very continuance of the species, it is obvious that the physical structure which created that intellect, and all those sagacious instincts, would be complete and entire at its first formation, or the animal could not have remained to occupy its place in creation. Even in the human race all that is necessary to the continuation and preservation of the species is not left to the gradual growth of intellect, but is made an instinct, like that of the inferior animals.

If this view of the case be admitted, the arbitrary distinctions which have been drawn between reason and intellect are no longer a stumblingblock. The "mind" of each is seen to be exactly the same congeries of functions, differing only in number and degree, but not in essence. The period of time allotted to man in this world, long as it appears to him who looks forward to it, is so small and insignificant a portion of the life of the race, that the gradual advances made by an individual of the species or of the whole race contemporaneous with him, form but a single and almost imperceptible link in the chain of progression by which we are to advance towards a more elevated state of existence even in this world; and the space between our present average and the degree of perfection it may be permitted us to attain may be vastly more extensive than from the state of the most ignorant and brutal savage to that of a Newton or a Kepler.

From time to time God permits a single individual to possess a brain endowed at once with a sagacity, an energy, and a virtue, which anticipates the slow progress of many generations; such men have their mission, and the complications of society which require their interposition are exactly those which call their talents into exercise. We see the human race, in civilized countries, under the guidance of such men, from time to time, take a sudden start and make a progress in one generation equal to that of many previous centuries, and we attribute the mighty change to some one grand event anterior in the order of sequence. No—the time was made for the man, as the man was adapted to the time; as in this, as in all other things, "all worketh together for good."

> "Nature and nature's laws lay hid in night,
> God said 'let Newton be,' and all was light."

I put forth the following observations as a pure hypothesis—a subject for the consideration of other minds; the limited experience and reasoning powers of one individual are not sufficient to establish the point, and it admits of none but inferential proof.

May it not be, that the distinction between mind and instinct consists in the parity or disparity of the two cerebra. If exactly equal and alike in every respect, does not the animal necessarily act uniformly from instinct? that is, from uniform unvarying impulse. Whereas, if unequal in power, and slightly different in function, the ideas of one brain may be weighed against the ideas of the other, there would then be comparison and judgment, and a progressional advancement in knowledge—and this, whatever be the shape of the organs of intellect. The first nest built by a bird displays as much of architectural skill as the tenth, because the same steady uniformity of impulse and *mode* of impulse would exist at one time as at the other; but the human being can set one brain to regard the other, can think of his own thoughts, can weigh in each brain reciprocally the testimony and the reasonings of the other, and thus, as the common adage runs, "two heads are better than one"—two brains are better than one. There is a steady advancement in the acquisition of knowledge during the whole period of our existence in this world—a world of external circumstances, obviously adapted to our organization, which is intended for the gradual reception of knowledge to an unlimited extent. The child is born, perhaps the most helpless and imperfect of created beings; but whatever its deficiencies, they are more than compensated by the superior intellect of its parent, capable of profiting by the knowledge stored up in a long succession of generations. Allowing only a slight difference in the power of the two brains, and a few of the subdivisions of the phrenologists, or even their three great divisions, the varieties of character which would result from the changes of the geometrical series are inconceivably numerous.

If it be contended that mind and instinct are essentially distinct qualities, what shall be said for the wonderful skill of the spider, for instance? I speak not of his accurate measurement of distances, his adaptation of the fibres of his net to the accidental arrangement of the parts to which it is attached, but to his knowledge of the habits of the creature he would entrap. See him at the first vibration of a line start from his place of concealment, and scan the animal that caused the disturbance. In an instant he decides that it is his appropriate prey, and he advances to weave his web around it. If the fly be so large that he has doubts if it may not overpower him, he leaves it to struggle till thoroughly exhausted before he attempts to gratify his appetite. If small, he kills it at once, and satisfies his hunger; but if a larger insect, a bee or a wasp, be entangled in his web, he sets himself instantly to work to liberate the captive, and cuts through his net with a skill and precision that could not be exceeded by a human artizan. Is not this reflection, comparison, judgment—in fact, *reasoning*? *My* intellect at least is not sufficiently acute to perceive the distinction; and when I see him roll himself up into a ball, or hang down by his hind legs as if dead and wait motionless in patience, hour after hour, that he may not alarm the creature he wishes to entangle, I cannot but call his mental process, thought, contrivance—in fact, *mind*. But as he makes no further progress in his skill with the accumulation of experience, I conclude that both brains (or both halves of nervous matter) being exactly equal, he acts from uniform impulse only, and call it instinct.

That animals are perfectly capable of following out a process of original ratiocination, I have witnessed numerous examples. I once offered an apple to an elephant, and let it drop at the moment he was about to seize it; it rolled out of his reach. He waited a moment to see if I would pick it up, and being disappointed in this expectation, set himself to blow violently against the opposite wall, and the recoil forced the apple to his feet. Now this was a trick which it was impossible that any one could have taught him, and it must have arisen from a process of reflection perfectly similar to that which takes place in the human mind. We have indeed examples of human minds not even capable of the degree of thought possessed in this instance by the elephant, yet performing, by a sort of automacy, all the ordinary functions necessary to their occupation. In some of the mechanical processes in our great manufactories where the minute subdivision of labour reduces the art of each individual almost to the very ultimate elements of muscular motion, I think that I have seen individuals incapable of a similar process.

As physical happiness is all that a large number of human beings are capable of appreciating, or in a position to enjoy, I have learned to cease to pity such animals as the artizan here spoken of, from the conviction that they are more happy and less unhappy than the discontented and envious educated mechanic.

I noticed a short time ago the following example of insect reasoning: A large grey spider established himself in a recess formed by a shed and a projection of the house, and taking his long line diagonally from the corner of the house to the eaves of a small building which was at the bottom of the recess, he then filled up the triangular space with a large and well-defined circular web. I had noticed with admiration during the day his wonderful skill, the accuracy of his lines and the equality of the spaces, and observed how carefully he pushed down his line and fastened it securely with his two hind feet to each radius in succession. When he had finished about two-thirds of his concentric circles, or rather of his helix, he went to the centre and swallowed a quantity of white, tenacious mucus, which he had deposited there at the commencement, having apparently spun himself out; he then proceeded to complete his work, which having accomplished and thus reduced himself to very small dimensions, he hung himself up by the hind legs, and I presume went to sleep. The slightest touch of a fly was however sufficient to make him start out, and having wrapped up a few of them in his toils and well stocked his larder, he again betook himself to repose.

In the mean time one of the smaller spiders, considering that the diagonal line of his neighbour was strong enough to bear two webs, began to attach his lines to it, and having so done in four or five places, proceeded to spin his own web. My older friend tolerated the intrusion very patiently, and acquiesced in the use his neighbour was making of the "party wall," though against *spider law*. By and by the new comer, having partly fitted up his own trap, and finding that no flies came into it, observing, I presume, the ample supply of food in his neighbour's premises, advanced along one of his own lines seemingly for the purpose of open burglary. My old friend had tolerated much, but this was a degree of impudence for which he was not prepared, and which he determined to punish forthwith. He proceeded to the centre of his web, and giving the whole framework a violent shake, hoped to shake the intruder down upon the ground. He did no more, however, than turn him round on the line, where he hung very patiently till the shaking ceased, and then resumed his march towards his neighbour's territory. Again and again, and with increasing violence, did the large spider shake his web—it was all in vain; there was the enemy advancing, and though so small as to be easily overpowered should he reach the mainland, the insult of the attempt was intolerable. On looking round, my elder friend saw that during the violent shakes he had broken two or three of his own short lines, and he left his opponent and set himself to work to mend them. Having completed the task to his perfect satisfaction, he returned to the burglar. The latter, when he came near, saw at once that he had been rash in provoking such an enemy, and hurried back to his own web. When his opponent saw him on his thin line in his retreat, he again set himself to his shaking fit, and made the most violent efforts to throw him down; it was all in vain, however, and he got safe home. After a moment's consideration, the other seemed to think that so audacious an attempt ought to be condignly punished, and he determined to retort the invasion. The thin lines of his diminutive antagonist, however, did not afford a sufficient support for his heavy bulk, and as he advanced he carefully spun a strengthener upon the other's tenuous cord. It was now the little one's turn to shake off the intruder, and twice did he break the thin part of the line and leave his enemy dangling. At last the latter gave up the attempt and went back to the centre of his own web, *after carefully detaching every one of the lines* which his neighbour had had the impudence to fasten to the long diagonal.

If this be not a process of reasoning, then I cannot understand the meaning of the word. Here was calculation of means to an end, and change of plan in consequence of unexpected obstacles. Had the human race spun webs, and dared one another to single combat, I do not see how they could have shewn more judgment and skill in the attack and defence. As I patiently watched the spiders, I could not but put words into their mouths, and fancy the conversation, although words could scarcely have added any force or distinctness to the pantomime I witnessed. The strengthening his own lines in order to bear the shaking, and the doubling his neighbour's lines while advancing to punish him, were really the strategy of an acute general; and I think I have seen more than one biped bearing the title, who was scarcely possessed of an equal amount of the power of ratiocination. The exploit of General Whitelock at Buenos Ayres certainly was not to be compared with it as a manifestation of intellect.

There must surely be a difference too in the *degree* of human responsibility; the houseless uneducated child of misery and vice, who has known nothing of civilization but its interference with the natural rights of savage life, who has been taught to look on the whole human race as the spider looks on the generation of flies; whose power of *thinking of his own thoughts* has never been cultivated to become an influential guide; who knows no motive to abstain from crime but fear of detection—surely such a being is not justly punishable to the same extent as another, who, born in the lap of wealth, and placed under the most favourable circumstances, has had all his evil tendencies repressed and his good ones created or encouraged; to whom every ennobling motive has been presented, and who has been confined in a great degree to associates similarly educated. Yet the specific offence which condemns the former to the utmost severity of punishment is often held in the latter to be an excusable freak of youthful indiscretion. It is the belief in a future state of existence where all wrongs will be righted, that can alone reconcile mankind to the unequal distribution of reward and punishment in this world, which is every moment obtruded on our attention.

But to return from a digression to which I hope to do justice elsewhere. Jacobi's opinions on the instinct or reasoning powers of animals are cited in a condensed form by Dr. Pritchard, from whom I quote them:

"It is a fact that among insects, if we take the different tribes collectively, manifestations of all the psychical [I propose the word *psychal*] qualities which we observe in mammifers and birds (regarding as a whole the properties divided among different departments), there may be recognised the most strict analogy. Attention, memory, the faculty of combining means to obtain ends, cunning, the desire of revenge, care of offspring, and all the other *psychal* qualities which have been traced in the former class of animals (mammifers), are likewise to be observed in the latter as typical or characteristic phenomena—sometimes in one combination, sometimes in another; or in different groups, sometimes strongly, sometimes more feebly expressed.

"Nor can it be maintained on any solid ground that phenomena so analogous depend on different causes, or that the lower tribes, and these exclusively, act on merely mechanical impulses, while their activity displays effects parallel to the manifestations of animal life in the higher orders. For what essential difference can be pointed out in the principle of action when we observe the young bee in its first flight from the hive, hasten straightways to the nearest meadow or sunny bank, and return home laden with wax and honey? And when the colt of the river-horse, foaled upon the land, after his mother has been killed, rushes from the spot and betakes himself to the water, which he had previously never seen—or when the young goat in the first hours of his life hides himself in the clefts of rocks which nature points out to him as his dwelling-place? Does *psychal* life display itself under a more limited or doubtful character in the flights of grasshoppers or dragonflies, than in the marches of lemings, so closely bound by the impulse which directs the course of their wanderings that they even attempt to gnaw the rocks that lie in their way rather than go round them; and follow each other, troop by troop, to their certain destruction, into the deepest rivers or the widest lakes? Does not the earth-worm endeavour to secure himself from the mole, who is provided with a well-formed brain, by making his way along the surface of the soil, where the latter cannot further track him, with as much cunning as the fox and the beaver display in acts which are typical or characteristic of their kinds? What difference is there between the skill with which the ichneumon and the anteater procure for themselves the same food, between that of the diving-spider and the corpse-beetle, and the arts displayed by so many birds and mammifers impelled to similar pursuits? Are not similar phenomena repeated in the economy of the beaver or of the alpine marmot? And if we must refer to manifestations of a higher and freer sphere of agency, in what tribe of sucking animals does such a power display itself more wonderfully than in the wars of conquest carried on by the different races of termites, in which the subdued become vassals to the victorious tribe, and serve their lords in laying up for them their stores and in watching and protecting their young?

"If we look but cursorily through the works of writers who have investigated the instincts, habits, and economy of insect tribes, we may well ask ourselves while contemplating this wonderful panorama, where *psychal* life (even in the same directions in which we trace it in mammifers, fishes, and birds) has taken a higher development, or when its phenomena are displayed collectively, displays itself in richer or more varied forms. In the interesting work of Kirby and Spence we find examples collected of the parental attachment and provident care which different tribes of insects evince towards their offspring—how the cimea griseus, like the hen, leads about her young brood, gathers them together, and exerts herself to defend them; how the earwig sits on her eggs, and when they are scattered collects them again under her, and after the young are hatched watches over them with equal care; how the aranea saccata watches over the sac in which she has enclosed her eggs, pines away with sorrow if she is robbed of it, and evinces the liveliest joy in regaining it; how she sustains the most valorous conflict for it against other insects, even to the sacrifice of her own life in its defence; how an ant, when cut through, ceased not to evince care for the eggs of her nest, and mutilated as she was, rescued ten of them from danger; how a throng of drones exerted themselves with energy, courage, and self-devotion, when their young had been placed by Huber in a situation of apparent danger; with what astonishing endeavours and apparent calculation of means, and with what varied art and contrivances the apis papaveris and apis centuncularis furnish their dwellings; how many water insects make use of the materials which accident throws in their way, to construct dens in which they dwell in the water. In order to become aware that *psychal* life displays its other manifestations among animals of all departments in ways nearly alike, we may read how wasps, as soon as new external conditions take place, which produce an essential change in the state of the organization, exert themselves with rage to destroy the very brood which, till then, they had watched over with the greatest care. How the working bees are at first so eager after the eggs laid by the female, that they consume them as fast as they can obtain possession of them, until the eggs, after a few hours, become changed in such a manner that the instinct of appropriation takes another direction, and they now tend the eggs and the larvae springing from them with inviolable fidelity; how some spiders, like some beasts of prey, cannot approach each other, even for the coupling, without danger, since amidst their caresses they are sometimes so powerfully impelled by a different direction of organic tendencies, that they fall suddenly upon one another, and one of them entangles the other and devours it.

"Now, if it should be established," says Dr. Pritchard, "that all those properties of animal life, approximating to (human) intelligence, or bearing analogies so striking to the manifestations of mind, which in one great division of the animal kingdom are assumed to be essentially connected with, and depending on, a particular system of organization, exist in another department, and display themselves in all the same various profusion, while the creatures belonging to this latter department are yet destitute of that system of organization, and of anything that bears resemblance to it, the advocates of phrenology will be obliged to abandon that broad ground on which they attempt to fortify their position. Within the more confined field, which the vertebrated tribes alone present, it will be more easy to maintain such an assumed connexion of *psychal* properties with a peculiar structure, or rather it is more difficult to disprove it when assumed. The general analogy which prevails throughout these tribes in the organization of their cerebral and nervous system affords no room for so decisive a contradiction to the relation which the phrenologists would establish."

For my own part I cannot consider the objections of Jacobi or of Dr. Pritchard to be perfectly conclusive as an argument against the truth of such a moderate phrenology as is professed by the more sedate portion of its defenders. If a large collection of examples, thoroughly authenticated, shew an uniform connexion between the external manifestation and the moral and intellectual qualities, and if these be not contradicted by any single example of the quality in excess without the corresponding external development, or (what would be still more conclusive) no example of the external manifestation without the corresponding character, then certainly we should be bound to put faith in the doctrines of phrenology as shewn by Cranioscopy; but till that be the case, the evidence is insufficient—the only thing which could make it completely satisfactory would be the correspondence between the loss of certain portions of the "mind" and the destruction by disease, of the part assumed to be the organ of that faculty or sentiment.

Still, as I have elsewhere remarked, whatever may become of phrenology, as the word is commonly understood, the division of the brain into parts ministering to different functions is an established fact, or at least inevitable inference from a consideration of the operations of the mind and the anatomical varieties of structure in the different portions of the brain, more especially at its basis; it is the location of the organs which constitutes one of the great difficulties—the very fantastic division of the portion round the eyes, for example, is so repugnant to common sense and so utterly impossible to be recognised if true, that, were it necessary to concede this point as a preliminary, every man of reflection would refuse to enter on an investigation founded on premises so utterly untenable and absurd.

The reason why the absence of anatomical proof of the connexion between the loss of a faculty and injury of the organ in which it is supposed to be located does not in all cases afford a valid argument against phrenology, is as I have before remarked, that the disease a man *died of* is not the disease he *lived with*. Changes have taken place, either as cause of death or concurrently, which may have entirely altered the character of the physical lesion. Indeed, if there be any foundation for the hypothesis that cerebral spasm is a frequent cause of insanity (as seems to be shewn by its occasional subsidence immediately before death), the want of correspondence between the moral and physical partial disorder would be accounted for and explained.

CHAPTER XXV: *Dr. Macnish, on the Philosophy of Sleep; Argumentative Dreams; Conscience; Somnambulism; Absence of Mind; Moral Apoplexy; Speech Given by Terror; Coma; Sudden Restoration of the Faculties*

Dr Macnish, in his "Philosophy of Sleep," gives the following account of some delusions to which he was subject during an attack of fever; the only thing at all remarkable is that he was perfectly conscious of the fallacy of his impressions during the whole period of their existence—otherwise, they do not differ from the common form of delirium in idiopathic fever. Indeed, similar delusions sometimes *accompanied* by consciousness are not very rare at the commencement of irruptive diseases, especially in children. Mr. George Combe cites the case, as if it were very extraordinary. Dr. Macnish says "the allusions did not appear except when the eyes were shut, or the room perfectly dark, so that I was obliged to keep my eyes open or admit more light then they could well bear. I had the consciousness of shining and hideous faces grinning at me in the midst of profound darkness, from which they glared forth in horrid and diabolical relief; they were never stationary, but kept moving in the gloomy background; sometimes they approached within an inch or two of my face, at others receded to a distance. They would break into fragments, which after floating about would unite, portions of one face coalescing with those of another and thus forming still more uncouth and abominable images. The only way I could get rid of these phantoms was by admitting more light into my chamber, and opening my eyes, when they instantly vanished, but reappeared when the room was again darkened or the eyes closed. One night, when the fever was at its height, I had a splendid vision of a theatre, in the arena of which Ducrow, the celebrated equestrian, was performing. On this occasion, I had no consciousness of a dark background like to that on which the monstrous images floated; but every thing was gay, bright, and beautiful—I was wide awake—my eyes were closed, yet I say with perfect distinctness the whole scene going on in the theatre: Ducrow performing the wonders of his horsemanship, and the assembled multitude, among whom I recognised several intimate friends, in short, the whole process of the entertainment as clearly as if I were present at it. When I opened my eyes, the whole scene vanished like the enchanted palace of the necromancers; when I closed them, it as instantly returned. But though I could thus get rid of the spectacle, I found it impossible to get rid of the accompanying music. This was the grand march in the opera of Aladdin, and was performed by the orchestra with more superb and imposing effect, and with greater loudness, than I ever heard it before—it was executed, indeed, with tremendous energy," etc. He goes on to say that the theatrical scene lasted five hours, and the whole delusion two days; and he then proceeds to account for it by asserting that the state of the reflecting organs was unchanged, but that certain other portions of the brain, which he calls idealty, form, wonder, colour, and size, were all in intensely active operation.

Now let us see if this assumption will bear examination, and whether we cannot give an explanation of the facts without the unqualified assent he requires.

It is agreed that the external object only gives *sensation*, and that *perception* is a subsequent act of the intellectual faculties. Whatever be the movement, undulation, vibration, concussion, circulation, or other act, which an organ of special sense takes on when the objects to which it is adapted are presented to it (odours to the nose, sounds to the ears, etc.), we know by multiplied experience it may take on spontaneously from disorder, and thus lead to *perception* as completely as the object itself. With only one brain, such false information given by a special sense must be credited, unless, by a long process of ratiocination, we at last prefer the testimony of friends to the evidence of our own senses. Without such testimony, and without the opposing evidence of other senses, the perception must be believed; but, if only one brain be the subject of disease, a very different process takes place in the mind; the recognition of the phenomenon as a delusion seems, indeed, positive proof that the other brain does not believe it. When the eyes were open, and real impressions made both on the sound organ and on the disordered organ, both together were sufficient to dissipate the erroneous impressions and prevent sensation and perception from creating belief; but if the eyes were closed, the false impressions being no longer counterbalanced by the true, the delusion continued, and it was only the comparison formed by the state with the eyes shut and the state with the eyes open which could raise a doubt. Had both brains been the subject of the disorder, it would have been the common form of delirium—there would have been entire belief in the reality of the scene represented by the disordered organs, which would have lasted till the disturbance of the organs had subsided into the natural state again.

There are few individuals accustomed to dream, who have not sometimes, when in that state, held a controversy apparently with another person. Like Dr. Johnson, they may have been overpowered by the greater prowess of their imaginary antagonist, and felt mortification at the superior wit of their collocutor. Dr. Johnson, in relating a dream of this kind, remarks, "Had I been awake I should have known that I furnished the wit on both sides."

I consider this process to be the action of two brains separately carrying on their respective trains of thought, and to be a state precisely similar to that of the madman talking to himself, or rather arguing with himself—one of the most common phenomena of insanity. The only difference I can perceive is, that in the case of the madman, one at least of the trains of thought is diseased, while in the dream each may be rational.

Perhaps there is a still greater analogy between the kind of dream I have described and the state of pervigilium which sometimes precedes madness. In all these cases the two cerebra are carrying on separate and distinct (even when not conflicting) trains of thought; it is a mere accident whether they shall take the form of an argument or not.

This form of dreaming is often an object of curiosity, and a source of much metaphysical mysticism. No one, that I am aware of, has ever attempted a physical explanation, yet, now it is suggested, I do not think that any one will hesitate to give a full assent to my theory of its origin. It is not long ago that I was myself annoyed with a dream of this kind. My *conscious self*, in possession of one of my brains, strenuously but vainly endeavoured to convince the other that certain acts I had committed many years ago were justifiable; the arguments by which they were condemned were so plausible that I awoke in very great anxiety at not being able to recollect the reasons for the condemned measures, but with a conviction that there were good and valid motives for them which had passed away from my memory. When thoroughly awake and able to exercise that most incomprehensible of all the mental faculties—*recollection*, I could have justified my conduct before any tribunal. There remained on my mind throughout the day a feeling like that which would possess a man who recalled, after an unsuccessful defence of a client in a court of justice, an overpowering argument which he had intended to use, but which had passed away from his mind at the proper time.

Memory may exist in each brain; but *recollection* is a conjoint act of two, and cannot, I believe, take place in a dream. I do not say that this explanation is probable; I do not say it is possible; yet I fully believe it. Let the reader consider the matter a while, and he will be of my opinion. It will appear to him fanciful and absurd perhaps, if I express my belief that the process here described as taking place during sleep, is only a modification of that which in our waking state we term conscience. Persons have felt remorse on the recollection of actions long passed; when at another time the motives of them would come spontaneously to the mind, and they would have the conviction that the actions they regretted were not only innocent, but praiseworthy.

Throughout these remarks I have endeavoured to avoid the use of figurative language, not from a belief that it is improper for the occasion, but from a doubt of my own skill in the management of this ornament to discourse, and thence a fear of conveying an erroneous opinion of my meaning. I am quite aware of the additional interest which would be given to the subject by a dexterous use of metaphorical and metaphysical language, more especially in addressing the public; but it is an attraction which must be sacrificed lest I convey false impressions, and thus raise objections to a theory which I believe to be absolutely true, and likely to lead to beneficial and important results.

For example, the word *conscience* is metaphysically and theologically considered by most men to be an internal sense with which we are specially endowed, in order to be a guide to us in our duties to our fellow-creatures. In this sense it seems to me to have no meaning. Do I deny the existence of conscience? certainly not; but I define it, *correct judgment of moral justice exercised by a healthy brain duly cultivated.* Is conscience possessed by the savage when he puts to death with every refinement of torture the victim of his instinct of pugnacity? By another who entraps the stranger into an ambush and murders him, to obtain possession of some glittering trinket? Did Burke and Hare, or the murderers of the poor Savoyard boy, possess a conscience?—No! Yet they possessed the organ which, if duly cultivated at an early period, before its form were fully defined, would have been enabled to exercise a conscience.

We may compare their apathy of conscience to the state of a muscular part of the body bound up in infancy until it had lost the faculty of obeying the commands of the will. The brain, which should judge of the morality of the actions, has been left in a state of torpor and its power is gone—a species of moral paralysis of the intellectual organs becomes established and the man is reduced to the condition of the inferior animals, or even below it, giving way to all his instincts without restraint, and not even attempting to exercise other control over his own volitions than that which is inspired by the fear of detection and punishment.

Original malformation may make a conscience impossible—disorder or disease may annihilate it when formed—defective or erroneous education may distort its decision, or it may perish altogether from desuetude. God has in this, as in other matters, given us the means, which it is our duty to cultivate into the results which shall be beneficial to society and to the individual.

It may be said, how is the individual to give himself this conscience, this moral sense, when it requires the *possession* of it, in order to know that it is necessary to *acquire* the possession of it? This is not expected of the individual, but of society. It is evident that the welfare of the world and its advancement were intended to be progressive—*why* this should be the scheme of creation is beyond our comprehension—it is so. The individual is formed with intellectual organs capable of cultivation to an indefinite extent, and the accumulated knowledge of successive generations is to be called into action to enforce this cultivation. In an advanced state of society I hold that there exists in the collective body of citizens an indefeasible right, and a paramount duty, to interfere *to any extent* in the education of the individual, to *ensure* this due cultivation of his mind in the knowledge of right and wrong, and the establishment of a *conscience.*

With all the care that can be exercised in this process there will still be a great number of human beings with intellectual organs (and therefore faculties) so feeble and imperfect that they can never be cultivated to such an extent as to overpower the propensities of the animal—at least not to exercise over them that continuous control which constitutes the good and virtuous man. Modifications of form and colour, of character and of instincts, in animals, are, however, produced by domestication; and it is probable that a universal cultivation of the intellectual faculties in man may in time produce a considerable amelioration in the species; that this amelioration may continue to be transmitted to the offspring, and thus the race be improved, till there be found very few brains quite incapable of acquiring correct moral principles and a reasonable degree of self-restraint—that is, A CONSCIENCE.

The phenomena of real somnambulism I conceive to be strictly analogous to those of waking reverie. I have seen a gentleman so entirely absorbed in thought, so completely *absent*, that he has gone on from time to time referring to a paper or a book, while his children have been talking, laughing, and playing tricks in the same room, being all the while utterly unconscious of their presence; they have even shaken their fists within a short distance of his face, and jocularly called him opprobrious names—he has neither observed them nor me, sitting by, and amused with the example of abstraction. I always noticed that when he was roused from his reverie suddenly, it was accompanied by a shock producing sometimes positive pain and headach, whereas (just like waking from sound sleep) if gradual, it was agreeable. In what does this differ from somnambulism but in degree?

The humorous character of Dominie Sampson shews that Walter Scott had closely observed these effects; and had that wonderful writer been acquainted with physiology, he might perhaps have thrown light on many disputed points of philosophical inquiry. I have known more than one example much more extraordinary than any that have been represented on the stage.

I can personally vouch for the truth of the following case of true somnambulism: The wine cellar and beer cellar were in separate parts of a gentleman's house; the latter was accessible to the servants, but the former could only be approached through the dining-room. A dinner party of gentlemen only was assembled, and as was the habit in those days, they were preparing themselves for a regular symposion, from which it would have been held disgraceful to the character of the giver of the feast had any one gone away sober; indeed to *go* away at all was humiliating, it shewed that the host was a stingy fellow, and grudged his wine; the true social etiquette of the day required that every guest should be *carried* away, or if that were impossible, be put to bed in the house. Then, indeed, the glorification was complete, and the giver of the entertainment took brevet rank accordingly—a rank he would retain till some other more noble amphitryon had succeeded in making a greater number *equally* drunk, or an equal number *more* drunk, when the honours passed over to the more worthy competitor

Heu! quantum mutati sumus.

On the occasion I speak of, a servant girl had been sent to

fetch something out of the wine-cellar (which was also used as a sort of store-room), and could not resist the temptation to steal a couple of bottles of wine. In her return through the dining-room, there being at the moment no one in attendance, she was ordered to do something at the table, and fearing that the bottles in her pocket might lead to her detection, she contrived to slip them out and place them each in a corner of the buffet—a sort of closet without a door, then in fashion. She made some vain attempts to approach the buffet again for the purpose of taking away the wine, but was compelled to leave the room without accomplishing her object. She was not able to make a pretext for going again into the room and was smartly censured by the man for wishing it, as "*she must know that by this time the gentlemen were pretty well up*," and that consequently a woman servant had no business to shew herself. She went to bed, and no doubt dreamt of her misfortune, and the danger of detection in the morning when the discovery of the two unauthorized bottles of wine would be inevitable.

In pursuance of the dream she came down stairs, in a fit of somnambulism, with no other covering than her shift, marched straight to the buffet and took away the two bottles of wine; made vain efforts to put them into imaginary pockets, and finding that there were none, carried them in her hands to her bed-room, and placed them under her pillow.

Every guest was so awestruck by the vacant stare and unconsciousness of the girl, that no one spoke a word, or made any attempt to detain her. The gentleman gave strict orders that she might not be told of the adventure, but that it should be left to him to explain it to her; the bottles were therefore gently taken away from under her pillow without awaking her, and she was left to her ordinary repose.

Whether the fun of the affair rendered it impossible for some of the servants to abstain from communicating the matter to her is not known; for, before the family were up in the morning she was gone, and was never heard of afterwards; in due time her clothes and wages were sent to her friends, and there ended the affair. She had either committed suicide, or had left the country.

I can see no difference between this state and the absence of mind of which I have given examples, except that a different set of muscles were employed; there was an equal abstraction and equal suspension of the functions of the special senses. In both cases I conceive that *the intellectual portion alone, of one brain only, was really awake*, and the remainder in a state of more or less complete and temporary abeyance, whether to be called sleep or torpor. In either case, a sudden shock would have restored the functions of all the organs of both brains.

The gradations in the exercise of mind are infinite—the absent man does not differ more from the man "with all his wits about him," than the man in a reverie, from the somnambulist on one side and the dreamer on the other. The state of sleep too, admits of every degree, from the intense and torpid repose of exhaustion, to that light and half-conscious state which we call dogsleep, or sleeping "with one eye open." In the former, there are no dreams, and external impressions do not produce corresponding perceptions. A pistol might be fired off without waking the sleeper. I have known a man sleep soundly between two embrasures of a fortress while twenty-four pounders were firing on each side of him. In the latter a slight impression on any of the special senses breaks the chain and instantly restores consciousness. There is another state, where we are asleep and dreaming, but yet possess just the degree of consciousness that enables us, if we wish to do so, to avoid waking and to continue the dream; and there is also a state where a dream of the most preposterous kind occupies the mind, accompanied by a conviction that it is only a dream. This last case, I think it cannot be doubted, on consideration, is the state of one brain as fully asleep as is compatible with dreaming, and the other brain in a state analogous to that where we are able to will the continuation of the dream—one brain half asleep, and the other almost awake, and capable of watching it.

If we go to sleep again after a short process of thinking we are afterwards unconscious that there has been any interruption of the sleep or the dream—we have not remained awake long enough to produce memory. Of this every married man's recollection must, I think, furnish him with examples, from the testimony of his wife.

The theory of two perfect brains, each composed of several organs, and each capable of all those functions of which the healthy aggregate is sound mind—this theory once acknowledged, we seem to have an explanation of a great number of the phenomena of sleep which have hitherto been inexplicable. In the state of languid reverie in the chair, which leads to the dream that almost always precedes sound sleep, I conceive that in the earlier stage one cerebrum loses its consciousness and begins to dream first, and the other is for a moment capable of watching it, till the gradual extension of the torpor to both brains porduces sound sleep and entire oblivion.

"Sleep may degenerate into a real disease," says Scipion Pinel. "I am attending, at this time, a young girl from the country, who, about every hour, falls asleep for three or four minutes, wherever she may happen to be. These attacks of sleep which only come on during the day (but even 25 or 30 times), are characterised by a profound calm—no hysterical shock, no acceleration of pulse, but a profound insensibility of the whole skin. After some minutes the girl wakes up as from a fainting fit, and resumes the conversation where she left off. I thought at first that there was a little simulation, or of acquiescence in epileptic hysteria, in these attacks; but in the end I was convinced that they were really and simply somnolence. The explanation does not appear to me very easy, for in my opinion, sleep is the effect of cerebral compression, probably the result of a regular afflux of blood into the pia mater, which stupifies the cerebral excitation; and during which, above all, is effected the nutrition of the cortical substance, which transmits it afterwards to the medullary. But how admit such congestions, repeated twelve or fifteen times a day, and only for a few minutes?"

What necessity for admitting anything so entirely gratuitous and unnecessary; there is not the slightest foundation for it.

Of all the men who have written on this mysterious subject, there is none whose omission to establish a true theory of sleep more surprises me than that of Bichat. There was something so peculiarly sagacious in the structure of his mind that I cannot understand how he, who did not fail to observe the completeness of the two organs of thought, but attributed his own strange character to the inequality of his two brains, could have overlooked the corollaries which so inevitably arise from that fact. The different degrees of somnolency in the two brains, and indeed the degree of somnolency of different parts of the same brain, are quite obvious to the cursory observer of a person who is falling off into sleep, when once the idea has been suggested; and we have, in the well-known occurrence I have alluded to, of dreaming, coexistent with a perfect consciousness all the while, that it is a dream, a complete proof (as it appears to me) that one brain is, strictly speaking, not asleep, but in a state capable of judging of the reality of the ideas passing through the unconscious other. It may even control them, as I have heard from others, and indeed experienced in my own person. The ideas which occupy the brain that is most asleep are felt to be wrong or criminal; a resolution is made not to indulge in them, and the whole brain having, before going to sleep, made a determination to check the process, the exercise of an act of volition by that brain, which is comparatively awake, can forbid and prevent it. On the other hand, every one must remember the occasions just spoken of, where one brain wakes up alone, and finding the train of images of its sleeping fellow to produce great pleasure, determines not to wake up the whole sensorium but prolong the agreeable delusion, fully conscious all the while that it *is* a delusion.

"It is important," says Dr. Holland, "in all our reasonings practical and theoretical, upon sleep, to keep in mind that it is not a unity of state with which we are dealing but a series of fluctuating conditions, of which no two moments perhaps are strictly alike. . . . These variations extend even from complete wakefulness to the most perfect sleep of which we have cognizance, either by outward or inward signs." In another place he observes, "Sleep, then, in the most general point of view, must be regarded not as one single state, but a succession of states in constant variation—this variation, consisting not only in the different degrees in which the same sense or faculty is submitted to it, but also in the different proportions in which these several powers are under its influence at the same time."

The strange mixture of rational and irrational acts and thoughts which present such curious phenomena in the somnambulist, are easily comprehended if we suppose one brain to be entirely asleep and the other intensely occupied with a single train of thought, as in a reverie, which is almost identical with somnambulism. The functions of the special senses are in such a case suspended—our eyes are directed to an object, but we do not see it, and are sometimes not aware that it presents an obstacle to our progress till we stumble over it; and so with the other senses, till some impression on one of them becomes sufficiently strong to wake up both brains into perfect consciousness, with correct perceptions and judgment.

A person may really die with symptoms of apoplexy where there is no apoplexy, but there is a sudden cessation of all the mental functions, producing effects resembling those caused by effusion of blood and consequent compression of the brain. Of this many examples are given by Abercrombie and Pritchard. There is also a moral apoplexy, from very strong emotion, of which the effect resembles the state of concussion, compression, or paralysis. Whatever may be the nature of the lesion, we cannot know it till further changes have taken place, obliterating the marks of the first, and destroying life. I have seen a conjuror take a large glass of jelly, and by a peculiar jerking blow on its edge, shiver the contents into fragments without displacing a particle. A close examination would shew that it is broken into minute angular portions, which were only visible from the refraction of the rays of light. May not something analogous take place in physical and moral concussion? Lord Clive, after inducing the minister of a native prince to enter into a treasonable negotiation to betray his master, and signing a treaty with him in which there was a clause duly stipulating for the reward of the treason, contrived in the act of signing to substitute another treaty which did not contain that clause. When this came to be publicly read before the sovereign, the minister found how he had been betrayed, and though a man of strong and remarkably acute mind, was in an instant struck with perfect idiocy, and remained for the rest of his life imbecile and childish. I do not stop to express the disgust and loathing excited by an act which may be palliated but can never be justified. Now there can be no question that both from physical and moral causes you may have every gradation of physical injury, reaching from that which instantly destroys life to that which scarcely produces a perceptible change. A state of torpor resembling that of physical concussion is well known, especially with the aged; in these cases a strong impression made on the organs of special sense has a great effect in re-establishing the functions of the brain. We observe that by speaking very loudly to a person in this state, and holding some stimulating odour to his nose, we can obtain a rational answer from him, although he is apparently in a state of entire lethargy, almost like death. How much more probable is it that you should produce a beneficial effect from such means, where one brain chiefly is in this state of torpor, and you are aided in your efforts by the influence, however imperfect, of the other. Here your physical means will be helped by the addition of strong motives—promises, rewards, or even punishment; and the violent effort of volition will sometimes re-establish the functions of the brain and its influence on the voluntary muscles.

I recommend very strongly in cases where the insanity partakes of the nature of mental torpor or imbecility, the use of black pepper as snuff; it has an extraordinary power of rousing the brain, and has even a considerable influence in slight coma from concussion; but in the senile torpor, almost amounting to coma, its effect is astonishing, and many a man may for a short time under its influence, be able to resume full possession of his judgment, and dispose rationally of his property. The powder sold under the name of Grimstone's Eye Snuff is almost exclusively black pepper; there is, I believe, a small quantity of tobacco or other substances put into it for disguise, but its beneficial qualities arise solely from the black pepper, and every addition is, *pro tanto*, injurious.

Were I desirous of establishing, for some interested purpose, the sanity of a patient affected with maniacal imbecility; and had the management of him during his examination by a committee "*de lunatico inquirendo*," I would certainly supply him with a large snuff-box filled with black pepper. Perhaps this may be borne in mind should I ever be again in that position.

I believe that in some other part of this work I have spoken of the importance of obtaining the signature of such a person, for the safety of his family. If the will thus made be rational and just, there is little danger of the law disallowing its validity. I reflect with satisfaction that I once saved a widow and children from the brutality of a vindictive heir-at-law by the stratagem I speak of.

There is a story of a youth whose tongue was suddenly unloosed at the sight of impending danger to his father, and doubt is often expressed as to the reliance to be placed on its truth. I can cite a parallel case. An export-merchant in the present day, whose immense establishment is one of the most conspicuous and remarkable in the city of London (and who consulted me, professionally, many years), had a son, about eight years of age, perfectly dumb, and the family had abandoned the hope that he would ever be endowed with the gift of speech. There was no defect in intellect, nor lesion of any other faculty. In a water-party on the Thames, the father fell overboard, when the dumb boy called out aloud, "Oh, save him! save him!" and from that moment spoke with almost as much ease as his brothers. Two of my intimate friends were present at the miracle, which was the subject of unbounded joy and congratulation. The young gentleman is now one of the most active and intelligent members of his father's firm.

This example, among many others, affords proof of the wonderful influence of a strong volition—or strong impulse, in restoring the functions of the cerebral nerves, and may explain some modern miracles, without the necessity of supposing a direct intervention of Providence. We are not justified in assuming a miraculous interruption of the laws of nature in cases which can be explained by the established laws of physiology.

Much curious speculation is suggested by such cases, and they afford confirmation also of many other things in cerebral pathology.

The following case I relate on the authority of the late Mr. Cleveland, a highly respectable practitioner in the City. It may throw some light on those subjects just treated of.

The son of a butcher in Leadenhall-market received a blow on the head from some object of no great weight, but the exact nature of which I have forgotten. The youth, about sixteen years of age, was rendered perfectly insensible; there was no fracture; coma came on, his eyes were insensible to light and his nerves to sensation. The father being a wealthy man, finding some discrepancy of opinion between the regular attendant and the hospital surgeon who was called in, determined to have a consultation. Three of the surgeons who stood highest in reputation in London at that period were added to those already in attendance. One of them was the celebrated Mr. Cline, and another (I believe) Mr. Pott; but the rest of the names have passed away from my memory. A full investigation was entered into, and for the credit of the profession I will not state some of the extravagant propositions that were made. No two, however, were exactly in accord; and when disputes had subsided into a sort of result, and the joint opinion (!) was about to be committed to paper, the father burst into the room from an adjoining closet and exclaimed to their great astonishment, "Gentlemen, I have been listening to you, and have made up my mind *nothing* shall be done, and I take all the responsibility on myself. My wife will pay your fees as you go down stairs, so good morning."

The gentlemen retired, with a determination no doubt that at the next consultation they would look into the closet! The boy remained either thirteen or seventeen days insensible, during which period he was very slightly fed by injection and by small quantities of food pushed into his stomach. No change took place, till one day the whole of the fire-irons, which had been place in front of the empty grate, were thrown down on the marble-slab by accident, making an extraordinary noise and clatter. The lad suddenly woke up as from a sleep, asked for food, and gradually recovered his strength, without any ill consequence from the blow or its effects. He lived to cite the anecdote to his friends for many years, as evidence of the wonderful sagacity of doctors.

Of course nothing of this kind could occur in the present day! "*Nous avons changé tout cela!*"

I hope the professional candour of the above will be duly

appreciated. It might perhaps have been more complete had I myself been a party to the consultation! But to be serious: Is it not worth consideration, whether the cases cited do not justify an experiment of the effect of a sudden shock in torpid insanity or dementia?

CHAPTER XXVI: *Dr. Brigham on the Effect of Mental Cultivation; Mind and Soul; Gradual Extinction of the Faculties by Pressure on the Brain; Restoration on Removing It; Summary of the Argument on the Distinction Between Mind and Soul*

In a very sensible and judicious little work entitled "*Remarks on the Influence of Mental Cultivation and Mental Excitement upon Health*," by Dr. Brigham of Hartford, Connecticut, there are some excellent observations on the injurious effect of too early cultivation of the mind. In proving (what it can only be necessary to prove to the public, and not to anatomists) that the brain is the sole organ of the mind, he remarks, "If the mind could be deranged, independently of any bodily disease, such a possibility would tend to destroy the hope of its immortality." This argument will probably have some weight with the religious public. Throughout most of the reasonings of this subject by writers, and especially theological writers, *the mind* is confounded with the *soul*. The former, every anatomist knows to be a set of functions of the brain—differing only in number and degree from the intellect of animals, but the soul is a very different topic for consideration. If mind and sould were convertible terms, there would be an end of all discussion.

"Teachers of youth," says Dr. Brigham, "in general appear to think that in exciting the mind they are exercising something totally independent of the body—some mysterious entity, whose operations do not require any corporeal assistance. They endeavour to accelerate to the utmost the movements of an extremely delicate machine, while, most unfortunately, they are totally ignorant or regardless of its dependence on the body. They know that its action and its power may be both increased for a while by the application of a certain force; but when the action becomes deranged, and the power destroyed, they know not what is the difficulty, nor how it can be remedied. Fortunately they do not attempt to remedy it themselves but call in the physician, who, if he affords any relief at all, does it by operating on a material organ. If medical men entertained the same views as the public they would, in attempting to restore a deranged mind, entirely overlook the agency of the body, and instead of using means calculated to effect a change of action in the brain would rely solely upon arguments and appeals to the understanding; for, if the mind may be cultivated independently of the body, why may not its disorders be removed without reference to the body?"

To desire that a curer of insanity act upon the mind independently of the body is to take your watch to the artist and tell him not to touch the works as it is the motion only that is wrong. It is true we cannot comprehend the nature of motion; that of the watch is composed of elasticity, momentum, and so forth; but we know nothing of the essence of elasticity and momentum. We do know, however, that a certain perfection of parts is necessary for correct motion; and an experienced artist, who understands the anatomy of a watch, can often tell, before he opens the case, the nature of the cause that interferes with the desired regularity; while at other times, he could know nothing without examination of the internal structure. So the physician. He knows absolutely nothing of the nature of mind; only that it is the result of certain machinery when perfect; but he does not confound this with the immortal soul, of which he also can know nothing but by revelation.

Is it not contrary to analogy, contrary to all we know and infer of the designs of Providence, to believe that the Creator's best and most glorious gift to man (as far as *this* world is concerned), the *mind*, should have been created liable to mutilation by the slightest accident; that when, in man, a bony case has been provided to contain the precious instrument by which it is manifested, and a development given to the organization of that instrument, which endows the animal with the highest privileges and rank in mundane creation—can it, I say, be conceived that the functions thus formed and thus protected, would be left to one single organ, so that the slightest casualty might deprive man of his guide and protector? The inferior faculties of our nature have two organs, to insure the due performance of inferior functions in case of accident or disease. I cannot think that the possession of an *immortal soul*, to render man a responsible being, is compatible with the existence of only one organ for the exercise of its subordinate agent, *the mind*.

The distinction between mind and soul, though clear to one who believes that a Revelation has been given to us, is so incomprehensible by the unaided reason, that it has been a subject of dispute from the commencement of history. "From the time of Xenophon downwards (as remarked by the writer, of whose work I have spoken as the direct incentive to this attempt) it was held, that men had two souls in a sort of antagonism, and that it was the due equilibrium between these which constituted his perfection."

To suppose the soul to be immediately implicated in, and dependent on, the functions of the brain, whose faculties may be either complete, imperfect, or annihilated, seems a contradiction. I should be sorry to speak with levity on so serious a subject, but the illustration I am about to give is not intended irreverently. Suppose a person afflicted with chorea (or St. Vitus's dance) to have an attack of convulsive movements, and overset the table every time he sat down to breakfast, would it be reasonable to infer that there was some mysterious connexion between chorea and broken tea-cups? *The soul*, as described to us by divines, or the authority of revelation, is *one*, *complete* and *immortal;* were it identical with *mind*, it would be sometimes wise, sometimes foolish—sometimes energetic, sometimes indolent—sometimes acute, sometimes fatuous and imbecile—sometimes courageous, and sometimes cowardly; its qualities changed by a few glasses of ale or wine—such we know is the *mind*. Surely such things cannot be predicated of the *immortal soul*, which might have an organ of thought in every part of the body without destroying its *oneness*. It is the confounding of two things so essentially distinct as *mind* and *soul*, which forms the same obstacle to our progress in the management of insanity and mental disturbance, as that the belief in the fixedness of the earth opposed to the reception of the doctrines of Galileo. The grey substance pervading the brain and nerves, now called neurine, is ascertained to be the seat of sensation and volition, and the medullary portion to be only the medium of conveying its orders to the various parts of the body, and *reflexly* sensations to the grey substance. But we do not suppose that neurine itself feels, till God has "breathed into it the breath of life;" and we might as reasonably be expected to abstain from all attempts at further astronomical discoveries, because we cannot either conceive limits to space or space without limits, as to abstain from carrying our researches to the utmost possible extent in the organs of mind, because we cannot conceive the nature of the soul. The sincere believer *acquiesces* with humility, and that is all that is expected of him. The drum must be broken before the child can search for the sound. The animal must be dead before we can examine his brain.

If mind and soul were identical, then the soul could not be an immaterial principle—for mind, we see, is a thing of gradual growth, increasing bit by bit, from less than that of the lowest quadruped to the exibition of the highest intellect. The infant just born has no voluntary power—no *will*, no reflection, no perception; it has scarcely sensation; yet all these come by slow degrees, and the accumulation of faculties which are ultimately to constitute *a mind*, may be retarded or entirely prevented by disease or want of cultivation. Some of these faculties may progress to the injury or extinction of others, or they may be all developed in due order and succession till they make the godlike gift of reason. Can the mind then be a thing, *per se* distinct and separate from the body? No more than the motion can exist independent of the watch; and all the arguments of theologians and metaphysicians on this subject are founded on the confusion of terms. Predicate what you please of the *soul*, you cannot exaggerate its exalted nature; but do not confound it with *mind*, which is nothing more than a collection, an *aggregate of functions*, and the word itself only a term to designate a set of processes, any one of which may be defective, excessive, or absolutely wanting, without destroying, and sometimes almost without materially impairing the reasoning faculties. No man possesses all of them in perfection, or he would be superior to humanity; few possess any of them in perfection; but a moderate degree of excellence in many of them may be attained by almost any one who is subjected to due cultivation, and they may almost all of them be lost by neglect and desuetude.

I have before spoken of the effect of pressure on the brain, and will here give the illustration a little more at large.

If I apply my finger to an opening in the skull, made, for example, by the trephine, and press gently on the brain, I gradually extinguish vision, hearing, and the rest of the special senses, and produce the effect called coma, or deep insensible sleep; the pressure continued longer and more forcibly, goes on to extinguish all mental faculties and manifestations, voluntary power, sensation, and perception, consciousness, memory, imagination, judgment, in fact the whole mind. The animal now possesses only organic life, and is utterly unconscious of its own existence; all the intellectual faculties are in abeyance, they are not annihilated. But we may advance still further in the process of extinction, as in the state of asphyxia from drowning; there is now scarcely a remnant of organic life, even—it is the left ventricle of the heart in which alone there is the slightest spark of vitality—it vibrates with a tremulous motion, and there alone *latet scintilla forsan*, and, if carefully fanned, may light up again into consciousness and power the whole congeries of functions which form the thinking man—but as yet, the body remains cold, motionless, unconscious, a mere clod, without any cognizable signs of life, even by a medical eye—it may be cut to pieces, or the bones broken, and no more pain will be inflicted than on a cabbage—it has not indeed, by any means, so much life as a vegetable—it is dead, absolutely dead in every sense, except that there resides, in the left ventrical, this germ of vitality; and restoration is still possible.

No theologian will surely allow that the *soul* has yet left its earthly dwelling, and can be called back by friction, warmth, and brandy—yet by such means we can restore the MIND, which no longer existed in any form or mode of being.

What, in fact, had I done by the pressure of my finger on the brain? I had not annihilated a single faculty, yet I had extinguished the MIND, and had the pressure been continued, it would never have returned; death and dissolution would have come, and the body would have been gradually resolved into its primary elements: into the hydrogen, nitrogen, oxygen, and carbon—the phosphorus, lime, and manganese—and the MIND of that individual would then be, indeed, annihilated.

Thus with the watch. I move a little point, and it stops; if I leave it there, the motion is suspended; does the motion continue to exist? The watch, like the body, will be gradually resolved into its ultimate elements by chemical action, and the *motion* of that individual watch is for ever annihilated. I take off the pressure from the brain and all the faculties resume their action, and the man becomes again a thinking, acting, sentient being. I move the little point of the watch, and the motion is resumed. I cannot see the slightest discrepancy in the reasoning process. To ask where the MIND is during the interruption to its functions seems exactly the same as to ask where the MOTION of the watch resides when I have placed the little spring against the great wheel, which prevents it from making its revolution. To speak of the mind, then, in this sense, as connected with the material world by means of the brain, has strictly no more meaning than to speak of digestion as connected with matter by means of the stomach.

The *divinely mysterious essence* which we call the SOUL is *not* then the MIND; from which it must be carefully distinguished, if we would hope to make any progress in mental philosophy. Where the soul resides during the suspension of the mental powers by asphyxia, I know not, any more than I know where it resided before it was united to that specific compound of bones, muscles, and nerves. Revelation here tells us nothing, and our own faculties could not even make us comprehend the existence of the soul, nor from any other source but Revelation can we form an idea of its nature or its destination.

Do not suppose, reader, that I would make a profane

comparison between the production of man's ingenuity, the watch, and the workmanship of the Creator; the difference is as great as between the beings who formed them. The movement is the result of the mechanism of the watch, but all the parts may be put together, and they will not set themselves in motion; the maker gives the first impulse; he could not even form the instrument on whose perfection he prides himself, unless God had bestowed on matter certain qualities, and established certain principles and laws of elasticity, momentum, and gravitation. It is the Almighty who confers the powers which set the watch in motion—without those powers, qualities, and principles, we could not form the watch; and the difference is not greater between the watch and the thinking quadruped, than between the quadruped and man: the only animal who has the power *to think of his own thoughts*, and consequently the only animal responsible for his actions.

Dendy, in his very curious volume, called the "*Philosophy of Mystery*," gives the following definition of mind and soul: "The mind is soul, evinced through the medium of the brain; and the soul is mind, emancipated from matter."

The ingenious writer of that sentence will, I think, if he consider the matter deeply, find that he has here used the word *mind* in two different senses; one of which is convertible with *soul;* and that the above definition is, strictly speaking, equivalent to the assertion that *soul* is *soul;* for if the mind be soul in the sense he uses it, then brutes have a soul as well as man. I do not *know* that this is *not* the case, but have no reason to believe it. We have no Revelation on the subject; and without Revelation we could not satisfactorily infer that man possessed a *divine incorporeal essence* distinct from matter and its properties. The reasonings of Plato and Cicero are mere guesses, and but a poor foundation for moral responsibility. Brutes, indeed, have their five special senses like man; very often in much higher perfection: they love and hate; are envious, irascible, placable, courageous, cowardly, vain, sober, haughty, humble, vindictive, generous, cunning, candid, or stupid, just like human beings. According to the division laid down by phrenologists, they possess self-esteem, benevolence, cautiousness, love of approbation, hope, wonder, comparison, and many other of the faculties possessed by man; there is scarcely one of the ingredients of MIND (in the sense I use the word in this work) which is not bestowed upon them; and they have perversions of the faculties from disease, like man; *they go mad;* and the mother destroys her offspring under the influence of puerperal insanity, as women do. *The wonderful faculty of thinking of our own thoughts, is bestowed on man alone.*

CHAPTER XXVII: *Double, or Alternate Consciousness; Double Identity; Four States of the Brain from Injury; Explanation of the Alternate Consciousness; Action of the Cerebral Fibres; Their Number; Powers of the Microscope*

The facts I am about to relate will perhaps be absolutely incredible by the non-medical reader—they are, however, established on evidence circumstantial, minute, and consistent, and derived from sources entirely devoid of suspicion. Were such testimony to be rejected, a man must go back half a dozen centuries in his store of knowledge, and reason on nothing but the evidence of his senses. These records are by competent and disinterested witnesses, and the narratives are beyond suspicion. We have examples then of persons who, from some hitherto unexplained cause, fall suddenly into, and remain for a time, in a state of existence resembling somnambulism, from which, after many hours, they gradually awake having no recollection of anything that has occurred in the preceding state—although, during its continuance they had read, written, and conversed, and done many other acts implying an exercise, however limited, of the understanding; they sing or play on an instrument, and yet on the cessation of the paroxysm are quite unconscious of every thing that has taken place. They now pursue their ordinary business and avocations in the usual manner, perhaps for weeks, when suddenly the somnambulic state recurs, during which, all that had happened in the previous attack comes vividly before them, and they remember it as perfectly as if that disordered state were the regular habitual mode of existence of the individual—the healthy state and its events being now as entirely forgotten, as were the disordered ones during the healthy state. Thus it passes on for many months, or even years. This is what is called *double consciousness*, but which I prefer to name *alternate consciousness*—the person being in a manner two individuals, as far as sensation and sense of personal identity are concerned.

But there is a state even more extraordinary than this, and which has been hitherto entirely inexplicable. No one has yet attempted even the slightest approach to an explanation, or given a suggestion leading to it.

In one form of these attacks the individual becomes a perfect child, is obliged to undertake the labour of learning again to write and read, and passes gradually through all the usual elementary branches of education—makes considerable progress, and finds the task daily becoming more and more easy, but is entirely unconscious of all that had taken place in the state of health. Suddenly she is seized with a kind of fit, or with a sleep of preternatural length and intensity, and wakes in full possession of all the acquired knowledge which she had previously possessed, but has no remembrance of what I would call her *child state*, and does not even recognise the persons or things with whom she then became acquainted. She is exactly as she was before the first attack, and as if the disordered state had never formed a portion of her existence. After the lapse of some weeks she is again seized as before, with intense somnolency, and after a long and deep sleep, wakes up in the *child state*. She has now a perfect recollection of all that previously occurred in that state—resumes her tasks at the point she left off, and continues to make progress as a person would do who was of that age and under those circumstances; but has once more entirely lost all remembrance of the persons and things connected with her state of health. This alternation recurs many times, and at last becomes the established habit of the individual—like an incurable ague.

It seems to me that I have a clear, complete, and satisfactory idea, in my own mind, of the nature and causes of this wonderful variety in human existence; whether I may be successful in conveying the same idea and the same conviction to others, is more doubtful—I will make the attempt.

The reader must bear in mind, that in deep sleep, the whole congeries of organs of both brains are in absolute unconscious torpor and repose, that in imperfect sleep and in dreaming the different parts are in different degrees of somnolency, or partial consciousness—that the accidental combination of the exercise of some cerebral organs or fasciculi of nervous fibres and the topor of others vary incessantly, and may often be guided by external sounds, or words imperfectly heard—that one brain may be asleep in its totality or in a large portion of its faculties, and the other brain sufficiently awake to observe it, as in the attempt to prolong an agreeable dream—or that both brains may be sufficiently awake to carry on a sort of contest, active enough to create memory, and to leave the effect of a dream, in which we have held an argument with another, (for whether in dreaming, in reverie, or in madness, we cannot by possibility suppose ourselves to be both the collocutors)—that these mental processes may be carried on while the body is physically sound asleep—all the special senses steeped in oblivion, and the mind entirely unconscious, not merely of surrounding objects, but of its own existence. All these things have been observed by every one. Many have attempted explanation; but the greater number of persons who have considered the subject confess that the phenomena are in their very nature inexplicable.

Now, before I proceed to the examination of these strange cases, I beg the reader to bear in mind and reflect on the following facts. It will require a patient attention to follow the reasoning.

[A] We know by innumerable examples, that a sudden physical shock or a blow on the head, shall reduce the healthy and acute brain of a profound scholar to a state wherein he has all the mental characteristics of childhood—is pleased or offended by trifles, so apparently insignificant that in his previous state they would not excite the most evanescent attention—his sensations and perceptions are still perfect, but his reasoning powers are gone.

[B] In other cases, a similar accident shall obliterate portions or the whole of his acquired knowledge—he will lose, for example, one language and retain others, or he may lose all; and, on his recovery from the physical effect of the accident, he has to begin his life again, and proceed to acquire information in the same mode as a child, though with a much slower progression.

[C] These effects arise sometimes also from a moral shock, such as the sudden communication of afflicting news: terror, detection in crime, or any other analogous cause, equally or indifferently whether the cause be moral or physical—the brain is either entirely spoiled, temporarily deranged, only slightly injured, or in gradation from one to the other—losing one or more of its functions, and one or more portions of acquired knowledge.

[D] After such effects have lasted a considerable time, and have or have not been accompanied or followed by any of the usual forms of mental aberration or of imbecility, the whole powers of the brain may be restored either gradually or in an instant—the watch may resume its motion.

All these facts are so familiar to medical men that for them it is unnecessary to cite cases; and other readers would find them tedious and difficult to understand; but if any one wish to examine for himself, he will meet with many such recorded in every work on insanity.

1. If then my doctine of the entire completeness and sufficiency of each brain as an instrument of mind be firmly established, it follows, so plausibly as to be almost certain that any of the states, A, B, C, and D, and many intermediate modifications of them, may spontaneoustly occur in one brain leaving the other entirely unaffected; we see an example of this in hemiplegia, or paralysis on one side only.

2. One brain may be subjected to one of these changes, and

the other brain may have its powers and functions changed or modified in a different manner.

3. One brain may be reduced to the state of childhood (state A), and the other remain in its ordinary state.

4. One brain may be in the state A or B, and the other may have its functions suspended or modified by a greater or less degree of torpor, as in sleep, catalepsy, ecstasis, etc.

5. One brain may be in the state of childhood, and the other torpid and unconscious.

Now, any of the states here described, or any modification of one or more of them may co-exist, or they may alternate. We see phenomena more or less analogous in intermittent insanity, where definite periods of excitement, collapse, and mental health follow in uninterrupted succession; the examples are numerous.

Suppose the lady whose case is spoken of as the second form of the malady of *alternate consciousness*, to be placed in the state No. 5 (a modification of that described under letter A). The only brain she now has at her command, is the brain in the *child state*; and, while the other remains in its torpor and *quasi extinct*, she must pursue her education as a child.

Let us next suppose the child brain to be in its turn seized with torpor, and the other to resume it functions with the use of all its previously acquired knowledge. Here, then, is the second state of the patient satisfactorily explained.

Strange and arbitrary as this hypothesis may seem, it is not difficult to shew that any one of the separate states here described as existing in one brain, or in portions of one brain, may exist in the whole brain (in the sense the word is generally used). Such phenomena are established by abundant evidence as consequences of blows on the head, moral shocks, disorder, or positive disease.

If, then, the *status* can exist in both brains, whether the derangement of functions depend on vibration, undulation, or circulation, or any other cause, it is a very natural presumption that the same *status* may exist in one only of the cerebra, in one only of the two entire and perfect instruments of MIND, which would at once solve the difficulty.

The wonderful powers of the microscope in its present state of perfection shew that the ultimate structure of a nerve or nervous fibre is a tube; that these nervous fibres contain a fluid, and it is asserted that it is to be seen in a state of congelation as well as in a state of fluidity; that this fluid circulates during life, and coagulates some time after death. How exceedingly minute are these nervous fibres or tubes can scarcely be conceived by the mind, although their diameter can be measured by the microscope as accurately as we can measure the threads in a piece of cloth. On the authority of Erasmus Wilson, I state the average size of the nervous fibres (which vary from fourteen to seven thousand according to their position) to be about ten thousand to the inch, which gives to a column of an inch square the amazing number of one hundred millions; and there are many square inches in the two brains.

We may conceive, then, that parts of the brain are in too active circulation or action, others too passive, modifications in the nervous fluid, spasm of certain portions, and other states for which we have no names; the mind in all its varieties may then be produced by the action of these fibres singly, or in determinate fasciculi, or in myriads of combinations, correct or erroneous, which so wonderful a structure may admit. Out of these combinations the states I have endeavoured to explain may easily be accounted for in health, as well as all the phenomena of insanity.

CHAPTER XXVIII: *Rev. J. Barlow on the Connexion Between Physiology and Intellectual Philosophy; State of the Brain When its Higher Faculties are not Called into Action; Reason Why There Should Be Two Organs of Thought; Mr. Hewitt Watson's Essay on the Use of the Double Brain*

The necessity of assiduously cultivating the higher faculties of the mind as a means of establishing self-control when the brain is in perfect health, and of enabling the healthy brain to exercise a pure tyranny over its brother when the latter is disordered or enfeebled, is the great duty of man—a duty he cannot neglect without injury to his interests, even in this world. It is this which makes the grand distinction between the civilized man and the savage, between the man of education and of virtue over the worse than savage of society—the ferocious unprincipled brute who gives way to his immediate animal instincts, like the beasts that perish; while the other "makes the past, the distant and the future, predominate over the present."

The Rev. Mr. Barlow, in his little book on the "*Connection between Physiology and Intellectual Philosophy*," has stated this admirably. In his 31st section he remarks: "Every bodily fibre acquires strength by exercise. None need be told how much muscular power is acquired by a constant and moderate exertion. The practised eye will see, the practised ear will hear, what these organs, when unpractised, distinguish with difficulty. Is it wonderful then, if the practised brain can also carry on its functions with greater facility and increased power? In savage life, where subsistence is hardly obtained and where danger is always at a point that keep the emotions that guard existence in constant exercise, men who have to struggle for their daily bread and defend themselves from their no less daily perils, require from the brain but a very small part of what it *can* accomplish; their greatest stretch of reasoning extends not beyond the connecting a bent twig and down-trodden leaf with the steps of their prey or of their enemy. In such instances we may easily conceive that the inexperienced faculties become as powerless as the limb of an animal which from the moment of birth had been restrained from movement. A child who had grown up with a limb so disabled would not be aware of its use, unless he saw it exemplified in others; and even if he saw its use, he would still find that in his own case the effort to make it available would be perfectly vain.

"Such I conceive to be the state of the brain which has never been called to exercise the higher faculties. The instinctive emotions are propagated through it with the almost delirious violence which characterises the brute creation, because the fibres destined to carry on the higher reasoning functions have remained inert till they have become powerless, and man is thus assimilated to the lower tribes, not because the organ of thought is wanting but because it has not been exercised. Christophe, the negro ruler of Haiti, was probably not removed above a generation or two from the African savage, yet his daughters were polished and accomplished women, fit to take their place in European society. A better proof could hardly be given of the improvability of all the races of men by education, even in one generation.

"I cannot pass over this part of the subject without drawing from it one useful lesson, upon the necessity of cultivating the higher faculties far more than is yet done, among the races calling themselves civilized. If the instincts, or as some will call them, the passions, assume so undue an ascendency in consequence of the inertness of the antagonist part of the brain, that man's whole moral nature falls into the morbid state of a convulsed, or finally, of a contracted limb, it is then no light crime in those who have the government of a family or a society of human beings, if they suffer the young to grow up without fully developing the powers of a nature, so admirable where its mental growth is duly proportioned, so tremendously capable of evil where it is not.

"It is from the depth of man's interior life," continues Mr. Barlow, "that he must draw what separates him from the brute, and hallows his animal existence; learning is no farther valuable than as it gives a certain quantity of raw material to be worked up in the intellectual laboratory, till it comes forth as new in form, and as increased in value, as the porcelain vase, which entered the manufactory in the shape of metallic salts, clay, and sand.

"Should my position, that the difference between sanity and insanity consists in the degree of self-control exercised, appear paradoxical to any one, let him note for a short time the thoughts that pass through his mind and the feelings that agitate him and he will find that, were they all expressed and indulged, they would be as wild, and perhaps as frightful in their consequences, as those of any madman. But the man of strong mind represses them and seeks fresh impressions from without if he finds that aid needful—the man of weak mind yields to them and becomes insane."

The foregoing observations of Mr. Barlow seem to me to go as far as the present knowledge of the mind will permit a man of strong reasoning powers to proceed. I believe, however, that the theory of two distinct organs of thought, which (at least) I have established, gives a much more satisfactory explanation.

The world is much indebted to this writer for the strong motives he has thus forcibly presented to exercise the most important of moral functions, *self-control*. If God intended this for a world of trial and progression, which every thing seems to shew, he must necessarily have formed us with instincts to be controlled. In making us, up to a certain point, absolutely parallel to the animals he has subjected to our dominion, he has bestowed on us all their impulses; but he has given us also an organization vastly beyond this—an apparatus to enable the soul to manifest its sublime powers. He gives to man, and to man alone, the power to think of his own thoughts, and to look to the past and to the future, instead of being, like the inferior animals, confined entirely to the present—to penetrate into the regions of space—to comprehend the will of his Almighty Creator, and to fit himself for a higher state of existence. But what shall control the controller? *quis custodiet ipsos custodes?* What shall control the intellectual power itself? What shall bound its wild and expansive fancies? What shall limit its researches to its proper purposes, and confine them to attainable objects? What shall check the growth of pride, arrogance, and presumption, and teach humility and submission? This is a widely different office from that of regulating the animal impulses; but is equally necessary to our welfare, to our sanity in this world, to our happiness in the next.

For this important purpose then I conceive that two brains were bestowed—two perfect organs of thought and volition—each, so to speak, a sentinel and a check on the other: to arrest audacious thought—to investigate and correct false conclusions, and to allow none to pass for settled convictions but those which have received the concurrent sanction of both brains. The two brains have a subordinate object, no doubt—to provide for the continued exercise of the intellectual functions when one of them shall be injured or destroyed by disease; but when this is the case the mutilated and helpless victim can scarcely be any longer considered a responsible being—he is redued to mere animal existence—he is dependent on the kindness of others for the very means of prolonging life—he enters into no presumtuous speculations, indulges in no wanderings into forbidden regions—he is incapable of sin, or he is mad—consequently, no longer a moral and responsible agent.

When this work was nearly ready for the press, and long after the "Propositions" had been published, my attention was called by Mr. Robert Cox of Edinburgh, to a communication in the *Phrenological Journal* (vol. ix, p. 608) entitled, "*What is the Use of the Double Brain?*" by Mr. Hewitt Watson.

There are some ideas in it well worthy of attention, as exceedingly novel and ingenious, although the writer has not fully and clearly stated any of them—except those which I have marked in italics; but the paper is short and interesting, and I think it but justice to cite the whole of it, that the reader may judge how far the writer has anticipated me in the matter. I will intersperse a few observations as I go on.

"Looking back to the very unsuccessful application of speculative theories in by-gone attempts to explain mental phenomena, it certainly behoves phrenologists to be cautious in resorting to this course. Nevertheless, in other sciences speculative explanations have been resorted to with great advantage, and have become of highly practical benefit, although incapable of direct proof. The atomic theory in chemistry, that of gravitation in astronomy, and the undulatory theory of heat and light, are familiar examples. In physiological and moral science we are almost compelled to resort to explanations which cannot be demonstrated, and the correctness of which must be assumed from their applicability to observed facts. I premise this observation, and adopt an interrogative title, more fully to impress that the following suggestions are to be regarded as questions or hints for the consideration of others, and not in the light of ascertained points. The subject seems likely to remain long open to discussion.

"I am unaware of any sufficient theory to account for the double brain, so universally found in animals, until we descend very low in the scale of organization and intelligence. Spurzheim writes: 'All the proper cerebral organs, like the other instruments of phrenic life, occur in pairs, or are double, from the medulla oblongata up to their expansion in the convolutions. This probably happens because of their importance, and to the end that the congenerate parts may supply each other's places should either of them chance to be injured.'—*Anatomy of the Brain* (p. 178). To me this appears an unsatisfactory explanation; the heart and stomach are most important organs, and yet there is no provision of a second, should one 'chance to be injured.' The following passage appears to afford a sufficient counter-quotation: 'From all the observations which have been made on animated nature, it may be inferred as an universal law, that whenever the Creator has bestowed two organs on an animated being, *the healthy condition of both is indispensably necessary to the production of their full effect on the economy of that being.*' What then is the full effect, in other words, *the use*, of the double cerebral organs?"

Now, this latter part of the quotation is obviously an entire fallacy; for I have shewn that one brain is sufficient for the manifestation of mind, even under the circumstance of the other being destroyed by disease, when the dreadful injury to the vital powers is necessarily productive of death. One ear also may suffice, or one eye. Each ear or eye may, in the common acceptation of the words, supply the place of the other should one of them chance to be injured. Had that remark of Spurzheim been known to me many years ago, I should have been tempted to enter on the subject much earlier. Spurzheim made nothing of it, but merely indicated that there was a statue in the block of marble, if any one would work it out. The rude notion on which Jenner founded his discovery of Vaccination had been known for ages; but remained unnoticed and useless, till he cleared away the rubbish and presented it in its due proportions—*Parva componere magnis*; mine is a similar labour, and I cannot but hope to be equally successful.

"The reply suggested in the work just referred to (continues Mr. Watson), is that *perception* being a lower, and *memory* a higher degree of functional activity, one sound organ may suffice for the former, though both may be required for the latter manifestation. This suggestion is not wanting in plausibility. [To me it seems utterly futile.] And may prove correct; yet I have some ground for questioning the entire correctness of it, which will appear at a future day. Meanwhile I proceed to my speculations.

"The human frame is almost a double; one side being nearly a counterpart of the other. But many of the double parts, from their use and constitution, act individually as well as jointly, and when acting in concert their actions are often different, and sometimes opposed.

"In walking, the legs move alternately; one being held more or less steady, while the other is in motion; and when both move at once their motions are usually different in kind and in degree. The hands, in like manner, are made to perform different motions at the same instant, and such are frequently antagonist motions. So also the eyes receive and transmit sensations singly at the same instant of time. Hence it appears like a matter of necessity that the internal organs which guide the hands, legs, eyes, and ears, as well as those which receive sensations therefrom or thereby, should also be double.

"But if it be necessary that the two legs and hands, the two eyes and ears, should be able to exert independent and even antagonist actions at the same time, so may the brain be required *to perform independent or antagonist actions at the same time*, and thus necessarily doubled throughout, *the two hemispheres being capable of acting singly or jointly*. [This is *a real and original thought*, and had it been dwelt on, would have led the writer much further.]

"I am not aware of any facts that can directly negative this suggestion; and although it will not suffice to explain all the peculiarities of consciousness [He will be of a different opinion, I hope, if he have the patience to read through the present work], yet it does appear reconcileable with several phenomena not to be accounted for otherwise. In players at chess, a person makes schemes and determines the movements of the pieces on his own side; to do this successfully, he must mentally play the game of his adversary as well as himself. Within his own cranium he must carry on the work of two brains—brains working in opposition to each other. [This illustration is of no value—a rapid alternation of thought would explain the apparently duplex reasoning; and, in fact, no man ever did anything requiring consideration without taking into account the obstacles as well as the facilities.] I take this game as an illustration of many of the schemes and movements of real life. [The writer has not read, it appears, that admirable little essay by Benjamin Franklin, called *Morals of Chess*, or he would be aware that the parallel had already been drawn.]

"It requires no argument to prove that we shape our conduct towards others, and have our feelings towards them excited, not in accordance with *their* actual motives and feelings, but in accordance with *our own* mental images of such, with the representations of their motives and feelings which we form or feign for ourselves. We do not see their ideas and feelings—we see only certain signs and symbols, the translation of which is made in our brains. It would hence appear that we must have the presumed wishes and ideas of others, as well as our own wishes and ideas pictorially present in the brain at the same instant. [This is a very loose employment of words.] But if our own ideas and feelings co-exist with the represented ideas and feelings of another, we are driven to conclude either that the two corresponding organs, manifesting any given function, work individually, or that each exists in two different states at the same moment. [The writer raises a difficulty out of nothing, and does not seem clearly and fully to state the question at issue—a little consideration will shew that there is not even the slightest analogy between this and a real antagonism, as of volition.]

"The only way of escaping this dilemma is by denying the coexistence of ideas, and attributing the apparent consciousness of it to the rapidity with which they succeed each other—an assumption not unreasonable, but fully as gratuitous. It appears to me that the coexistence of ideas is most reconcileable with observed facts, and that the existence of two connected brains thus becomes necessary. [I hope that my proofs depend on reasoning more consecutive, or there would be little chance of producing general conviction.]

"According to this view, mental communication with others, as it is commonly expressed [I do not understand this], may be just a self-communing between the hemispheres of our own brains, accompanied by sounds and signs addressed to the senses. If so, we must have the power of dividing the consciousness of the two hemispheres to a certain extent, so as to make one of them represent the mind of another person, more or less divested of the ideas familiar to ourselves. This I apprehend to be really done while in conversation with others [Only in insanity]. It is rendered more apparent in those confabulations and self-communings which active brains are ever carrying on when awake, and not fully occupied by impressions arising from the external senses; and it becomes still more evident during dreams, when consciousness is so completely dissevered, that, in idea, we make ourselves into two parties, one of which is always *self*, more or less changed. The very remarkable case of twofold personality mentioned in '*Combe's System of Phrenology*' (page 519, of the 3d edition), appears to be a more exalted degree of the state of brain during sleep, and was ushered in by somnolency and dreams. [I hope that my endeavour to account for this very rare and curious mental phenomenon will be deemed more satisfactory.] Many cases of insanity look like intermediate states, between the vivid pictures and dialogues of active or excited brains while awake, and the more completely divided consciousness in dreams. The divided consciousness of the insane does not appear to be complete. Though an individual pronounces and seems to believe himself to be a Deity, many of his actions have still, necessarily, a reference to his own proper self and nature; and there is often a betrayed anxiety lest others should detect mortality in assumed divinity. [One brain believes and the other disbelieves—a very common phenomenon in insanity.]

"Were this supposed individual action of the hemispheres an established point [it seems to me that I have established it, beyond the possibility of cavil], it might lend some aid towards explaining states of mind or consciousness which have much puzzled metaphysicians. In such case, for instance, I should be induced to regard perception as the active state of either of the corresponding intellectual organs. *Attention might be supposed to rest in the combined activity of the two organs directed to the same matter* (we *see* with either eye, we *look* with both). The sense of resemblance might depend on the two corresponding organs co-existing in the same state, though individually excited. Sympathy would arise when the same occurred to the affective organs. The sense of contrast and discord would imply the opposite state. Memory seems nearly allied to comparison. I will not, however, run off too far in the application of a merely speculative theory until the essential part of it has been tested by other minds; the essential part, I consider to be, *the capability of independent activity in the two hemispheres.*"

The mere act of walking is, if deliberately considered, an absolute proof of "the capability of independent action in the two hemispheres." The right brain has no command over the right leg, nor the left brain over the left leg; whenever the right brain is paralyzed there is no power whatever to move the left limb, yet the left brain moves the right as well as ever —consequently, the brains *are* capable of independent action

—the proof is complete. The operation of putting the legs forward alternately was one of the very first things which attracted my notice thirty years ago, when I thoroughly comprehended the structure of the brain—but, to the best of my belief, Mr. Hewitt Watson is the only writer who has ever drawn any inference whatever from the fact. In truth, there is not a single act or function of the body that is not a key to undiscovered treasures of knowledge, if duly considered and thought *at*. I hope that I have proved a great many things besides the alternate influence of the two brains on *muscular motion*.

The passages I have put in italics shew that the writer *had* an idea of the truth, but it was smothered by fixed notions as to the nature of ordinary mental operations.

I feel satisfied, however, that if he should read these pages he will become a valuable auxiliary in the dissemination of a great and important truth, and no longer feel himself under the necessity of clothing his ideas in the language of conjecture. I am inclined to attribute much of the obscurity of his statement to a sort of conviction that the new doctrine could not be reconciled to some phrenological theory previously fixed in his mind; for, had the idea of the duality of the mind suggested itself to him in its naked simplicity, as a necessary consequence of perfect duality of the brain, it is apparently impossible that he could have escaped the conviction which has taken complete possession of my own mind, and of which it seems to me that I have given super-abundant proof. If Mr. Watson's paper had fallen into my hands before my own was so far advanced, I should certainly have communicated with the writer, and asked his aid in establishing the truth of his very important hints as to the true physiology of the brain. Had he entertained clear ideas and decided notions on the subject, I think he would not have objected to the suggestions of Spurzheim, which he has cited at the beginning of his essay.

CHAPTER XXIX: *Power of Abstaining from Evil; Calvinist Doctrines; Great Concert of Nature; Effect of the New Theory if Adopted; Quotation from J. B. Rousseau; Change by Conversion; Proposal of Early Restraint in Insanity; Amendment of the Criminal Law; Concluding Parable*

It is certain that God intended that disease or malformation should sometimes give rise to erroneous judgment, since he permits the existence of moral insanity and of depraved imbecility. In such cases we do not hold the unhappy patient responsible for his actions, however much they may deviate from the recognised standard of virtue. In the minor degrees of moral aberration we are justified in inflicting punishment —not for vengeance, but for example to others, and for the reformation of the culprit; but after all, we cannot know how far the tendency to evil was or was not an irresistible impulse; and no doubt many a man has escaped the punishment of voluntary premeditated wickedness, while others have been subjected to the highest penalty of the law for acts they had no power to abstain from.

> What's done ye partly may compute,
> But never what's resisted.

If we concede the existence of a future state of reward and punishment, there is no longer injustice in the dispensation allotted to this, one of the smallest of the planets revolving round perhaps one of the smallest of the myriads of suns which we denominate stars. In some other state of being we may be recompensed for sublunary sufferings, and the errors of man's feeble judgment may be rectified. In giving us two brains of unequal power we have the materials of every diversity of character which distinguishes the human race, and constitutes the moral world such as it was intended to be; as we have the foundation of all the struggles which dignify our humble nature. From time to time a missionary is sent into the world to teach us our duties, and endowed with faculties vastly above the average of humanity, to give effect to his doctrines; but it is not in our present state of existence that the divinely mysterious essence connected with our bodily organization—the special gift of the Creator to the human race alone—can be comprehended in all its magnificence and sublimity. There is no ground therefore for objections to my doctrine, that it tends to a kind of fatalism, and that if our actions and our thoughts depend on the structure and health of the brain, there is an end of moral responsibility—that man is directed by inevitable impulse, and that his actions are consequently neither good nor bad as respects the agent. Some theologians, it is true, seem to take this view of the matter, and to believe that God brings the whole human race into existence with an innate propensity to evil—that it is only in favour of a small number, termed the elect, that he specially interposes to save them from the consequences he has himself ordained—that the immense majority of his creatures he leaves to the operation of an organization which inevitably ensures their destruction, and subjects them to endless misery and inconceivable tortures—that he foresaw the consequences that would necessarily result from this organization, which he *deliberately intended and pre-ordained*, and that having so ordained, he is himself bound by his own resolve and cannot interpose to save them! "*Non meus hic sermo.*" I will hope, however, that no reader of this book subscribes to so atrocious a doctrine, which took its rise in the brain of a madman, and must have been adopted by others *implicitly* and without examination, through a mistaken reverence for the authority on which it was promulgated.

We listen to a distant band of music and feel delighted when a full chord of masterly harmony bursts upon the ear; the wind carries it away and the next sound which reaches us is perhaps the shrill note of the fife; then comes the booming of the double drum—the exquisite melody of a voice which thrills in the inmost recesses of the soul; we are enchanted, and inwardly praise the admirable skill of the composer and of the performers. There are intervals when we hear nothing, and the concert seems to have ceased. We are next aware of a series of the harshest discords and we retract our praise of the author and wonder at his want of taste and judgment; but have scarcely time to express disapprobation when another gush of harmony turns the current of our feelings into breathless admiration, and we lament our fate to be thus debarred by distance from the fulness of enjoyment. He who is familiar with the art doubts not that were he near enough, he would find it acceptable to the senses; but he who understands the *science* of music knows that the discords offend only because we do not comprehend the whole, and that they were as necessary to the perfection of the concert, as the exquisite melody which delighted the uneducated ear.

It is thus with the great concert of the universe and its Almighty Contriver. We cannot comprehend the whole and we alternate between admiration and discontent, according as the few and distant sounds which reach us please or displease our limited and imperfect senses. In some future stage of existence we may be permitted to understand the vast scheme of Divine government in this world; and even now, a partial cultivation of the faculties bestowed upon us will produce the satisfactory assurance that "all worketh together for good," and that (to carry on the metaphor) the discords which offend the uncultivated judgment will be in due time resolved into one universal burst of harmony, filling up every sense with perfect satisfaction.

Conclusion

And what then is proved by all these arguments and examples? *Cui bono*? What is the result the effect, the benefit of the discussion? I reply, first of all, *the establishment of a new fact*, in the firm belief that every truth involves sequences beneficial to society, although the mind that makes the discovery be incapable of perceiving them. A conviction that no truth is sterile but the parent of innumerable other truths that seem in no way to spring from it, but which could not have had existence had not the first led to them, by exciting the interest and curiosity of fresh minds. I just catch a glimpse of corollaries to be hereafter drawn from the premises I have endeavoured to establish, which are so important as to be absolutely startling from their novelty and extensive influence, but to which I dare not even allude at present lest I should cast discredit on my theory.

In the next place, I think that the new doctrine may lead to further advances in the road of improvement as to the management of the insane, and may also lead to the anticipation and prevention of the diseases of which that disorder of the understanding is the consequence.

Thirdly, that it may excite compassion for the wicked, and induce society not to rest satisfied with the punishment alone of the guilty, but to make greater efforts to reclaim them, and to remove the causes which give rise to the acts of criminality. That it may also establish the conviction, that in the great majority of cases it is not voluntary intentional depravity which leads to crime, but ignorance and imbecility, from the want of development of all the higher portions of the intellect by early cultivation of the brain; that it was God's pleasure to give mankind not a perfect, but a cultivable mind, and that all its best and highest qualities are the result of education; that without such moral instruction as it is the imperative duty of society to enforce, we have no right to exact obedience to the laws, or to punish the breach of them. That man has no valid claim even to the accumulation and conservation of wealth, but by concurrent endeavours to accomplish these objects; that it is as much the duty of the State to furnish education as to furnish food, and as great a crime on the part of society to let any of its members perish for want of teaching, as to let them perish for want of physical nourishment; and that till a man has been placed in a position to learn his duties, it is tyranny to punish him for the neglect of them; that the mind in its natural state is a collection of the lowest instincts, in no respect better than those of brutes, and that the natural development of intellect, unaided by education, is nothing more than the animal wisdom called cunning, devoted solely to the gratification of the animal propensities. But in this wilderness of weeds that spring up and choke the neglected garden lie the germs of the noblest plants, which, had they been early cultivated, would have fully occupied the ground, and left no space for the noxious plants that now disfigure the soil.

There is little danger that this mode of thinking should lead to too great indulgence towards criminals: the comfortable conviction which occupies the mind of every one who has been exempted by his position and education from temptation to commit the grosser crimes—the more than inadequate indignation excited by the offences of the uneducated—the very disgust and detestation we have been taught to feel for the crimes we could never be in a position to commit. These things are quite enough to ensure at least a sufficient degree of severity in our judgments of others, and there is little danger of becoming too lenient towards any faults but our own. The Divine founder of our religion felt no anger, no hatred, no scorn, no indignation, towards the wicked, nothing but sorrow and compassion. Let us imitate the feeling as far as our imperfect nature will admit, and think more of implanting good sentiments as motives to good actions than of deterring from bad ones by the extravagant severity of punishment, which never yet accomplished its intended object.

But one of the most important of all the consequences of my theory, if on investigation it be found worthy of entire confidence, will be the establishment of a merciful feeling towards the great number of unhappy beings who have one brain requiring incessant control; who, with all their efforts, lose their hold from time to time, and commit acts of extravagance and folly inconsistent with the habitual tenor of their lives and their own deliberate feeling. Hundreds of thousands of human beings pass their whole existence in the incessant struggle between two volitions; making the most heroic efforts to overcome their tendency to evil and to error, and sinking from time to time into despair when they have had the misfortune to incur the censure of their fellow-creatures by some ungovernable act of imprudence, contrary to their deliberate will and resolve. Such men, if society at large could be aware of their mental struggle, and duly impressed with a correct notion of the physical cause, would be objects of sincere compassion, and meet with the encouragement which alone is wanting to turn the scale in their favour: it is already nearly balanced by their own virtuous resolves; but when involuntary faults and follies have drawn upon the unhappy possessor of such a brain the extremity of censure from his fellow-creatures, he loses heart, gives up all efforts to recover his own self-respect, and lets himself go to perdition.

I speak now more especially of the young and of the poor; at least of those of straitened circumstances, who have not the means of waiting to redeem a lost character. I believe vice to be almost always the offspring of mental imbecility, and that some of the early wicked may, by the gradual development of the intellect, become so continuously conscious of right as to lose all tendency to wrong. Crime is the child of folly, or of ignorance, which is of itself the cause of folly—

Je le soutiens—Justice et Vérité
N'habitent point en cerveau mal monté.
Du vieux Zénon l'antique confrérie
Disoit tout vice être issu d'ânerie;
Non que toujours sottise de son chef
Forme dessein de vous porter méchef;
Mais folle erreur, d'ignorance complice
Fait même effet, et supplée à malice.

JEAN BATISTE ROUSSEAU

How many men have I known filling a high station with honour, and dispensing a large fortune with discretion; a blessing to all around them; who in early life committed acts of folly and wickedness, which had they been poor, would have cut them off from the world in shame. Can the most virtuous among the *undetected* lay his hand on his heart and say with the Pharisee, "I thank thee, O Lord, that I am not as this man." Can he declare with truth that he never committed the sin for which he is now condemning a fellow-creature to punishment? Or if, indeed, he have always had such self-command, or such timidity and continuous fear of detection as to abstain therefrom, can he conscientiously declare that the wanderings of imagination have never contemplated such a sin with complacency? And had opportunity and impunity combined, does he feel *certain* that he could have resisted the temptation? If such a man there be, it is time he were dead; this world is not worthy of him; he has been sent to the wrong planet in mistake. Perhaps in Jupiter or Saturn he may find congenial spirits.

I believe, however, that there *are* such human beings, and that in the other sex they are not even of great rarity; but here the conventional state of society deprives them of early temptation. A moral atmosphere is made for them to breathe, from which every noxious ingredient is carefully excluded. A tone of religious feeling is cultivated, which there is nothing to interrupt or destroy, and the practice of virtue in the absence of temptation is not a very difficult task. But this negation of vice is necessarily unaccompanied by that development of intellect which is the result of the incessant conflict of two fierce volitions in the other sex. For men, we cannot make a moral atmosphere; they must fight the world as it stands; and it is the ultimate triumph of the good or the bad propensities, after the struggle, excited and sustained by a virtuous education, which is to stamp the permanent character.

I have lived long enough to see men whom I had known in youth desperately wicked, redeemed by affluent parents from the consequences of their follies and crimes, and in their further progress arrive at honours and reputation; when, had there not been wealth to remedy the effects of their wickedness, they would have perished in infamy by the violated laws of their country. It is more especially among the exalted members of the aristocracy and the church that this has been exhibited—men who had held a distinguished rank and were universally recognised as models of piety and zeal, the latter portion of whose career was passed in strenuous exertions for the welfare of their fellow-creatures; yet who had in early life committed serious crimes, and had the veil been then stripped off by poverty, must have sunk into infamy and obscurity. They had been converted; at least such is the explanation given by some persons of the change, and I do not attempt to controvert it. If their subsequent acts and sentiments were sincere, they were most exemplary men. God alone can know if they deserved the character.

> For neither man nor angel can discern
> Hypocrisy,—the only ill that walks
> The earth invisible—except to God
> Alone. MILTON

The physical cause of the crimes of the young is an object worthy of research—if such a cause exist, it is not merely deserving of the most ample investigation, but the investigation is an imperative duty. I believe myself to have made some advances in this direction, and that I shall be able to point out a mode of greatly modifying, and even sometimes of removing it. I do not allude to the development of the sexual propensities, which alone has been assigned as the exciting cause of their ungovernable impulses to evil; but of a state of brain *recognisable* and *removable* by medical means—means which if generally adopted, might save many a family from distress and misery. This work, however, has already extended much beyond the limits I had proposed to myself, and the subject of which I now speak being complete in itself, and not directly connected with the present inquiry, I pass it over to a more convenient season. If the public think my present speculations worthy of notice, I may be induced to offer it on a future occasion.

The reader will perhaps object that the arguments I have adduced go to remove the dread of punishment, and thus to encourage the commission of crime. Such is by no means my belief, and it cannot of course be my intention; on the contrary, I believe the fear of *proximate* (not *excessive*) punishment to be the strongest motive which can be presented in aid of the exertion of self-control. With the young there is no correction so influential as bodily pain. I think that in our present administration of the criminal law we give way greatly too much to the maudlin sensibility of the day. The infliction of severe corporal chastisement is the fitting punishment for the great majority of crimes in the young, and almost the only punishment which does not give rise to evils serious nearly as those it removes. I do but allude to the subject here, and must leave to others to draw what seem inevitable inferences from premises I propose hereafter to lay down.

There is yet another among the beneficial results which would follow the adoption of my theory, and that is, an early, a very early, interference with the actions of men who, although they cannot be pronounced absolutely insane, yet are clearly unfit to be entrusted with the control of their property and the government of their families. Whether anything could be devised sufficiently in harmony with our free institutions to obtain the general assent of the people at large, must be decided by men conversant with legislation. If such a measure could be guarded from abuse, and a man in the stage of transition to insanity could be stopped short before he had ruined or disgraced his family, and without the publicity and permanent disqualifying consequences of a commission of lunacy, it would be an enormous blessing to thousands who are now watching with trembling anxiety the moment when the most afflicting certainty shall terminate intolerable suspense. Many of the acts of infamy which have disgraced individuals of the higher classes have been foreseen and foretold to the friends by the medical attendant, but there have been no means of arresting the calamity. The pathological physician sees clearly the point at which the patient either *can not* or *will not* control the disordered brain by the sound one, or the propensities by the intellect: the former is a justification of restraint in every respect as valid as the latter—they are in fact virtually the same.

The right to remove altogether from society those who are incorrigibly bad, who have resisted every attempt to reform them, who deliberately prefer and determine to exercise the indulgence of their own bad passions regardless of the injury to their fellow-creatures—the right to remove altogether such beings even from the list of the living (if no other mode of disposing of them could be devised) seems to me as evident and as indefeasible as to destroy the vermin that infest the earth—the continued existence of such beings is an intolerable evil to mankind, and ought to be removed. It seems to me, however, that without the infliction of death, such persons may be not merely adequately punished, but made in some considerable degree to compensate their fellow-creatures for the evils of which they have been the cause—that incessant and painful labour, and the infliction of corporal chastisement, would in almost all cases, if accompanied by proper instruction, reclaim the sinner; but that solitary confinement *without education and occupation* can do nothing but aggravate the imbecility which led to crime, and terminate in positive insanity. After much observation of the management of criminals in various countries conducted on a variety of benevolent theories, the plan which appears to me to have the greatest effect in deterring from crime, which is accompanied by the least injury to the intellectual faculties, which avoids the greatest number of evils, which is least expensive, and above all, the most merciful, is short imprisonment and the infliction of corporal chastisement, graduated according to the crime; light for the first offence, and increasing in severity on repetition till it become truly formidable, and an object of permanent terror.

We must always bear in mind that the cases of real insanity, exclusive of connate imbecility, are only a thousandth part of the whole number of human beings, and therefore complete exemption from the full penalty of crime can be but rarely deserved—that every intermediate state is left to the discretional punishment of society—that it is probable that by better education and moral discipline, even these cases may be so diminished in number as to allow a vast improvement in the moral structure of the world; yet that, although there can be no question of the right of society to punish a violation of the laws for example sake, the main and most satisfactory object is the reformation of the criminal; that, in like manner as we are justified in applying the red-hot iron to cure a disease of the hip, we are justified in inflicting such a degree of corporal punishment on an offender as will, by the recollection of it, aid his own imperfect self-command; but that it is our duty to obviate every thing that can tend to produce the moral disease, as it is our duty to enforce, if necessary, the healthy discipline which shall prevent the disease of the hip, by removing the constitutional tendency which gives rise to it; and especially, that legal punishment, however severe, should always be inflicted in the same spirit that the surgeon performs a painful operation.

Whether the feelings of society would permit the adoption of this system is doubtful. In the present day we do not make the laws we deem the wisest, but the laws which will be most acceptable to the temporary frame of mind in which the great mass of the population is placed; because we know that in our form of government it is impossible to enforce an obnoxious regulation. Whether this influence of the people on legislation by attended by more advantages than evils, I leave to wiser heads to determine; it exists, and we are compelled to frame our measures accordingly.

Some of the alterations of the law, as to the infliction of the punishment of death for certain crimes, were delayed long after an almost universal conviction that the change was necessary and essential to its due execution, but no one dared to propose a specific abolition for specific crimes; and it was only by an evasion that this just and necessary change could be brought about. I know that some of the most active promoters of that reform were of opinion that severe corporal chastisement was the most appropriate punishment, and that simple imprisonment was by no means adequate to the offence, but they dared not come forward and advocate their own convictions when their arguments were to be spread all over the world, and their names inseparably connected in imagination with the crimes for which they were legislating.

If, in spite of the pains I have taken to avoid offence, some who have not read my work with attention, or who have not the preliminary knowledge necessary to the clear understanding of it, be inclined to draw inferences from my doctrine which it does not justify—I enter a protest against the proceeding, and defend myself by the following parable:

A certain man, about to leave his country, pointed out to his children the poppies which were the natural and uncultivated produce of the soil; called their attention to the graceful form of the leaves, and the wonderful variety and beauty of the flowers; recommended the seeds as a wholesome and agreeable article of food; and shewed how to make from them a bland and benign emulsion for the relief of sickness. He advised that they should be satisfied with these pleasures and blessings, and leave untouched all other parts, which he assured them were unwholesome and injurious. He was no sooner departed than his children wounded the skin of the capsules and extracted the opium, and thus obtained the means of intoxication, disease, and death.

The father is not responsible for the mischief caused by the wilful disobedience of his children; he could not remove the poppies, for they were the spontaneous growth of the soil. He gave the advice which might have rendered them a blessing, and he would have pointed out even the beneficial qualities of the drug they had abused could he have calculated on their discretion and self-command in the use of it. It was their own perverse disposition which converted the blessing into a curse.

APPENDIX I: *On the Influence of Religion on Insanity*

Having been much occupied in investigating the origin and progress of insanity in Catholic countries, I have been struck with the rarity of religious madness in that sect as compared with our own. I have no wish to express any opinion whatever on the peculiar tenets of the two great divisions of Christians; they are entirely out of the province of the physician, who, in estimating the influence of different modes of faith on the intellectual functions, has rather to consider the usages than the dogmas.

The *practice* of the clergymen of the two sects is, however, so diametrically opposed in the management of that state of mind which precedes religious insanity as to exercise great influence on the progress of the disease. Some Protestant clergymen, when first made acquainted with the doubts and embarrassments of their young and fragile-minded communicants, enter into explanatory discussions, recommend the study of the Bible, and of works of theological controversy. The patient, at an age when the brain is expanding perhaps faster than its bony covering can make room for its growth, enters upon the investigation of subjects so abstruse that they have disturbed the intellect of the most able and energetic men. The poor girl (for it is most frequently, though by no means exclusively, in that sex that these doubts and delusions take root) becomes more and more bewildered. If it be only one of the brains in which the disease is beginning, the sound one, instead of performing its duty of acting as a sentinel and controller, is taught to dwell constantly on the same morbid train of thoughts which occupy its fellow, and thus confirmed insanity is established, where a different mode of treatment would perhaps have restored the disordered brain to a healthy state.

It is not to be expected that the clergyman should possess medical knowledge and tact to see the commencement of mental disease in an apparently increased acuteness of the reasoning powers, or many might be saved from destruction, who fall a sacrifice to well-meaning but mistaken views of duty. If one of these gentlemen, with more sagacity or better information than the rest, should discourage the further prosecution of theological studies in the applicant, there is risk of his incurring serious censure, and its painful consequences, for his presumed indifference to the tenets of his sect and the welfare of an immortal soul.

The practice of the Catholic clergy is exactly the opposite. They give their communicants a large quantity of ceremonial devotion to perform, and prayers to be recited, and forbid all controversial or doctrinal reading. The incessant repetition of these prayers and observances has the soothing effect of all monotony, and tranquillizes the morbid emotions of the brain.

It is also a principle with the Catholic clergy to confine the study of theology to themselves, and entirely to discourage it in the laity. Thus one large source of mental disturbance is superseded. I have sometimes wished, when hearing flippant young girls discussing the abstruse doctrines and mysteries of religion, that a similar practice prevailed in our church with the young.

I cannot shut my eyes as a medical man to the mischievous consequences of such studies to every brain whose delicate structure tends to insanity, nor to the advantage (medically speaking) of a system which puts such brains in repose.

Yet no one can be more convinced that without the influence of religion on society at large, the number of maniacs would be vastly increased, as was seen in France during the horrid Revolution, at the time Esquirol first gave his sentiments to the public. The increase of insanity was frightful, when no longer checked in its beginnings by the judicious control of the clergy, and by the calm influence of a tranquillizing faith. At the same time the form of *religious mania* was become so rare that, in three hundred and thirty-seven patients admitted into the private establishment of that gentleman, only a single case could be attributed to that source.

For one person rendered mad by fanaticism, half-a-dozen are reduced to that state for want of religious consolation. I will here venture to relate an example of what I call (medically speaking) judicious conduct on the part of a clergyman, the dignitary of whom I have already spoken.

A woman of the upper class of artizans came to him one evening and asked permission to consult him in a serious religious difficulty, on the ground of being a parishioner, although not of the same faith. He listened very patiently to her story. She told him with the greatest naïveté and simplicity her interesting tale of virtuous self-denial and benevolence. She had been on the point of marriage to the man of her heart when her sister (a widow) died and left six children totally destitute; she at once resolved to break off her projected marriage and devote herself to the orphans. Having a small independence, she was enabled to accomplish this—had brought them all up virtuously and happily, and having established them in the world, was now waiting patiently the time when she should be called to render an account of her stewardship. She had been happy and contented, and had always found a source of consolation and of hope in the good deeds she had been enabled to accomplish.

Some pious Protestant ladies, belonging to a society which in the zeal for religion violates rather too boldly the sanctity of the homes of the poor, had forced themselves upon her, and by dint of iteration had almost convinced her that the Catholic faith was the broad path to eternal destruction.

In her embarrassment and despair she had applied to this gentleman, from a knowledge of his benevolence and sagacity, and requested him to direct her into the right road.

The clergyman, who was one of those active and useful men that make themselves acquainted, as far as possible, with all their parishioners, listened with great patience and attention to her history, which he knew to be true—told her to return home and cultivate tranquillity of mind—to rest quietly in confidence, that the God who had thus enabled her to triumph over her own feelings in the prosecution of her duties would ultimately receive her into eternal happiness. I believe that a different advice would have driven the poor woman to the madhouse.

These examples of splendid virtue among the lower classes

are much more common than will be credited by those of more elevated station—*how* common, is known only to clergymen, and those medical men who practice among the poor.

I may mention, parenthetically, that on relating this anecdote to a family of influence in the same parish, I was rather surprised to find that it excited strong feelings of indignation.

Wishing to see the effect on the opposite sect, I related the story the same evening in a Catholic family of rank, and heard on all sides, the exclamation—Oh! what a good man—he will be converted to the true faith, no doubt. He is a Catholic at heart, and God will not suffer him to perish.

If the office of medical adviser and spiritual guide were united in one person, and if the whole cycle of sciences necessary to be acquired in order to constitute an efficient director in either department were compatible with an equal proficiency in the other, the task of managing and of curing insanity, when curable, would be comparatively easy; such a combination of knowledge is, however, not to be expected, for the professors in each department will agree, that to attain moderate excellence in one of them is quite sufficient to occupy all the life and all the faculties of man. Neither of them can convince the other that his own is not by far the most difficult and the most important science, and it is rare that either will concede that his own opinions in the other department are worthless. The reason is obvious: he knows the difficulties of his own set of sciences, because he has gone through the long and laborious task of conquering them; but he makes a very inadequate estimate of the difficulties of the other, and believes that common sense and common application could easily master them.

In the management of the insane, the sincere co-operation of the two is essentially necessary. If I say that (*caeteris paribus*) the clergyman should always give way to the physician, it will be very naturally attributed to professional prejudice. If, however, insanity be as strictly a physical disease as fever, dislocation, or fracture, it is certainly more within the province of the latter; and the clergyman should only be called in at the times and under circumstances indicated by the physician. It has always seemed to me a desecration of the office of spiritual adviser to set him to the task of convincing a person who is incapable of correct ratiocination. The soothing effect of ceremonial devotion is a very different affair—like the benevolent gentleness of manner, now so generally adopted towards persons of deranged intellect, it is a moral medicine, calculated to produce a physical effect—but it would not be adopted by the patient, nor, if adopted, beneficial, unless the practice were sanctioned and recommended by the clergyman.

I do not presume to give an opinion on the disputed dogmas of religion. The general principles running through the two systems of devotion of the two great divisions of Christians are the claim of the right of individual judgment on one side and absolute submission to authority on the other—that is, discussion and acquiescence. It is the antagonism of these two principles which constitutes the essence of the controversy between Protestantism and Catholicism. Each is excellent in moderation; but eternal discussion of principles leads to universal Pyrrhonism and Sceptism, while uniform acquiescence without discussion as naturally tends to the prostration of the intellect. Enlightened and good men on both sides take a middle course. The general character of the two sects is, however, that which I have stated, and the great majority of the members of each party are so convinced, and so strenuous in their zeal, that they will not hear of a compromise. With one party nothing can be done without discussion, with the other, nothing must be discussed.

As a sincere Protestant, I cannot acquiesce in the latter dictum, because, looking at the whole course of the history of religion, it seems to me to lead to infinitely greater evils than its opposite. A Catholic will tell me that I am of this opinion because I was from infancy furnished with a pair of Protestant spectacles; that these spectacles are coloured, and that all I see is tinged by them. It may be so; I do not think so, but I may retort the accusation with equal plausibility.

It is very different, however, when called on to decide medically on the physical effect of the religious ceremonies and practices of the two sects, and I beg that my recommendations may not be attributed to any other motives than those I profess. The unhesitating acquiescence in religious dogmas, and the obedient performance of ceremonial duties, are much better adapted to soothe and to calm the disturbed functions of the brain, than the attempt to follow out a train of reasoning. The former may not be permitted to a Protestant divine to prescribe; but it must be evident that the latter will tend to aggravate the disease, and that it is in fact a real degradation of the sacred science.

It is with the usages of the religious sect that we have to do, not with their theological tenets, when speaking of their influence on cerebral disease.

How many examples have I seen of innocent and virtuous girls who, if intended for nuns, would have been cured during their novitiate, and would have returned to the world to become happy and respected mothers of families—how many such have I seen injudiciously encouraged to pass their time in studying the mysteries of sanctification, regeneration, redemption, till they have rapidly progressed into positive insanity, and taken refuge from intolerable terrors in suicide. How often have I felt anguish of heart at witnessing these horrors and being utterly unable to prevent them. I have heard these pure and innocent creatures accuse themselves of impossible crimes, and die in the agonies of despair, while the bystanders attributed the unnatural accusations to remorse at having ceded to the instigations of the devil.

At the risk of becoming tedious I must dwell a little longer on this topic, for the influence of the form of religion in promoting or preventing insanity is likely to become a subject of compulsory attention. The rapid extension of the Catholic form of worship since the alteration of the laws affecting the members of that church, makes it impossible to evade the consideration of the important subject; and although it is obviously impracticable to discuss the matter comprehensively in a work of this nature, I may facilitate to others the acquirement of a competent opinion, by shewing some of the physical considerations which must be perpetually borne in mind by theologians, if they would arrive at a satisfactory conclusion.

In a very deliberate and interesting conversation at Rome with a physician of great acquirements, and an ecclesiastic of rank and great attainments in literature and science, the latter remarked that he should not be surprised to hear that England contained a proportion of insane many times greater than Italy, for that the discussion of theological subtleties by the uneducated was more calculated to disturb the understanding than all other causes put together. I endeavoured to shew the superior advantages of free investigation, and that a result arrived at after ample examination was more satisfactory than one accepted from blind deference for authority.

To this he replied, that the mass of mankind had neither time, education, nor intellectual development sufficient to put them in a position for examining the foundations of their faith, and therefore to them the permission to investigate was a nullity, and on them the duty of examination could not be incumbent. "When a poor afflicted creature comes to you, sir, and states his sufferings and his symptoms, would you say to him, consult Hippocrates and Galen? His answer might be: are these books written in my own language, for I do not know any other? You reply, No, but there are translations. And are all the translations agreed? Certainly not; but there are numerous commentators. And do all these accord in their opinions? O No! on the contrary, you must reply if you act honestly, they are of all possible opinions, and give the most contradictory explanations of almost every proposition; but you must read them all, and then form an opinion for yourself. But, sir, I have not time—I am ill—my brain is disturbed, and I am not in a condition to investigate even if I had leisure and education, and I come to you on the presumption that you have studied all these things and will give me the fruits of it. You may reply, perhaps, that the habit of study strengthens the mind, and that the task becomes daily more and more easy, and that, if every one were to study, the average of the nation's intellect would be higher. To all which the poor man replies, I am ill, and before all this can take place I shall die. Give me the result of your knowledge and experience—cure me—and I will leave the rest till I am in health.

"It is exactly so, sir, with our penitents. I listen to the story of a sinner. I find that, although he knows that he has sinned, he is endeavouring to persuade himself that he has a hundred excuses and palliations; he has repented perhaps of his crime, but has not made restitution; he is still enjoying the fruits of his iniquity and most unwilling to relinquish them. Shall I send such a man to the Bible? He will dwell only on those passages which he can twist into accordance with his depraved wishes, or distort into palliation of his sins. It is my duty to strip off the covering which his diseased mind throws over his derelictions and shew him his naked soul in all its deformity —not to set him to judge himself after his own fashion, with the judging faculty perverted by prejudice and self-love till he can persuade himself of anything which can minister consolation to his depravity. I tell him the true nature and extent of his wickedness—the necessity of repentance and the endurance of expiatory punishment—of relinquishment of all the profits, all the comforts, all the indulgences, he has wrongfully acquired and would fain retain. I compel restitution and recompense to those whom he has injured, and I insist on a firm resolve to lead a new life.

"And you also, sir," added he, "you do the same. You do *not* send your patient to Hippocrates and Galen—although you do not forbid the man of eduction from studying their works if he please; at the same time you tell him that in order to judge correctly of their advice, he will need a great deal of preliminary instruction—you give him the result of your own knowledge —you tell him what to do, and what to abstain from—and you, above all, command an entire change of habits, and the relinquishment of all those vicious indulgences which you know to have been the cause of his disease.

"But it is especially amongst persons of imperfect minds—of beings who have but a glimmering of the real nature and consequences of sin—whose weak intellects, in attempting to comprehend things beyond their mental powers, have lost all self-control, and, if not stopped short in their endeavours to comprehend the incomprehensible, rapidly pass on into a confusion of mind which must end in insanity. To set such persons upon a task which requires all the faculties in health would be destruction. They have not lost their feelings of devotion, which are, perhaps, in excess—they are not incapable of self-control in the absence of excitement. To these unhappy beings we prescribe a course of prayers and ceremonial religious observances which tranquillize their minds, occupy their time and thoughts, and produce the soothing satisfaction of duties fulfilled—and thus they escape the insanity which would have been the effect of permitting theological studies by disordered minds."

I endeavoured to shew that judicious clergymen of the Church of England took the same view of incipient insanity; but my collocutor denied that such a plan could possibly be practised by Protestants, and said that the statistics of England shewed the contrary.

It is evident that much must depend on the discretion of the clergy of both systems; but with ignorant preachers, amongst the uneducated especially, every medical man must have seen examples of quiet delusion transformed into confirmed insanity and fanatical devotion (the result of cerebral disturbance) encouraged by such men as a manifestation of Divine Grace. I am sorry to say that some of the clergy take a similar view of the matter in discussion, and that they concur in opinion of the utility of the study of theology by such persons, than which nothing can be more fatally mischievous. I have some hope that the remarks on which I have ventured may tend to convince them of the danger of such undue excitement of brains requiring absolute repose. It must be evident from the whole scope and tenor of my work, that I am a sincere friend to the Establishment, and hold the clergy in the highest veneration; my sentiments, therefore, ought to have some weight. My predominant wish, indeed, in writing this book, was not merely to avoid offence but to induce them to take it up as an auxiliary and introduction to the study of moral philosophy, to which, in fact, it seems to me that a correct (even if *limited*) knowledge of the functions of the brain in health and disease is an essential preliminary.

APPENDIX II: *Conjectures on the Nature of the Mental Operations*

In the preceding pages, while deprecating every attempt to describe the nature or mode of action of the SOUL, which indeed can be comprehended or even conceived only by direct revelation, it is, I think, proved, that the production of MIND is not only through the instrumentality of the brain, but that every manifestation of the mind is immediately caused by a direct and physical action of that organ, however difficult it may be to conceive the mode of such action, still more to assign a name to it from any analogy with the actions known to us—as contraction, dilatation, vibration, oscillation, circulation, and many others; or even to such as are less obviously material, as electricity, galvanism, and magnetism. However difficult it may also be to describe or to name such action, it is clear that *some* action, *some* movement, *some* change, *must* take place on these occasions. That such action takes place, not in the *whole* brain, at every impulse, thought, reflection, or idea, is also evident; because we see that injuries of different parts of the organ, and different degrees or kinds of injury, distort or destroy *parts only* of the mind, leaving the remainder in the ordinary state, and capable of the ordinary functions. One kind of blow on the head shall annihilate the knowledge of a language—another shall produce a permanent irritability—another a torpid and almost imbecile amiability; one kind of injury shall change love into hatred—another transform a sober, steady, and wise man, into a vain and chattering fool; one shall excite all the mental functions into undue and brilliant activity and power, while another shall annihilate all the higher intellectual faculties, and leave none but the instincts of the animal. Disease in a very small and circumscribed portion of the brain shall utterly distort the judgment and the power of combination and comparison; or leave all these perfect, except on one single topic. All the varieties of insanity—the absurd reasoning—the base and disgusting propensities—the ferocity of the beast of prey—the extravagant and incongruous feelings of devotion or sexual fondness—all arise from the mode of action of the organ, or rather organs, which create the mind.

The *soul*—the immortal, immaterial principle itself, cannot be sometimes good and sometimes bad, sometimes vicious and depraved, sometimes amiable and virtuous. It is the gift of the Creator! and did it not leave the hands of the Maker pure and perfect, it would be tyrannous to exact from us a good and virtuous life. Revelation tells us its exalted nature, and that it is man alone who dims its lustre and destroys its original brightness.

This, however, is a subject too profound to be discussed in a work like the present. It is for theologians alone, and to them I leave it.

The modes and manifestations of *mind* are strictly within the bounds of physiology and pathology, and belong specifically and exclusively to the medical philosopher. The immediate physical movement of the intellectual organs by which they are enabled to manifest their specific functions, it is not only permitted, but it is a *duty* to investigate; and let us push our researches as far as we may in the ascending series. We shall never arrive at the first principle, the *primum mobile*, by any other road than a Revelation.

The many forms of imbecility and insanity which are permitted to exist by the will of the Creator, and which it would be monstrous to subject to reponsibility, are proof incontrovertible that the due and proper influence of the soul upon intellect and moral conduct can only be exercised through a healthy brain; and that when, from any cause, that brain is incapable of correct reasoning, all the *future* actions of that individual are absolutely exempt from moral responsibility. For the acts which *led* to that state of brain as, for example, intoxication and gross indulgences, the individual is, however, justly answerable. The investigation of the physical action of the brain in producing the effects we call *mind*, is then not only a laudable effort, but a very important aid to religion, and the physician who enters upon it ought to receive every encouragement from the professors of the sacred science; for, if he can point out the physical state which leads to vice and crime, it is reasonable to believe that he may essentially aid in anticipating or removing it.

I beg the reader to bear in mind the title of this chapter: CONJECTURES. It is only as conjectures that I offer my speculations on this mysterious subject. I do not expect them to be accepted, but I do expect that they may lead others to a much more advanced position than that occupied by the suggester; just as the "Scantling, No. XCV," of the Marquis of Worcester's "*Century of Inventions*," led distinctly and clearly to the discovery of the steam-engine.

Preparatory to an attempt to expain the *modus operandi* of the brain, I will beg leave to introduce a trivial anecdote which may tend to facilitate the comprehension of it by analogy.

I was sometime ago at Liverpool, and in consequence of the excessive heat of the weather, passed a considerable part of the day in going backwards and forwards across the river in the steam-boat, where alone the atmosphere was breathable.

A man on board was engaged in amusing the company by ventriloquism, and depended on the casual pence of the passengers for his remuneration. He took out of his pocket a little doll, dressed as a sailor, and in a low and vulgar dialogue of much wit, so completely established the deception, that I observed several persons approach the man who did not dare to touch the puppet, because of the screams which were uttered the moment a hand came near him. I had heard Alexander, and many of his predecessors, but none of them came up to the startling fidelity of this entirely uneducated man. I watched him with the closest attention for a considerable time, looked about for some pipe which might have conducted the voice of another person to the spot, and was long before I could assent to the truth of the wonderful performance.

A narrow slit between his lips, not an eighth of an inch wide, gave passage to the voice, but the lips themselves were as absolutely motionless as if they had been carved in marble—not the slightest tremor in them could be detected by the closest examination.

In the course on conversation with him I discovered that he was a man on whom I had formerly conferred some obligations, and he readily lent himself to a minute examination; he took off his cravat, and I examined the movement of the muscles of the glottis, which, though slight to the eye, was very sensible to the touch. The muscular fibres, and consequently the nerves used on this occasion, were certainly not those which are by nature obedient to volition; they had been brought under the command of the will only by long and strenuous efforts. I asked how he had acquired the art, and he was evidently desirous of telling me, for he could not dread a rival, and I tempted him by the offer of money. His reply was in nearly these words: "I can only explain it by saying that I was always *trying*—my master gained his living by the art, and I watched him as closely as possible, but it was all in vain; I never could gain any hint from it—he would have dismissed me immediately had he supposed I was endeavouring *to learn the business*, so I *tried* when I was alone; I went on *trying* for some hours every day, for years together, for I was *determined to conquer* (the true mode of overcoming a difficulty). At last, one day, it came to me all at once like a flash, and I could do it better than my master."

"And now," said I, "if you had a son whom you wished to place in your shoes before you die, how would you set about teaching him?"—"I could only tell him to *try*," said he; "I could give him no further instruction; I don't believe anybody knows how he does it—*it is by trying.*"

It is this strong impulse of volition which suddenly confers on nerves of a class not obedient to the will, the same power we possess over those which are strictly voluntary. It was this which gave men power to control the action of the heart—which enabled the dumb youth to speak when his father fell overboard—which formed the milk in the breast of the man in South America, whose case is related by Humboldt, and in the instances of others equally authentic. It is this strong impulse which enables the bed-ridden cripple to escape from a fire, and it is this which we have all seen to aid in restoring a paralyzed limb. To use a vulgar expression, "No man knows what he can do till he tries;" and every man can, under adequate excitement, do a vast number of things which in his state of torpor and apathy he believes to be impossible. There are a few things which cannot be acomplished by a vigorous determination, as we have innumerable opportunities of observing in works of extraordinary and unequalled skill.

Now this effort, this impulse, although applied to a purpose clearly physical, is as much an operation of the mind, as the discovery of fluxions or logarithms. It is equally the influence of the grey substance of the brain on its nervous fibres, which leads to the solution of an arithmetical problem, and to the guidance of the hand in a new and delicate surgical operation. We can go no farther back in the process, and we resolve all the rest into the great *principle* with which we are endowed by the Creator, and which it has not pleased Him to give us faculties to comprehend—all abuts on this—we are at the end of our tether, and all the progression we can make is circular, and leads us round again to the point from which we started. The rest may perhaps be known to us in some future state of existence.

An attentive consideration of the foregoing will, I think, enable us to form a tolerably clear notion of the nature of the mental operations.

In thus *completing* the power of a nerve, which ought to have been obedient to volition originally (as in the case of bestowing speech on the dumb), in *restoring* the power of a nerve (as in the paralyzed limb), or in *creating* the power in nerves not formed for the purpose (as in controlling the heart's action). In all these cases it must be the establishment of the circulation, vibration, oscillation, or whatever it may be called which thus bestows or renews the function, and this must first begin in the brain.

The phrenologist groups contiguous cerebral fibres into certain specific fasciculi or bundles, and calls them organs. He believes that one of these groups gives the feeling of benevolence, another of veneration, another of a tendency to destroy, and so on. It may be so. I have as yet seen but a very small and insufficient portion of the evidence which would be necessary to establish the fact in defiance of anatomy; but I will for the nonce concede all this, and allow that all the impulses, instincts, or propensities, are exercised always by the same fibres in the same combinations.

But when we advance to the reasoning powers, I see not a tittle of evidence to shew that the aggregations of the cerebral fibres in their myriads of possible combinations are always the same. On the contrary, I think we have the strongest presumption that they are of unlimited variety. My conjecture is that these fibres can be used either singly or in fasciculi, or in combinations of fasciculi, or in combinations of different and distant single fibres, or combinations of single fibres with fasciculi of fibres, in the innumerable millions of millions of arrangements admissible in a geometrical series composed of at least a thousand millions of single fibres. If this be the mode in which *mind* is formed, how small a portion of the whole is all the knowledge which the greatest man that ever was created has possessed—*and yet there is a limit, however distant.*

I conceive, then, that the cerebral fibres do naturally fall into certain groups more readily than into others, and that it is these spontaneous groups which form the ordinary mind of the uneducated, and of those who deviate little from the common standard of common humanity.

I conceive that it is in the power of almost every man to produce new groupings, combinations, and aggregations; and that, if in the complicated processes he chance to hit on one or more which have never before been formed, he *invents*.

I conceive that the object of education and training is to establish such habitual combinations of cerebral fibres (that is to say, opinions and sentiments), as experience has shewn to be most beneficial to the individual and to society; and that this can be done with a large, and an almost unlimited proportion of human beings, but that there are still many whose spontaneous combinations are so strong, that the good or the bad qualities which are produced by these combinations can never be changed, even by surrounding circumstances and a moral atmosphere the least adapted to their peculiar virtues or peculiar vices—that is to say, that some individuals are permanently by nature foolish or wise, virtuous or vicious, benevolent or malignant, irascible or tranquil, active or idle, courageous or timid, etc.

I conceive that artificial combinations may be made so enduring, as to influence even the progeny, and give them a facility for falling into similar combinations; and that by a careful arrangement of circumstances, as in the complicated ceremonial system of the Jews, the establishment of caste in India, the education of Mahommedans, and others which might be cited, this early and consistent grouping of the cerebral fibres in their *mind-producing* action becomes permanent and unchangeable. That it is possible to teach a man to think in certain modes, to walk in certain intellectual *ruts*, to reject every inducement to deviate therefrom, and to despise all who wander freely over the field of knowledge. When we disapprove any one of these modes of mind, we call it prejudice, bigotry, or fanaticism.

I conceive that this consists in establishing certain arbitrary combinations of cerebral fibres in which only a limited number are used; and that the attempt to use other fibres left in habitual desuetude, or to make new combinations, is attended by a species of cramp exceedingly painful or disagreeable, and therefore readily rejected.

I conceive that where a man has been left to form his own sentiments and opinions (that is, has received no education), they will generally be bad and vicious—they will have reference only to the proximate gratification of the individual, regardless of the welfare of the species; and that a very large proportion of the human race are not fitted, and were not intended, to be the inventors of their own cerebral combinations, but to follow in the track of others who have been specially endowed with more than average power, in order to exercise the office of guides and instructors.

I conceive, nevertheless, that an occasional example is met with, where the unpruned tree assumes a shape of vigour and beauty which no pruning and guidance could have produced, that such men are fitted for the office of lawgivers, and have a tendency to assume that office; but that of the many who are thus qualified, the great majority either sink into oblivion, or fall victims to the ignorance and brutality of their fellow-creatures, who are not sufficiently advanced in knowledge to appreciate their services.

I conceive that the process of invention—whether in things absolutely and essentially new, as logarithms and fluxions, or in new arrangements of known powers, as in the steam-engine—results from a forcible rearrangement (for the moment) of the cerebral fibres—that by thinking *at* a thing, as Sir Isaac Newton; by *trying*, as the ventriloquist, etc.; we virtually *make innumerable new combinations, till we accidentally hit on exactly that which produces the desired result.*

I conceive that every man of fair powers who will set himself strenuously to disentangle erroneous combinations (prejudices), and allow his mind to luxuriate freely in considering almost any unsettled subject, will make important advances; and that the attempt alone, persevered in, will give him a conscious increase of mental power, which will be a source of great pleasure, and lead to advances in other departments with which his previous attempts were in no way connected.

I conceive that the immense majority of mankind must always be led, and that the combinations they have been taught are those which must guide them through life—that they will generally follow those who will spare them the trouble of thinking; and that the confidence bestowed on the priest, the doctor, the general, and the political leader, is merely the dislike or the difficulty of forming cerebral combinations for themselves.

"Men will always *act* for those who will *think* for them—they love to cast their cares, as well as rest their hopes, and pin their faith upon others. The priest, the physician, the steward, and the lawyer, know this; so does every officer who deserves to hold a commission."—*Quarterly Review*, vol. xli, p. 386.

But I fear to be tedious. Those who have gone through the drilling of a liberal education will see innumerable other illustrations, whether they attribute them to the same cerebral cause or not.

I have no faith in sudden changes of character; and have never known a sudden reformation unless accompanied by a moral shock equivalent to physical *concussion*, under which circumstances, perhaps, habitual aggregations may be destroyed and new ones may be formed.

In this view of the functions of the brain, we see the paramount importance of forcing, at an early age, the habitual grouping of the cerebral fibres in their mind-producing action, into such combinations as experience has shewn to be most conducive to the happiness and welfare of the species. Not to trust to the accidental arrangements which may result from the undirected efforts of the individual. It is possible that one in a million might unaided discover a new arrangement, superior to most of those which have hitherto satisfied mankind; but it is not safe to trust to so remote a contingency. When it occurs, the man thus gifted probably becomes the teacher and the law-giver of his fellow-creatures, either in morals or in science; more rarely in the latter, where it is necessary to avail himself of the previous labours of others. But how many men thus capable of benefiting the world must have been disheartened, and turned from their task by the brutality of the remainder; so that ages would elapse before the concurrence of a new power to guide, with the disposition in any considerable portion of the mass to be guided, would lead to a material amelioration of the habits and feelings of mankind. The general character of a wood is better for the lopping, pruning, and training, although we sometimes see a tree left entirely to nature, exhibit a beauty and perfection of form unattainable by art; but we do not, in the hope and expectation of so rare an occurrence, leave the whole of our plantations to run wild, unpruned, and unguided. We know, by the experience of many generations, *which* of the many forms we can give to the young tree is best adapted to its health and growth, as well as to the specific purposes to which the timber is intended to be applied, and we establish its form accordingly. It is thus in the moral world.

Individuals have been permitted to arise in states of society which would seem to render their labours futile and abortive, yet their high cerebral endowments have enabled them to overcome all obstacles, and to be the benefactors of the human race. No doubt they have been specially endowed for these high purposes; and when the laws they have laid down are seen to be in harmony with all the best and holiest impulses of our nature—when they manifestly tend to the happiness and the virtue of the race, it is our duty to enforce the knowledge and the practice of them—even of those which we know to be merely of human origin. In the daily progress of society do we not see men who obviously *have their mission?* Were not Clarkson and Wilberforce created for the abolition of slavery? God works in this world only by human means. I see around me those whom, as living, I can hardly venture to name, who seem to me as absolutely made for the time, and the time for them, as the sun to produce the blossom and fruit, the germination and the harvest.

When, however, this drilling of the mind is guided by ignorant and bigoted instructors, how lamentable is the effect! We see it in the prejudices of caste in India, and in the overwhelming fanaticism of some Mahommedan nations, and indeed among Christians, in days whose record is written in letters of blood.

As, then, it is possible, we see, to fix the cerebral combinations till the individual shall firmly resist all attempts at conversion, how overwhelmingly important is it that these combinations be such as enlightened reason approves. For this purpose, and to give a liberal and periscopic faculty to the mind (of such at least as are to act the part of guides and directors), it is essential that it should be familiar with the productions of the human intellect, as developed in several modes of society. It is for this reason, I presume, that the enlightened teachers who have the management of clerical education in this country (and whose entire belief in Christianity cannot be doubted), send their pupils, nevertheless, for the larger portion of their instruction to the days of Paganism—and no man is thought to be well educated whose mind has been drilled only in the literature developed under the influence of his own religion.

I once more remind the reader, that these ideas are put forth entirely as conjectures, in the hope that they may be suggestive of new trains of thought in other men of greater mental power and higher education, who may establish from them results which I can but dimly discern.

APPENDIX III: *On the Management of Lunatic Asylums*

The following remarks on Asylums for the Insane were written with the view to publication in a periodical. The tone is scarcely sober enough for the topic, but it is a subject on which I, at least, cannot write with patience. The absurdity, inefficiency, incongruity, and mischievous effects of the present arrangements, are enough to drive to despair a philosophical thinker and physiologist, were it not that he has so often seen how large a cairn may be produced by the contribution of single pebbles, and that the strongest cable may be picked asunder, fibre by fibre, by the feeblest hands.

The present most absurd plan cannot be continued; and the steps which have been taken in Ireland shew so strikingly the benefits that would be derived from an extensive change of system, that I am desirous of attracting notice in all ways and in all quarters to the anomalies of that which is now in action, in the hope of hastening its overthrow.

The reader will, I hope, excuse the rather intemperate tone in which they are written. I was appealing to the masses, without whose aid nothing can be accomplished in the present day. I did not study refinement of expression, being desirous only of stating my thoughts forcibly, and in such a way as to be comprehended by persons of limited education and strong prejudices. Readers of a different class however will, I hope, find the real objections to the present mode of governing Lunatic Asylums to be succinctly and fairly stated; and I can assure them that were it not for the dislike felt by a *gentleman* to point out specific examples of mismanagement, and thus excite odium towards individuals when the fault is in the system which puts such persons into such positions, I could give very startling examples of all that I have asserted. If any results are to be obtained from modern discoveries on the nature and management of Insanity, it can only be by cautious, patient, and humane experiments in public establishments, unfettered by ignorant control.

To those who are entirely ignorant of the structure, functions, and disorders of the organ of thought, and intend to remain so, yet are desirous of exercising authority over the unhappy beings who are the subjects of mental derangement from the disturbance of the *functions* of that organ, I recommend an attentive perusal of the first half of Dr. Conolly's work on the "*Indications of Insanity*," and a little book by Dr. Pritchard, "*On the different Forms of Insanity.*" They will then know as much of the matter (if they have read with great attention) as a man can know of a new language who has not yet learned the alphabet, they will just know that they know nothing—a large step in the progress towards knowledge. It is true that another, who has not merely made himself familiar with the shape of every letter of the language, but knows the grammar of it by heart, may yet make mistakes from a want of familiarity with all its multifarious idioms and inflexions, but in spite of his deficiencies, he would be perhaps better qualified than the first to settle a difficult point in philology. Few will dispute this assertion, or contend that when the master of the language I have supposed has been convicted of a breach of syntax, he should be superseded by the other who has certainly never committed a solecism, because he has never learned even the alphabet. Few perhaps on the strength of this superiority would propose that the latter, rather than the former, should be placed at the head of a school of which the new language formed the chief part of the instruction.

Now the judicious management of the insane demands an infinitely greater amount of mental cultivation and exact knowledge than the acquisition of a language; it is nevertheless held to be quite proper to invest the most ignorant man (provided he is wealthy) with authority and control in the management of a lunatic asylum; and when a doubtful point of intellectual grammar is raised in a court of justice, the persons elected and selected to decide it—to make, in fact, one of the most important decisions in jurisprudence, namely, whether a man be or be not responsible for his actions—whether he be or be not fit to be trusted with the custody of his own body and the management of his own property—whether he shall breathe the free air of heaven, or be shut up in prison. The persons, I say, selected to decide these points, shall be chosen solely from those who know nothing whatever of the organs of the mind, of their condition in health, or of their diseased manifestations, and who are consequently not merely incapable of taking a rational and comprehensive view of the whole case, but who are often still further disqualified by gross prejudices, the result of ignorance and fanaticism. That all those who know something of the brain (however short of the complete knowledge which might be directed to the case) shall be carefully excluded from the jury, and that the men who are acquainted with the structure and functions of the organ of thought shall have no voice in deciding the real point in issue, namely, *the health and perfection of that organ on which the whole matter depends.*

But medical men are so prejudiced! And prejudice is a frightful thing! So, when it is doubtful whether the shoal lies to leeward or to windward, do not let us leave it to the pilot who knows the harbour and understands navigation, because, with all his knowledge, he last year lost a ship; but let us put it to the vote, and take the sense of the majority of the crew, or rather the passengers, who are entirely unacquainted with the port and utterly ignorant of seamanship.

So also when a foreigner is accused of crime in a court of justice, how much better would it be to omit the examination of witnesses and the formality of an interpreter; for these men are sure to be prejudiced either in favour or against the prisoner, and the interpreter may give false translation. Now, by excluding all these sources of prejudice, we shall certainly have an *unbiased* verdict, whether it be a correct one or not. Should this happy suggestion be acted on, the law will at least have the merit of consistency.

But I cannot continue to use sarcasm on so serious a subject. My heart aches at the reflection—how many of my fellow-creatures might be cured of insanity in its early stage—how many might be turned aside from the road which inevitably leads to it—how many families might be saved from destruction and despair—how many suicides of the sane might be prevented—how many wavering minds re-established—how many desolate hearts rendered cheerful—how many atrocious crimes superceded—how many an irreproachable character might be preserved—how many souls might be saved—if the whole management, medical, moral, social, and economical, of the insane, and of that vastly greater and infinitely more pitiable class who are wending their downward way to insanity, were placed exclusively in the hands of a body of enlightened medical men—*a medical jury*—exempt from the necessity, the suicidal necessity, of adapting their measures and their explanations to the ignorance and prejudices of the public.

It would not appear a wise proceeding, if the officer in command of a vessel were not allowed to steer its course till he had made the crew and passengers comprehend his reasons and acquiesce in their validity. He might object perhaps that five in six of them did not even know the meaning of the words latitude and longitude, that still fewer could understand the use of lunar observations, and that all were ignorant of astronomy and navigation. These would be thought reasonable objections, the matter would be left in his hands, and he would conduct the ship to its destination, if such an issue were possible; nor, if the vessel were lost in spite of his care, would it be thought better another time to place the next ship in charge of a man who was confessedly ignorant of all these things, and perhaps had never been to sea.

Yet this is done daily with the insane—nay, it is worse. Not only are men appointed to the control of these establishments on the strength of possessing a certain amount of income, or the reputation of it, but men are placed in that position because of their presumed knowledge of other branches of education, in no way connected with it—lawyers and clergymen—the former perhaps because their want of success in their own department leaves them leisure for the new calling, and the latter because of some vague theories of the mind, which (for lack of preliminary knowledge in physical science) tend to distort still more their judgment in the matter. It is more easy to put into the right road the man who has not yet set out upon his journey, than the man who has made some advances in the wrong one. It is a desecration of the office of a clergyman to place him in such a position, where the greater his talents the greater his errors; and with respect to lawyers, we have not even the test of legal knowledge, since they are not subjected to the examination which decides the qualifications of the clergyman and the physician. Any man becomes a barrister on the strength of eating his commons and paying his fees; and the practice is defended on the ground that, though he may be stupendously ignorant, he can do no harm, for nobody will employ him—so he has leisure to become governor of a lunatic asylum.

And it is under the mischievous activity of such men—the more zealous, active, and sincere, the more mischievous. It is under the guidance of such men that our lunatic asylums are placed; for virtually it is to such guidance alone that these establishments are subjected. The really well-informed and benevolent gentlemen who form a large portion of the body of governors, more especially at a distance from the metropolis, where the *novi homines* are not so readily admitted into the magistracy—such men do not put themselves forward, but conscious of their want of the specific knowledge required, are easily led by noisy and conceited talkers, who boldly proclaim their own sufficiency, and who argue something after this fashion: "My horse is strong—brandy is strong—and I give my horse brandy to make him stronger, for it stands to reason that two strongs must be stronger than one." I will give another illustration, rather coarse perhaps, but emphatic, and much within the truth. I have known similar but more absurd arguments respecting insanity from men entrusted with the management, or I should rather say, *the control of the management*, of the insane. Had they the real management, the fallacy of their reasonings would be evident even to themselves.

The master of a coal brig, I will suppose, who has spent a large portion of his life in coasting between London and Newcastle, becomes rich and a ship-owner. A captain is recommended to him for a voyage to India, and applies for a chronometer, to which application the ship-owner replies, "Nonsense, sir, I have no faith in such jimcracks—won't your own watch tell you the time?" "But, sir, we cannot reckon our longitude without a chronometer." "Pooh! pooh! sir, haven't I been sailing these twenty years without one, and never met with an accident? I believe it to be all prejudice, and that a chronometer does not *contribute to the safety of a ship*; and as a proof of it, wasn't that great ship lost the other day with a dozen chronometers on board?"

Now, a large portion of the Governors of Lunatic Asylums are much more profoundly ignorant of the intellectual management of the insane, than the imaginary master of a coasting-vessel of the voyage to India; and with the best intentions *they will not allow the use of the chronometer!* The Superintendent may double Cape Horn if he think proper, but he must on no account go below fifty degrees south latitude.

There are, no doubt, many excellent men among these Governors; sincerely desirous of doing their duty, and actuated by the most benevolent motives. They are sagacious on all subjects that are within their competence; but in attempting to form an opinion of insanity, they run either into metaphysics or religious mysticism, or else consider the whole affair a simple matter of common sense, and that the professional caution of the practitioner is only a refinement of quackery. "Is the man mad, or is he not?" I have heard from the lips of a judge, apparently indignant at being trifled with in a case *so easy of decision!*

But the best and most reasonable set of Governors that ever were assembled, is liable to one overpowering objection; they form a *mutable* body; the regulations that are laid down by one set of men may not meet the approbation of another set. "The infusion of new blood, " as Lord Chatham called it, may spoil the whole constitution; change in a few weeks a machine, which the skill, patience, suavity, address, and forbearance of the medical superintendent had brought into a *working condition*, may change it into an unmanageable mass of discordant volitions—agreeing in one thing only—to thwart and vex him with contradictory, impracticable, or mischievous suggestions.

If there be one collection of human beings in the world for whose welfare a *Monocracy* is absolutely essential, it is the inmates of a lunatic asylum; and till the whole management of these establishments be taken into the hands of the Government, and the medical superintendent invested with full power to carry out his own ideas, it is vain to hope for any substantial reform in the treatment of the insane. I will beg leave to introduce an anecdote which bears on many other assemblages besides the Governors of a Lunatic Asylum.

The late Lord Bagot had a pack of hounds which were the admiration of the country; the perfection to which their discipline had been brought by the skill and patience of the *whipper-in*, was the theme of unbounded panegyric; the docility of the hounds, a topic of wonder. A word—a sign sufficed, and their governor sat in his place of authority with a glow of affection for the animals whose obedience and attachment conferred on him so much honour.

In an evil hour a new dog was introduced; he was received at first by his fellow-brutes with almost cordiality; and the day passed in tolerable harmony. Towards evening there were symptoms of discussion and dispute in the kennel, and there was reason to fear that the new dog was a sad dog, and resembled that idle and profligate scoundrel found in every village and every parish in the kingdom, who always calls himself "the people," and whose sole office it is to convince his fellow-creatures that they are miserable, though they know it not, and to set them together by the ears. At the approach of night the disturbance subsided, and short angry growls alone indicated, from time to time, that the assembly was not in its ordinary state of perfect tranquility.

Soon after midnight the patriot of the kennel had succeeded, it is supposed, in convincing his fellow-subjects that they were oppressed and injured; had translated, no doubt, into dog Latin the "*Hereditary Bondsmen;*" the whole pack renewed the uproar with an energy and determination that compelled the whipper-in to leave his warm bed, and advance to the vindication of his hitherto undisputed authority. Nothing doubting that his whip, the symbol of his office, would instantly produce the desired submission, he entered the kennel like a sovereign. His voice was heard in tones of violence and anger, but at last it ceased, and the affectionate partner of his bed, tired of waiting for his return, betook herself again to repose.

In the morning, the cranium and spine, the thigh bones and a few of the ribs, were all that remained of the Dog-Compeller, as Homer would have called him. The dogs, formerly so peaceable and submissive, had agreed in nothing but in hostility to the "superintendent," and found him, no doubt, a much nicer meal than the carrion to which they had been accustomed.

By concessions which ought never to required or made by the Superintendent of a lunatic asylum—by respectful feelings towards him as an individual, entertained by the body of governors—by a sincere desire on their part to forward the objects of the institution, such establishments make *some* advances, and preserve comparative tranquillity; but they are utterly incapable of being made available for all the high purposes for which they are fitted. They might be the means not merely of alleviating the sufferings and promoting the welfare of their inmates, but of testing and deciding a great number of important points in medicine, morals, and jurisprudence, which still remain in mischievous suspense.

The medical head of a public establishment for the insane is not even permitted to select his subordinate officers; the instruments he is to use in his most delicate operations are not even of his own choosing; he is neither allowed to have sharp and well-adapted tools, nor to decide himself on their fitness for purposes which he cannot make comprehended by the Governors. His agents, who ought to be in all cases of his own selection, and largely paid to make the risk of dismissal a serious motive for obedience, are not even of a class which gives presumptive evidence of their fitness, and they are taught to look up for patronage not to *him*, but to a mutable body of governors, confessedly ignorant of the very rudiments of medical knowledge, and of every thing connected with the medical treatment of the insane—a body of men, by its very position and composition, in a state of perpetual antagonism with the medical superintendent. Should there be a "sad dog" among them, he acts like an acid dropped into milk, and curdles the whole mass.

If I dwell on this subject unduly, I hope to be pardoned; it is one of paramount importance, and another Session of Parliament ought not to pass without an alteration of the present very absurd and mischievous regulations. Until the public become more enlightened on the subject, there is but little chance of their abandoning an interference which is destructive of its very object. The entire management of a lunatic asylum should be under the sole and absolute control of the medical superintendent, to whom, and to whom alone, every person in the establishment should look up for the *fiat* and *non fiat*. No one but he can be aware of the whole scope of his plan and the object of many of his regulations; and it would be as reasonable to expect every one who is to be guided by a chronometer to understand its construction, as for the subordinate agents in such an establishment to comprehend the gist of many of his nicest rules. He and he alone knows that the countenance which inspires disgust or even repels confidence —the gesture which excites anger, or the tone of voice which creates interest—the flowers which grow in the garden, or the dominos which amuse the leisure—the odour which pleases or offends, or the wine which creates excitement—that all these are as much medicines to be used or avoided as the strychnine or the veratrium, the opium or the calomel.

Even supposing that he could make the nicest operations of mental physiology comprehended by the Governors, the tax upon his time and thought, how to let himself down to their level in a matter of pure science is a serious drawback on his efficiency. He ought to have no such cares upon his mind; but having arranged his machine to his satisfaction, so as to move with the slightest possible effort and the least possible friction, he should have the entire disposal of his time, and ample leisure for the philosophical reflection which would enable him to draw the inferences that a large experience would afford. Some persons seem to think that no portion of the medical superintendent's time is devoted to his duties, but that in which he is going round the establishment or prescribing for the patients; that when there are *so many bars rest* the musician ought not to be paid as if he were playing—that the long course of reflection which ends in deciding *to wait* is so much lost time.

To accommodate even his language to the comprehension of men utterly ignorant of the structure, functions, and diseases of the brain, is a miserable waste of the physician's mind. He fancies he has made a case clearly comprehended, when in fact, his words have been taken in a sense totally different from that in which he intended them to be received. "My liver has been secreting bile again," said a lady-patient to me, "but I hope you will be able to fetch it out, I shall never be well till it is gone." Now here, perhaps, I had been myself to blame in using a word technically which had another meaning in ordinary language—but in the disorders of the mind—that is, in the derangement of the cerebral functions, we have, unfortunately, none but figurative language to make use of; for though common words used by medical philosophers have very clear and specific signification when applied to mental processes natural or perverted, it is utterly impossible to make the public comprehend their meaning—they have not the preliminary knowledge which would enable them to follow the explanation. The carpenter knows perfectly well what a circle is—that it is easily formed by sticking one leg of a pair of compasses into a board and moving the other round it—and he very naturally listens with contempt to the jargon of the mathematician who is attempting to demonstrate its properties. He thinks it all *learned nonsense*, intended to mystify a simple matter, easily understood by any man of common sense who has got eyes, hands, and a pair of compasses.

It is thus with some non-medical Governors of Asylums—many of them make a true estimate of themselves, and do not put forth their crude opinions; but if there be one noisy and vivacious disputant among them, too utterly uninformed on the subject to know that he knows nothing, he can often lead a party of more modest men who are conscious of their own deficiency, and be a constant obstacle to the good intended by the medical officer, whom he keeps in a state of irritation and suspense which materially injures his efficiency and renders his life thoroughly miserable. Let us hope that in a short time we shall be able to "reform it altogether."

Should the plan I speak of be adopted, the medical superintendent will be able to execute his important duties properly and effectively, and he will escape the harassing visitations of his numerous taskmasters. The irritation caused by one visit having scarcely time to subside before it is renewed by another. His mind can never be tranquil nor his energies fully exerted till the whole is entrusted to his sole and uninterrupted care. Instead of issuing a prospectus of his wishes for the consideration of a body of governors, he should promulgate a set of orders to be obeyed, and then he might justly be held responsible for the success of his treatment. An absolute division should be made between those who are received in a state of hopeless disease or idiocy (that is, with brains spoiled by nature or by accident), and recent cases admitting of curative treatment, for the present mode vitiates the statistics and renders them useless. Were this done, then, by comparing the number of cures in the different establishments, we might form some estimate of the merits of the different modes of treatment. The present plan is like building a hospital for the cure of lameness, and putting therein all who have lost a leg.

Surely the expense of such a plan ought not to be an obstacle to its adoption. The contributors should know that the tax they pay is but a slight acknowledgment for their own blessed exemption from the dire calamity.

There are some men specially qualified for the full responsibility I speak of, and they ought to be largely paid. Such men deserve a higher remuneration than the mere barrister, who may or may not be even a man of fair education in his own department—yet, when employed by Government such men are always paid double the sum which is supposed to be an adequate reward for the highest medical philosopher—a thing utterly disgraceful and scandalous.

There is one man so pre-eminently fitted to preside over the whole system, that if the profession were polled he would be almost unanimously elected. To leave men of this stamp unused to the full extent of their powers, is a crime of *leze-humanity.*